General and comparative endocrinology

an introduction to
General and comparative endocrinology

E. J. W. BARRINGTON

EMERITUS PROFESSOR OF ZOOLOGY, UNIVERSITY OF NOTTINGHAM

SECOND EDITION

CLARENDON PRESS · OXFORD

1975

Oxford University Press, Ely House, London W. 1

GLASGOW NEW YORK TORONTO MELBOURNE WELLINGTON
CAPE TOWN IBADAN NAIROBI DAR ES SALAAM LUSAKA ADDIS ABABA
DELHI BOMBAY CALCUTTA MADRAS KARACHI LAHORE DACCA
KUALA LUMPUR SINGAPORE HONG KONG TOKYO

CASEBOUND ISBN 0 19 854120 1
PAPERBACK ISBN 0 19 854131 7

© OXFORD UNIVERSITY PRESS 1963, 1975

FIRST EDITION 1963
SECOND EDITION 1975

PRINTED IN GREAT BRITAIN BY
THOMSON LITHO LTD., EAST KILBRIDE, SCOTLAND

Preface to second edition

We read that the traveller asked the boy if the swamp before him had a hard bottom. The boy replied that it had. But presently the traveller's horse sank in up to the girths, and he observed to the boy, 'I thought you said that this bog had a hard bottom'. 'So it has,' answered the latter, 'but you have not got half way to it yet.'
Henry D. Thoreau (1854). *Walden*.

I have been told that I was lucky in the timing of the first edition; if I had left it only a little later, remarked a candid friend, I could not have hoped to have covered the field.

Undeterred by the implied warning, and fascinated as ever by the subject, I have attempted a revision. This has been no simple matter, for the advances during recent years have been immense. An explosion of new information has led to the overthrow of some hypotheses, while others have been strengthened, and new ones brought out for scrutiny. A great deal of the text of the first edition has therefore had to be reworked, and much new material incorporated. Similar treatment has been accorded to the illustrations. Many new ones have been added, while most of the others have been redrawn and relabelled. Here, as in all aspects of the revision, I am greatly indebted to the unremitting care and skill of my publishers. There have also been a few major changes in the organization of the book. Nevertheless, the fundamental plan is still the same. It is organized to provide an integrated account, but this remains, of necessity, highly personal in selection and balance.

I hope that students will find it a pathway into an endlessly attractive field, and that senior workers in many countries will feel it not unworthy of their own achievements, without which the writing of it could not have been justified.

Alderton, Gloucestershire.   E.J.W.B.
1975

Preface to first edition

All that Mr. Wright, the rubber estate manager, ever knew of the business was that an army patrol had ambushed a band of terrorists within a mile of his bungalow, that five months later his Indian clerk, Girija Krishnan, had reported the theft of three tarpaulins from the curing sheds, and that three years after that someone had removed the wheels from an old scooter belonging to one of his children. As it never occurred to him to look for a possible connection between the three incidents, he remained unaware even of that knowledge.

Eric Ambler (1959). *Passage of Arms*. Heinemann, London.

The science of Endocrinology has its roots set deep in clinical observations, supplemented by experiments on convenient laboratory mammals, but it has never neglected other groups of animals. This has not been merely a matter of Bayliss and Starling's Christmas goose or the goitrous trout which, in the hands of Marine, made a significant contribution to our understanding of the consequences of iodine deficiency. One is thinking rather of investigations into the reproductive endocrinology of birds, or into thyro-pituitary relationships in amphibians, or into the regulation of colour change in the lower vertebrates, investigations that are classical in their own rights and which have made fundamental contributions to the establishment of the science.

Endocrinology, in fact, has always been a branch of biology, and not merely a specialized section of mammalian physiology, and recent years have seen a remarkable growth of interest in the extension of its principles throughout the greater part of the animal kingdom. It is the more regrettable, then, that the student who wishes to discover how the subject is developing at the present time is confronted with a formidable literature into which there is very little access except through specialized review articles and symposia reports, excellent in themselves but discouraging reading for the newcomer.

Banting is said to have remarked that he would never have undertaken the isolation of insulin had he known how much had previously been published in this field, but this anecdote sounds apocryphal, for it is difficult to believe that anything at all could have damped down that particular surge of energy. In any case, the volume of publication relating to a particular problem may well be a tribute to its interest and importance rather than an indication of exhausted possibilities, and there is no need for the young researcher to be depressed by it. In 1922, at the very beginning of modern studies on the endocrinology of colour change, 150 papers dealing with the problem in amphibians had already been published, yet entirely novel contributions are still appearing. In 1949 a review of the literature relating to the pituitary gland of a single species of toad (admittedly a famous one, for it was Houssay's *Bufo arenarum*) listed no less than 197 titles in the bibliography, yet who could claim today that we are near to a complete understanding of the functional organization of that gland in any vertebrate group?

It is clear that those who really demand sympathy in this situation are the teachers who would like to see this absorbing subject fully incorporated into contemporary biology and the students who need a path of entry so that they can explore for themselves, and it is for these groups that this book has been written. Rigorous selection and elimination have gone into its composition, for it aims to set out some of the main themes of endocrinology rather than to describe the endless variations that nature has worked upon them. These themes are explored primarily from the standpoint of the comparative physiologist, but I do not believe that such a treatment can be effective, at least in the present state of development of the subject, unless it is founded upon a clear exposition of the principles that have been derived from the study of man and other mammals. By virtue of the inclusion of this foundation the book becomes General as well as Comparative, and I hope that in consequence it may be of value to students of medicine and physiology as well as to the zoologists whose needs were my initial stimulus.

The result is probably a highly personal one, for it must be supposed that half a dozen different writers setting out with the same aim would have produced half a dozen very different books. I have myself borne in mind that I am dealing with a rapidly growing subject, and I have therefore devoted some attention to the way in which hypotheses have been developed, and have even at times followed the rather unusual course of mentioning some of the mistakes that have been made, for I believe that it is helpful to judge the present position against the background of past experience. I have also ventured into speculations and I must ask for these to be accepted in the spirit in which they are offered; there is nothing, I believe, for which some support could not be found somewhere, but they do not necessarily represent a majority viewpoint and they are intended primarily to extend horizons and to form bases for discussion.

One particular difficulty that faces all writers in this field is the problem of nomenclature, and here I have had to make one or two decisions. For example, I have rejected a good deal of the alphabetical jargon that is essential shorthand for the specialist but merely irritating to the general reader, and I have preferred the suffix 'tropin' to 'trophin' because it seems to me to be a better expression of the implied relationship. In dealing with various alternative names I have drawn comfort from the knowledge that a gathering of experts, confronted in 1959 by a motion that 'the term ICSH should henceforth be used instead of LH

with respect to one of the pituitary gonadotropins' were unable to do better than produce ten votes against it and nine in support. I have felt obliged to be more selective in the disposal of my own favours, and in making my choices I have tried to take counsel from that useful legal fiction, the 'reasonable man'. If at times his influence seems less obvious than could have been wished, I can only plead that 'where reason cannot instruct, custom may be permitted to guide'.

In a book that has partly grown out of lecture material it is difficult to make proper acknowledgement of all its sources, nor have I wished to crowd the text with references. I have therefore provided suggestions for further reading, as selective as the book itself, but containing publications which have been particularly useful to me and which should be equally useful to readers if, as I hope, they accept this book as truly an introduction and not a complete statement. I am glad to express my own indebtedness to the writers concerned, and to the personal discussions which are such a pleasant feature of contemporary science. I am grateful also to my friends Mr. T. E. Hughes and Dr. A. E. Needham, who were so kind as to read the whole of the manuscript; they are not responsible for what I have written, but they have improved it a great deal, and it has been helpful to draw on their wide experience in the teaching of comparative physiology to undergraduates.

Finally, I must express my appreciation of the care and skill which my publishers have brought to the preparation of the book for press. This stage, however, would never have been reached without the tolerant acceptance by my wife and family of the insatiable claims that the writing of it has made upon my time.

Nottingham   E.J.W.B.
1962

Acknowledgements

Barrington, *Hormones and evolution* (English Universities Press, London); Barrington (ed.), *American Zoologist* **15** (suppl.); Barrington and Jørgensen (eds), *Perspectives in endocrinology* (Academic Press, New York); *Brain Research* **6**; *British Journal of Pharmacology* **3**; *Cancer Research* **15**; *Diabetologia* **3**; *Endocrinology* **69**; *Experientia* **18**; Ganong and Martini (eds), *Frontiers in neuroendocrinology* (Oxford University Press, New York); *General and Comparative Endocrinology* **8, 12, 14, 15, 17, 18, 20,** and supplement **3**; Gorbman and Bern, *Textbook of comparative endocrinology* (John Wiley & Sons, New York); Highnam and Hill, *The comparative endocrinology of the invertebrates* (Edward Arnold, London); Hoar and Randall (eds), *Fish physiology,* Vol. 2 (Academic Press, New York); Idler (ed), *Steroids in nonmammalian vertebrates* (Academic Press, New York); *International Encyclopaedia of Pharmacological Therapy,* section 41, Vol. 1 (Pergamon Press, Oxford); *Journal of Endocrinology* **31, 43**; *Journal of experimental Biology* **40**; *Journal of experimental Zoology* **157**; *Journal of the marine Biology Association, U.K.* **38**; *Journal of Morphology* **106, 116**; *Journal of Physiology* **155**; *Journal of Zoology* **148, 150**; Lentz (ed.), *Primitive nervous systems* (Yale University Press); Moore (ed.), *The biology of Amphibia* (Academic Press, New York); Pecile and Müller (eds), *Growth and growth hormone* (Excerpta Medica, Amsterdam); *Philosophical Transactions of the Royal Society, London, B* **250, 263**; Pincus, Thimann, and Astwood (eds), *The hormones,* Vol. 4 (Academic Press, New York); *Proceedings of the Royal Society, London, B* **157, 170**; *Proceedings of the Zoological Society, London,* (1937); *Quarterly Journal of microscopical Science* **97**; *Recent Progress in Hormone Research* **24, 26, 28**; *Review of Canadian Biology* **1**; Lefebvre and Unger (eds), *Glucagon* (Pergamon Press, Oxford); Waring, *Colour change mechanisms in cold-blooded vertebrates* (Academic Press, New York); *Zeitschrift für Zellforschung und mikroskopische Anatomie* **78**.

Contents

x Contents

1

Introduction

1.1. Chemical regulation

Whatever the circumstances under which life first evolved, living organisms must at a very early stage have developed the capacity for responding adaptively to stimulation both from within and from without; for reacting, that is to say, in a manner most likely to ensure their survival. We may assume that such reactions of chemical systems would have been mediated by chemical means, and that for this purpose use would have been made of suitable substances which were present in the environment or which were arising as by-products of the organisms' own activities.

Certainly we see evidence of this at the present day. Water from crowded cultures of *Hydra* has the capacity for inducing sexual differentiation in this animal, an effect that is apparently a consequence of the high carbon dioxide tension in the medium. Whatever the significance of this may be for the normal life-cycle of *Hydra*, we have here an illustration of members of a species being able to influence each other through a chemical substance which in this instance is one of their waste products.

Towards the other end of the animal scale we find that the growth rate of frog tadpoles is sharply reduced if they are placed in water in which crowded tadpoles have previously been living. This effect of crowding is a result of the presence in such 'conditioned' water of a substance which is non-dialysable and which will not pass through Whatman No. 1 filter-paper; its property is destroyed by heating or drying it, or by subjecting it to ultraviolet irradiation. The origin of this substance is not understood. It may be that it is a product of micro-organisms growing in the culture (although the property is said to persist in the presence of penicillin and streptomycin), but it is interesting to speculate that it might also be a metabolic product of the tadpoles themselves, adaptively modifying the metabolism of other tadpoles in such a way as to limit their growth while permitting their maintenance.

It has been argued that such chemical interactions are a widespread phenomenon of nature, dependent upon the excretion by organisms of active metabolites, and upon the readiness with which water permits the interchange of these substances, and it may well be, as Lucas has suggested, that they are a basis for far more subtle ecological relationships than those between organisms and their physical environment, or between predator and prey. For example, the presence of certain carbohydrates in water directly stimulates the pumping action of oysters. The significance of this is obscure, but the substances concerned are thought to be the products of plant metabolism, so that theoretically there is here a means by which feeding activity could be integrated with changes in the composition of the surrounding water and of the organisms in it.

Chemical interactions between organisms may also serve to synchronize the spawning of invertebrates. For example, the sperm and testes of male oysters contain some chemical which evokes spawning in the females; these induce spawning in other males which then induce it in other females, so that a chain reaction develops. Similar although less elaborate relationships have been described for worms; thus isolated females of the polychaete *Platynereis dumerilii* will spawn spontaneously, but males will only do so in the presence of females, a situation which presumably depends upon the release of a chemical signal from the latter.

Such signals also operate as part of the regulatory machinery within the body of a single individual. A familiar example is the influence of the carbon dioxide pressure of the arterial blood in controlling the rate of ventilation of the lungs in mammals, but such mechanisms must have been operating before the evolution of vascular systems. Sponges, which lack both blood and nervous systems, depend upon chemical diffusion from cell to cell for such very limited powers of co-ordination as they possess, and this may still be important in the platyhelminths.

The planarian *Dugesia tigrina* occurs in a sexual and a non-sexual strain. If the anterior third of a member of the sexual one is grafted on to the posterior two-thirds of a member of the other, it will induce in the latter the development of testes and copulatory organs. Of course, this might be due, at least in part, to the migration of cells from the sexual portion into the non-sexual one, but the appearance of accessory organs as well as testes certainly suggests that the diffusion of some chemical factor is involved.

Such relationships need much more thorough investigation, and the interpretations applied to them are often somewhat hypothetical, but there is no doubt of their reality in vertebrate embryos, where they underlie the phenomenon of induction. This is essentially the control of differentiation by the passage of cues, or signals, from one group of cells to another, an example being the induction of neural structures in the ectoderm by the chordamesoderm which lies beneath it. The signals are chemical, involving the transfer of material, as can be shown by labelling the chordamesoderm of urodele embryos with [^{14}C] glycine. This is followed by the preferential accumulation of the label in the cells of the induced neural plate.

The principle of chemical communication in the vertebrate body is not restricted in its operation to early development. On the contrary, it is carried further in the fully formed animal, with transmission over greater distances, and with use of the blood stream as the transmitting medium. One example of this is the control of the regeneration of the liver. After part of this organ has been removed the remainder will embark upon growth and differentiation until the original total mass has been approximately restored. The regulatory agent concerned here is believed to be a substance, perhaps a protein of the blood plasma, which is released from the liver into the blood stream and which is believed to have an inhibitory action upon the synthesis of fresh intracellular protein. If the total mass of the liver is reduced, so also is the concentration of this substance in the blood stream; thus, with the reduction of its inhibitory influence the liver is freed to increase its own mass until, with the restoration of its normal size, the concentration and inhibitory action of the substance are restored to normal.

This principle is not peculiar to the liver; such systems of chemical intercommunication and control are widespread throughout the animal kingdom, and we shall see many examples of them. In this particular instance the system provides what is called a feedback cycle, in which the activity of a process is regulated by information that arises out of that activity and is passed back, directly or indirectly, into the originating organ. However, the interactions may be of a more generalized character, or they may involve a direct stimulating action of one organ upon another in what has been called the shot-gun type of relationship. In the latter case the stimulated organ is often referred to as the target organ, the response of which depends upon its possession of a specialized receptor mechanism, able to trap the activating substance. That substance, if an analogy is required, might perhaps be compared with a coded missile, the relationships between it and its target becoming one of mutual adaptation. Whatever the exact nature of these interactions may be, however, it is likely that there are few cells in the body which are not involved in them; indeed, it is clear that cells are organized to function in an environment of mutual interaction, as is shown by the way in which they may often lose a great deal of their characteristic metabolic machinery and synthetic capacity when they are cultured *in vitro*.

1.2. The content of endocrinology

The study of endocrinology is concerned, in the classical use of the term, with hormones, which are particular and specialized components of the communication systems which we have been considering. Hormones are chemical substances which are produced in particular regions of the body, usually in specialized glands, and are discharged into the blood stream. This is the process known as internal or endocrine secretion. They are then carried in the circulation to other parts of the body where, in minute quantities, they produce specific regulatory effects.

The concept of hormones arose gradually, for the idea of the production of internal secretions was already current in the eighteenth century. However, it was first formulated in clear terms by Claude Bernard in 1859, for he had realized that the functioning of certain organs involved the discharge of their products into the blood, and he had referred to the passage of glucose out of the liver as an example of this. It has been customary to regard such early speculations as being of too generalized a nature to be directly relevant to twentieth-century endocrinology, and they were certainly far removed from current concepts of the close interweaving of the neural and hormonal components of regulatory processes. Nevertheless, it will prove helpful to approach those components as part of the wider system of chemical interrelationships which we have outlined above.

Thus, it is possible to make some distinction between the regulatory influence of the nerve cells, precisely localized in space and time, and the much more diffuse action of hormones, but we shall find that both are equally products of secretory activity. Indeed, we shall learn that nerve cells may have specifically endocrine functions, and that they may even have given rise to the first fully differentiated endocrine organs. It is possible, again, to make some distinction between the diffuse action of hormones and the localized action of embryonic inductor substances, yet both of these effects may sometimes be produced by secretions that are closely similar, if not actually identical. Moreover, substances resembling established hormones, or chemically related to them, are widely distributed in nature, and it is possible that the evolution of endocrine systems may have involved the utilization of such substances. Thus the tracing of the evolutionary history of highly specialized secretory products may help us to understand their nature and their mode of functioning

As for hormones in the classical sense of the term, the development of endocrinological research has led to the acceptance of a series of criteria (listed below) which need to be met in order to justify the interpretation of a particular secretion as a hormone, and hence of its gland of origin as an endocrine organ. Collectively, they constitute an ideal which may not always be attainable. Nevertheless, each one may yield significant information, and we shall see that with some hormones the criteria already satisfied are sufficiently complete to be as convincing as could reasonably be demanded.

(a) *Histological and histochemical studies by light microscopy.* It should be possible to identify in the organ its secretory cells, an ample blood supply, and the absence of secretory ducts. Secretory products or their precursors should be visible in the cells, and it should be possible to correlate variations in their appearance with variations in the activity of the organ. These variations might be natural ones, or experimentally induced. Histochemical observations, based upon known chemical reactions, should be correlated with the chemical data mentioned below. Immunohistochemistry should permit the identification of the cells of origin of many hormones.

(b) *Ultrastructural studies.* These will often define, more precisely than is possible with light microscopy, the characteristic features of the secretory products and of the biosynthetic machinery. The differences between protein-secreting cells and steroid-secreting ones (p. 107) are an example.

(c) *Physiological studies.* The hormone must be identified at its site of origin, and shown to have specific actions at sites other than this one. These effects must be shown to persist after all nervous pathways between its site of origin and sites of action have been eliminated, and some at least of them should therefore be demonstrable *in vitro*. Reduced activity of the gland of origin, or its complete absence, should produce a clearly defined complex of symptoms (syndrome), observable clinically in human subjects or experimentally treated laboratory animals. These symptoms should be alleviated by replacement therapy, which can include treatment with extracts of the organ, or with the pure hormone, or by introducing implants of the organ.

(d) *Chemical studies.* These are aimed at the purification of the hormone, followed by its chemical characterization and by its synthesis. This should permit determination of its pathways of biosynthesis, and the course of its metabolism and excretion. Knowledge of the molecular structure of the hormone should contribute to elucidating its mode of action.

(e) *Assay procedures.* The strength of preparations and extracts must be measured before their effects can usefully be analyzed or compared. This involves either direct chemical assay, or bioassays in which use is made of living animals or of tissues removed from them. Techniques of competitive protein binding, including radioimmunoassay (p. 51), are amongst those which have greatly facilitated the determination of minute amounts of hormones.

(f) *Blood studies.* The classical concept of a hormone as a substance transmitted through the blood stream (we shall have to examine this concept further in due course) requires that it should be identified chemically or immunologically in the blood. Further, it should be possible to demonstrate the release of the hormone into the blood under specific physiological conditions, and to be able to determine the concentrations at which it circulates. Ideally, it should be shown to be present in the venous effluent leaving the supposed endocrine gland, and, to give assurance that it has actually been secreted from that organ, it should be possible to show that its concentration is higher in the venous blood than in the arterial blood entering the organ.

(g) *In vitro and transplantation studies.* In addition to the possibility of demonstrating endocrine action *in vitro*, the maintenance of endocrine tissues in suitable incubation media makes it possible to study such aspects as the ability of the organ to continue functioning independently of the action of other hormones, and the factors that may influence its secretory output. There are, however, limits to the extent to which the activities of an explant can be accepted as a guide to its activities in the complex internal environment in which it normally functions. As a variant of this type of study, it is possible to examine the behaviour of tissues when they are transplanted to other parts of the body (ectopic transplants), where they may be free from local or neural mechanisms that normally regulate their activities.

1.3. The comparative method

Endocrinological evidence tends to be found at its most secure in the field of mammalian studies, for many technical difficulties arise when experimental investigations are extended to other groups. Nevertheless, we shall find encouraging examples of these difficulties being overcome, so that comparative studies are developing their own independent strength, and are beginning to clarify problems of mammalian endocrinology by revealing something of the origin and history of mammalian adaptations. It remains necessary, as in all branches of comparative physiology, to avoid generalizing too optimistically in advance of appropriate evidence, and to resist the temptation to accumulate detail for its own sake. Yet it would be much more difficult today for W. M. Bayliss to say of comparative physiology, as he did in his great treatise on *Principles of general physiology*, that it was 'sometimes apt to become in great part a description of functions peculiar to certain lower organisms, even when they throw no light on the activities of the human body, which are, after all, the most vitally interesting and important problems presented to the physiologist. . . . In treatises on comparative physiology, copious details of alimentary or digestive mechanisms will be found, but no discussion of the general nature of the action of enzymes'. In the present account there will be no room for copious details. What we shall do, however, is to compare hormone with hormone, and system with system, first within the mammals, for that group provides at the present time the foundations of our understanding. We shall then extend our analysis to other groups of vertebrates, and to those groups of invertebrates that have been investigated most thoroughly. Our comparisons therefore will be developed on two fronts, the hormonal and the taxonomic. As a result we shall hope to extract from the variability that is so characteristic of animal life some statement of general principles, which will be

reinforced by excursions into evolutionary speculation. Thus we shall hope to show, amongst other things, that the comparative treatment of animal function can contribute to an understanding of human physiology and, indeed, is ultimately essential if that understanding is to be reasonably complete.

Such was clearly the opinion of William Harvey. We can see him still, through the eyes of Aubrey, wearing his dagger, 'as the fashion then was which he would be apt to draw out upon every occasion' (not offensively, as a more recent biographer insists, but merely in the way of gesticulation!), and we can hear him answering those 'who say that I have shown a vain-glorious love of vivisections, and who scoff at and deride the introduction of frogs and serpents, flies, and others of the lower animals upon the scene, as a piece of puerile levity, not even refraining from opprobious epithets. To return evil speaking with evil speaking, however, I hold to be unworthy in a philosopher and searcher after truth; I believe that I shall do better and more advisedly if I meet so many indications of ill breeding with the light of faithful and conclusive observation'. Elsewhere, in an Epistle Dedicatory to the 'learned and illustrious the President and Fellows of the College of Physicians of London', he expressed the essence of the matter when he observed that nature was the best and most faithful interpreter of her own secrets; 'and what she presents either more briefly or obscurely in one department, that she explains more fully and clearly in another'.

It is worth examining why this should be so. The issue has been cogently discussed by Pantin, who, in reference to the nervous systems of crustaceans, cephalopods, and vertebrates, asks how it is that 'not once but many times a highly complex mechanism to meet the requirement of behaviour has been built up on principles so similar that valid information about the one can be obtained by study of the other?' He finds the answer in the fact that natural selection does not work upon an unlimited range of random variation. On the contrary, animal organization has limitations which are inherent in the properties of the materials of which it is composed, and which are a consequence of all living organisms sharing certain common molecules and metabolic pathways established during the chemical phase of evolution. This imposes upon them a fundamental unity of plan.

We shall see many examples of this unity. We shall find, for example, that arthropodan neurosecretory systems are exploitations, in different contexts, of the same principles as those involved in the evolution of the vertebrate pituitary gland. This is why studies of the organization of one group can contribute to our understanding of the organizations of very different ones. However, if our comparative studies are not to yield bitter fruit, it is important that the interpretation of them shall be based upon a grasp of the classical concepts of homology and analogy.

An organ in one animal is said to be homologous with an organ in another when the two organs resemble each other in their development, and in their morphological relationships with other organs, and, to some extent, resemble each other in their structure. The organs may also have similar functions, but this is not a necessary condition of homology. Indeed, divergences of function may lead to divergences in structure, so that the homology is more evident in early development than in the fully developed animals.

The concept of homology originated in pre-Darwinian biology, but it is now seen, in evolutionary terms, as a consequence of the derivation of the organs concerned from a common ancestral organ. However, the concept must be extended to include also resemblances between organs which were not themselves derived from an organ in a common ancestor, but which have developed independently, by parallel evolution, in related groups. This parallel evolution is attributed to the possession by these groups of similar genotypes, which, under the influence of similar selection pressures, have given rise to similar phenotypes in the course of later evolution. Such resemblances are sometimes termed homoplastic instead of homologous, but the distinction is obviously a fine one.

Homologous organs are contrasted with analogous ones. The latter are organs that resemble each other because they have similar functions, but which did not have any common evolutionary origin. In the light of what we have said, however, their similarities may well be due to the possession, by quite unrelated groups of animals, of similar molecules and biochemical pathways. To this extent, we animals are all one, and this is why, to quote Pantin again, we have to learn to handle, in our comparative studies, 'a morphology with new and unfamiliar rules'. Our analysis needs, therefore, to be approached cautiously, yet without restricting the intellectual exhilaration which flows as naturally from comparative endocrinology as from other branches of contemporary biology.

2

Hormones and digestion

2.1. Gastrin and the regulation of gastric digestion

It is a mistake to suppose that the introduction of new ideas into a science is a logical and tidy process, evolving naturally as older ones are discarded or modified in the light of new discoveries. Biological problems are so complex that too close an application to what appears to be logical reasoning may actually impede the acceptance of new facts. The result of this is that empiricism and intuition prove to be essential tools for the investigator, provided always that their use is based upon wisely informed experience. The truth of this, which will repeatedly appear in our survey of comparative endocrinology, is well illustrated by the progressive unravelling of the physiological principles that are involved in the regulation of the digestive processes of vertebrates.

The alimentary tract of these animals is essentially a tube connecting the mouth with the anus, and bearing certain localized outgrowths. It is lined by an epithelium which secretes enzymes, absorbs the products of digestion, and contributes hormones to the regulation of various aspects of digestive activity. In mammals (Fig. 2.1) the food passes down the oesophagus into the stomach, after some preliminary treatment by the saliva. Within the stomach proteolytic digestion is initiated by the secretion of hydrochloric acid and pepsinogen from the chief glands of the antrum, while mucus is added from the lining epithelium and from the glands of the cardiac and pyloric portions. Most of the digestion, however, takes place in the small intestine; the first section of this (the duodenum) receives secretions in part from the liver and pancreas, and in part from Brunner's glands and the crypts of Lieberkühn. These crypts are distributed throughout the small intestine, while Brunner's glands, which are probably related phylogenetically to the pyloric glands of the stomach, are confined to the duodenum.

The next part of the small intestine after the duodenum is distinguishable in some mammals as the jejunum, but the greater part of it is the ileum, and

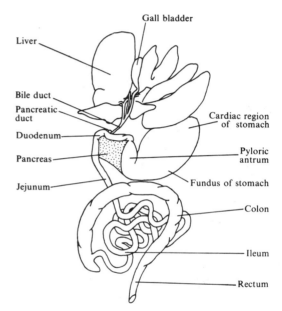

FIG. 2.1. The alimentary tract of the cat in ventral view. (After Mivart.)

it is here that the digestive processes are largely completed. Water, however, is absorbed through the wall of the large intestine, while a specialized microflora in either the stomach or the caecum has an essential role to play in many herbivorous mammals. We may follow Pavlov in comparing such an alimentary canal with a chemical factory in which food is processed in preparation for its absorption. The necessary reactions take place in stages, sometimes in separate compartments, and always through the agency of secretions which are discharged in a co-ordinated way in the right place at the right time and in the appropriate quantities.

The mammalian salivary glands are regulated by impulses transmitted along reflex pathways of the autonomic nervous system; the endocrine system plays no part. This is understandable. The requirement here is for a rapid and often quite brief response to the presence of food in the buccal cavity, and for this the nervous system is well suited. Elsewhere in the alimentary tract, however, where the situation is more complex, regulation is effected by an elegant interaction of nervous and endocrine pathways. The importance of hormones in this regard was first made clear in studies of pancreatic secretion, but it will be more convenient to follow the passage of the food, and deal first with the control of gastric digestion.

activities of the main stomach, and these can in consequence be analyzed by collecting the gastric juice produced in the pouch. A valuable adjunct is an oesophageal fistula, which permits sham feeding, in which the ingested food can stimulate taste buds but cannot pass on into the stomach (Fig. 2.3).

An important later development was the application by Ivy and Farrell of the technique of auto-transplantation, so called because the organs remain in the animals from which they originate.

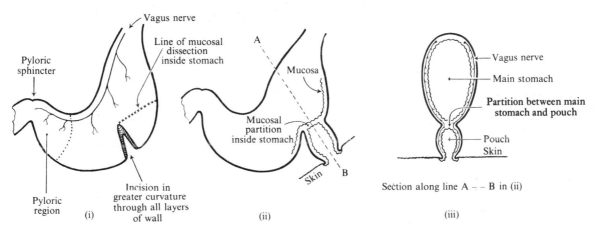

FIG. 2.2. Diagram illustrating Pavlov's operation for making an isolated pouch of the stomach. Note that the pouch has the same nerve and blood supply as the main part of the stomach. (From Bell *et al.* (1956). *Textbook of physiology and biochemistry*. Livingstone, Edinburgh.)

Up to the end of the last century, and largely as a result of Pavlov's brilliant exploration of the physiology of digestion, it was supposed that co-ordination throughout the alimentary tract was exclusively provided by the nervous system. Pavlov's studies of gastric digestion had been much influenced by the pioneer observations (by the American Army surgeon Beaumont) upon Alexis St. Martin, a French Canadian trapper who was left with a permanent gastric fistula after unexpectedly surviving the effects of a serious gunshot wound in the abdomen. Much of our later knowledge is drawn from chronic experiments (p. 11) carried out upon dogs with a surgically prepared gastric fistula, or with a gastric pouch, the latter being a portion of the stomach completely or partially separated from the main organ and arranged to open to the exterior. Heidenhain devised a pouch that was deprived of its vagus nerve supply, but Pavlov (aided, it is said, by his ambidexterity) developed a technique for preparing a pouch (Fig. 2.2) that retained its full innervation. Events proceeding in this Pavlov pouch may be expected to parallel closely the secretory

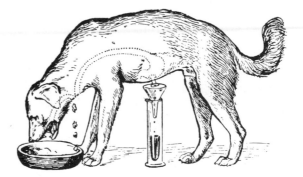

FIG. 2.3. A demonstration of the nervous phase of gastric secretion, illustrating Pavlov's experimental methods. The food consumed drops out of the open end of an oesophageal fistula without entering the stomach; the gastric secretion evoked by feeding is collected through a gastric fistula, consisting of a tube flanged at each end. (From Winton and Bayliss (1937). *Human physiology* (2nd edn). Blakiston, Philadelphia.

This technique, as applied to the study of gastric secretion, involves moving a portion of the stomach, with its nerves and blood vessels intact, to a new position under the skin, the mammary region being selected because of its rich vascularization. Here the transplant, formed into a pouch, develops a new blood supply and, when this has occurred, its nervous and vascular connections with the main organ are severed. Secretion is collected from the pouch through a fistula, and it can be assumed, as with the auto-transplanted pancreas, that stimulation of its secretory epithelium can only be effected through the blood stream.

With these and other techniques it has been established that the secretory response of the stomach to feeding takes place in two stages, known as the cephalic phase and the gastric phase. Both are regulated by the co-ordinated action of the nervous system, mediated by the discharge of acetycholine at parasympathetic nerve endings in the stomach wall, and by gastrin, which is a polypeptide hormone released into the blood stream from the mucosa of the pyloric antrum.

The cephalic phase is essentially a preparatory one, producing what is often referred to as 'appetite secretion'; the need for promoting it provides physiological justification for beginning a meal with what is disagreeably called a 'starter'. 'Now good digestion wait on appetite, and health on both!' Evidence for the action of the nervous system in this phase was established by Pavlov in experiments of the type indicated in Fig. 2.3. These show that the secretion is released either in response to the stimulation of taste buds, or, as a conditioned reflex, and with the higher nervous centres participating, in response to stimulation of other receptors, such as the eye and nose. The gastric juice so produced is very rich in pepsin, and in agreement with this it is found that faradic stimulation of the vagus will result in depletion of the granules of the chief (peptic) cells.

The gastric phase is initiated by the presence of food in the stomach, and depends upon signals transmitted by vago-vagal pathways; that is, centrally by afferent fibres, as a result of stimulation arising within the stomach, and then peripherally by efferent ones. It was from the study of this phase that evidence for hormonal involvement first emerged, although it is now realized that this involvement influences both phases. The evidence, however, was slow to win acceptance. First reports of it followed shortly after the discovery by Bayliss and Starling (1902) of 'secretin', a fundamentally important development that will be discussed later. Edkins, who was evidently much influenced by that discovery, found in 1905 that intravenous injection into cats of extracts of the pyloric region of the stomach would evoke the secretion of acid and of pepsin, whereas extracts of the fundus had no such effect. This was far from being a complete proof of chemical regulation. Nevertheless, Edkins felt justified in postulating the existence of a chemical principle which he named gastrin. Later in the same year, when Starling introduced the term hormone, he applied it to gastrin as well as to 'secretin'.

This ready acceptance of what later came to be known as the gastrin theory proved, however, to be premature. Certainly it received some experimental support. Particularly convincing evidence was obtained from experiments upon dogs in which, in addition to the preparation of an auto-transplanted gastric pouch, the main stomach was also denervated and transformed into an isolated pouch. Liver extract placed in the latter pouch evoked secretion both in it and also in the transplant, but would not do so if the lining of the main pouch was first treated with procaine. It could be inferred from this that the gastric lining responds to the presence of the extract by releasing a chemical factor into the blood stream, but is unable to do so if it is first anaesthetized.

The difficulty, however, was to establish that this factor was a specific hormone. 'Looking back now', writes Gregory of Edkins, 'we can appreciate how cruelly unlucky he was'. His ill-luck was the discovery by Dale and Laidlaw in 1910 of the ubiquitous histamine, with its vasopressor activity, and the later demonstration by Popielski that it was present in the antral mucosa, and that it had a powerful secretagogue action upon the oxyntic cells. This action, overlooked by Dale and Laidlaw 'because', as Dale later explained, 'we did not look for it', is the one major secretory effect of this substance. The demonstration of it led inevitably to the conclusion that histamine was the agent discovered by Edkins, and that no specific hormone was involved. Indeed, it was uncertain whether or not the action of this substance upon gastric secretion was of any physiological significance at all, and this doubt remains to the present day.

Interest in gastrin lapsed, until the problem was reopened in 1938 by Komarov, in Montreal. He was then able to show, only two years before the death of Edkins, that the original proposition was correct, and that Nature had set one of the traps that become so familiar to biologists. Histamine is present throughout the body, but in the antral mucosa it co-exists with gastrin. Both must have been present in Edkins's extracts, but Komarov separated them by precipitating the hormone with trichloracetic acid. He had rightly suspected that gastrin, like 'secretin', might be a polypeptide, so that precipitation of a protein fraction would be an essential step in its separation. Injection of this fraction into cats (Fig. 2.4) elicited secretion of gastric acid, but not of

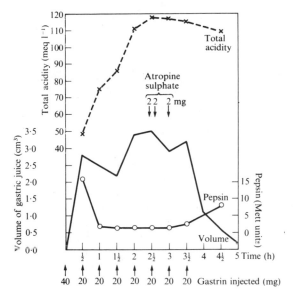

FIG. 2.4. Demonstration of the action of a gastrin preparation, using a cat under chloralose–urethane anaesthesia, with both vagus nerves cut. Gastrin was injected intravenously at $\frac{1}{2}$-h intervals; it was shown in another experiment that such injections had no effect on blood pressure. The injections evoked the secretion of a highly acid gastric juice, with only a low concentration of pepsin after the first injection. The volume and composition of the gastric juice were not influenced by atropine, indicating that there was no parasympathomimetic material in the extract, and that the hormone was acting directly upon the acid-secreting cells. (Modified from Komarov (1942). *Rev. Can. Biol.* **1**.)

pepsin, just as had the extracts of Edkins; in this case, however, the material was free of histamine.

Purification studies have led to the isolation, characterization and synthesis of gastrin, defined as the hormone, extracted from the antro-pyloric mucosa, that stimulates gastric acid secretion. Two closely related peptides (gastrin I and II) are present in the stomach of various mammalian species, including man, the pig and the dog. These are heptadecapeptide amides, gastrin II (Fig. 2.5) having

a sulphate group attached by ester linkage to the single tyrosyl. Interspecific differences lie in the centre of the molecule; they have not been associated with any differences in properties of the molecules, while the significance of the sulphation is also unknown. Larger molecules, called 'big gastrin' and 'big big gastrin' have also been described, and await full exploration.

The availability by synthesis of gastrin itself, as well as of analogues and fragments of it, has made possible a full exploration of the physiological properties of the molecule. This has confirmed earlier suspicions that its most obvious effect, which is the strong stimulation of acid secretion, is not its only one. Much variation is found, both between species and also dependent upon the conditions of the experiment, but it seems that the hormone also evokes a weak stimulation of volume output of the pancreas (in the dog), a strong stimulation of pancreatic enzyme output, and a weak stimulation of the flow of bile. All of these actions (apart from a slight action upon the pancreas) are properties of the COOH-terminal tetrapeptide, and almost all activity disappears when the terminal amide group is removed. It is significant (and we shall return to this matter later) that the terminal sequence is not subject to interspecific variation by amino-acid substitution.

Chemical synthesis has also contributed to the solution of a long-standing problem of alimentary endocrinology, which is to determine the source of the hormones concerned. Often, there is no serious problem in locating the cellular sources of hormones; indeed, in the development of vertebrate endocrinology the recognition of an endocrine gland has often preceded the identification of its hormone. The digestive hormones have been an exception to this, for the cells secreting them long eluded identification. Now, however, several of the cell types concerned have been identified by immunohistochemical procedures. For example, the source of gastrin has been demonstrated by using antibodies raised to a synthetic human gastrin comprising residues 2–17. When these antibodies, labelled with fluorescein, are applied to histological sections of the stomach,

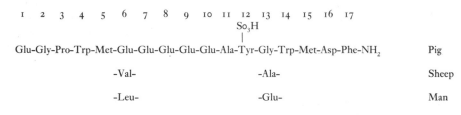

FIG. 2.5. Gastrin II of pig, sheep, and man.

they react immunologically with clearly defined cells lying in the antro-pyloric glands at about the middle third of their length, depositing on them a fluorescent precipitate (cf. Fig. 3.4(d); p. 28. These cells, which have also been identified by light and electron microscopy show formalin-induced autofluorescence and other properties that characterize them as cells of the APUD series (p. 154).

We can now summarize present understanding of the regulation of the two phases of gastric digestion. The cephalic phase is regulated by vagal reflexes, cholinergic stimulation evoking the release of enzyme from the fundus glands, and also of gastrin from the antrum. The hormone, passing into the blood stream, evokes secretion (primarily of acid) from the fundus glands, and has also the other effects already noted. The gastric phase is regulated through vago-vagal pathways, being initiated by the presence of food in the stomach, and particularly by antral distension. As in the cephalic phase, cholinergic stimulation results in the liberation of enzyme and of gastrin, the latter then mediating the liberation of acid. Local reflexes within the stomach wall may also contribute to the cholinergic stimulation.

It remains to add that gastric activity is brought to an end by an autoregulatory device, the accumulation of acid in the antrum inhibiting the further release of gastrin. Gastric activity is also inhibited by certain duodenal polypeptides, the precise physiological status of which is not always clear. They will be referred to again later (p. 20).

2.2. The discovery of 'secretin'

Pancreatic secretion, like gastric secretion, is controlled by the interaction of neural and hormonal mechanisms. Pavlov demonstrated the direct involvement of the nervous system in experiments with dogs that had permanent pancreatic fistulae, with the pancreatic duct opening to the outside of the body; the rate of discharge of secretion could thus be directly observed. After prior preparation of the cervical vagus nerve, he was able to show that no (or very little) secretion occurred while the animal was resting; however, if the nerve was electrically stimulated, a flow of juice began after a latent period of some two minutes, and continued for four to five minutes after the end of the stimulus. Thus it appeared, in his words, to be 'definitely settled that the vagus is the secretory nerve of the pancreas'.

What, however, was the normal stimulus which brought the cervical vagus into action? When food enters the duodenum, it carries with it the acidity of the gastric secretion. It seemed possible, there-

fore, that the acid might signal the need for the release of pancreatic secretion, and experiments showed that some such device was, in fact, used. If 150 ml of 0·5% solution of the acid was introduced into the stomach of a dog with a pancreatic fistula, there resulted, after 2–3 minutes, an increased outflow of secretion from the duct. Pure gastric juice had a similar effect, but an equivalent amount of alkaline water did not, while if the contents of the stomach were neutralized at the height of the normal digestive process, when pancreatic juice was flowing freely, this flow ended. So, again in the words of Pavlov, it seemed possible to conclude that 'this powerful influence of acids upon the pancreas is one of the most securely established facts in the whole physiology of the gland'.

Thus it might well be that the increased outflow of juice from the pancreas during normal digestion was mediated through the vagus as a result of acid stimulating the intestine. Even so, however, it remained to determine the actual connection between this stimulus and the discharge of impulses through the nerve, and it was at this point of the analysis that difficulties appeared. Popielski showed at the beginning of the century that the stimulating effect of the acid could still be demonstrated even after all connections of the alimentary tract with the central nervous system had been destroyed by section of the vagi and of the splanchnic nerves, together with removal of the solar plexus and destruction of the spinal cord. He therefore concluded that the pancreatic response must depend upon a peripheral mechanism rather than a central one, and that it must be mediated by local reflexes operating through nerve cells in the pancreas and the intestinal wall. This view was plausible, although it remains uncertain how far the neural organization of the alimentary canal actually provides for such local reflexes. In any case, however, a more rigorous analysis was to show that this was not, in fact, the only possible explanation. The credit for this belongs to Bayliss and Starling who, in resolving this problem, established one of the major landmarks in the development of endocrinology.

Their achievement in breaking through the established preconceptions that were hindering progress was the more remarkable in that their studies of the movements of the alimentary canal had led them to the view that peristaltic contractions might be mediated by local nervous connections in Auerbach's plexus. This was, of course, substantially the explanation postulated by Popielski to account for the regulation of pancreatic secretion, but Bayliss and

Starling perceived in the literature indications that the explanation was not wholly convincing in this particular context. Wertheimer and Lepage, for example, had shown in 1901 that the introduction of acid into a portion of the jejunum would evoke pancreatic secretion even when this portion was completely severed from both the duodenum above it and from the rest of the intestine below it. It is curious that they did not carry this experiment to its logical extreme by cutting at the same time all the possible nervous connections, but Bayliss and Starling saw the necessity for doing this and made it the basis for their crucial experiment.

This was carried out on 16 January 1902. Using an anaesthetized dog maintained under artificial respiration in a warm saline bath, they removed the ganglia of the solar plexus, cut both vagi, tied off a loop of jejunum at both ends, and cut the mesenteric nerves supplying it; the loop was thus connected to the rest of the body only by its arteries and veins. (Such an experiment, in which the animal is necessarily killed at the end of it, is referred to as acute, while those in which the animal remains alive, as in the pancreatic fistulae experiments already mentioned, are described as chronic.) With a cannula inserted into the pancreatic duct, and with the blood pressure being recorded from the cartoid artery, they introduced 20 ml of 0·4% hydrochloric acid into the duodenum. This (Fig. 2.6(a)) evoked a well-marked pancreatic secretion of one drop every twenty seconds, lasting for some six minutes, after an initial latent period of about two minutes. Such a response merely confirmed previous work, but they went further and introduced the acid into the loop of jejunum, and found that this, too, evoked the discharge of pancreatic secretion. This might have been a result of the acid stimulating the pancreas directly after it had been absorbed into the circulation, but Wertheimer and Lepage had already shown that the injection of acid into the blood stream did not produce a secretory response. Bayliss and Starling therefore concluded that the presence of the acid was causing the jejunal mucosa to discharge some chemical excitant into the circulation, and that it was this that was stimulating the pancreas. To quote the words of C. J. Martin, who was present at the time, 'I remember Starling saying: "Then it must be a chemical reflex." Rapidly cutting off a further piece of jejunum, he rubbed its mucous membrane with sand in a weak HCl, filtered, and injected it into the jugular vein of the animal. After a few moments the pancreas responded by a much greater secretion than had occurred before. It was a great afternoon.'

This important experiment (Fig. 2.6(b)) was one of the major steps in the evolution of the fundamental concept of internal secretion. As we have already seen, this was not a new concept at the time, nor is it usual for such a novel idea to arise, as it were, ready made. Bayliss and Starling, however, were dealing with a particular type of internal secretory activity in which a product of one tissue was co-ordinating the functioning of another tissue by acting as a chemical messenger. To the secretion which they had shown was produced by the intestine they gave the name 'secretin', which we shall continue to place within inverted commas for a reason that will become apparent later. After much search for a general term for such secretions they adopted the name hormone, which had been suggested to them by W. B. Hardy, and which we have already defined (p. 2). This word is less apt than could have been wished, for it is derived from the Greek *hormaein*, which merely means 'to impel or arouse to activity'. Bayliss, in recounting at a later date the history of this event, therefore found it necessary to emphasize that 'although the property of messenger was not suggested by it, it has been generally understood as carrying this meaning'.

2.3. The hormonal status of 'secretin'

The demonstration that signals could be transmitted from the intestine to the pancreas through the blood came as a shock to the workers in Pavlov's laboratory, but his own reaction was as dignified as might have been expected. He asked for the experiment to be repeated in his presence, watched the result, and disappeared into his study for a brief interval. On his re-emergence, he remarked that of course Bayliss and Starling were correct. 'It is clear that we did not take out an exclusive patent for the discovery of truth.'

Nevertheless, it was natural that this important finding should have been subjected to searching examination and criticism by contemporaries. Thus it was argued that the nervous connections of the pancreas with the jejunal loop had not, in fact, been as completely severed as the investigators had claimed. This was fair criticism, in so far as it was impossible to be sure that no nerve fibres were reaching the loop in conjunction with the blood vessels that were supplying its circulation, but Bayliss and Starling replied that the possibility of such fibres being present did not alter the fact that by assuming their absence they had been led to the discovery of 'secretin'. The demonstration of such fibres, even supposing that they were present, could not invalidate that discovery. It could not be denied,

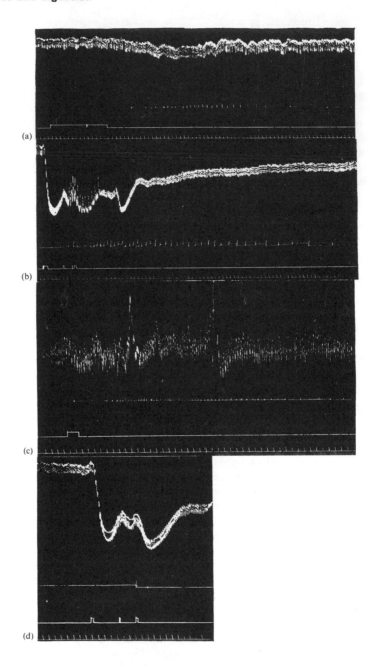

FIG. 2.6. Tracings illustrating the discovery of 'secretin' in the dog. Upper curve, blood pressure; uppermost of the three lines, drops of pancreatic secretion; middle line, signal indicating injection; bottom line, time in 10 s intervals, and level of zero blood pressure.

(a) Effect of injection of acid into duodenum after destruction of spinal cord; a marked flow of pancreatic juice occurs after a latent period of about 2 min.

(b) 'The crucial experiment'—the injection of acid extract of jejunal mucous membrane into a vein; the effect is a considerable fall of blood pressure, followed after a latent period of about 70 s by a flow of pancreatic juice.

(c) Effect of injecting 'secretin' prepared from mucous membrane extracted with absolute alcohol; there is a powerful effect on the pancreas, but no fall of blood pressure. (Blood pressure zero is here at 21 mm below the time marker.)

(d) Effect of injecting acid extract of lower end of ileum; there is a fall of blood pressure but no effect on the pancreas. (From Bayliss and Starling (1902) *J. Physiol.* **28**, 325–53.)

however, that such an important new principle would appear in a much more convincing light if all possibility of nervous control were actually eliminated, and this assurance was subsequently given as a result of ingenious surgical procedures that were developed in the United States by Ivy and others, utilizing dogs as experimental animals.

In essence, they auto-transplanted a portion of the pancreas and its duct, and also portions of the jejunum, into new positions beneath the skin. As with the gastric transplant already discussed, they acquired a new circulatory supply from the cutaneous vessels, and when this had happened their original supply was cut away. They were now vascularized solely from the skin, and there was no possibility at all of their newly developed vessels conveying into them nerve fibres which might connect them with each other or with organs from which they had been separated. In these circumstances it was found that when dilute hydrochloric acid was passed through the isolated jejunal loop there resulted a discharge of secretion through the duct of the auto-transplanted portion of the pancreas. This response could only have been evoked by the transmission of some substance from the loop to the pancreas through the blood stream.

This experiment, incidentally, goes a long way to demonstrate that the supposed hormone does actually circulate in the blood in normal physiological conditions. To this point attention was given as soon as Bayliss and Starling's first results had been published, and within a year other workers had shown that the transference of blood from a dog with acid in its intestine into another dog would cause the pancreas of the latter to secrete even though no acid was present in its own intestine. Further evidence came from Matsuo, who, in 1913, devised a cross-circulation experiment in which two dogs were placed together head to head with a carotid artery of each connected by glass tubing with a jugular vein of the other, and with separate cannulae inserted into their pancreatic ducts. After this common circulation had been maintained for ten minutes, during which time no secretion was discharged from the pancreas, 30 ml of 0·4% hydrochloric acid were introduced into the duodenum of one of the animals. In 5 minutes the pancreas of this dog began to secrete, and after another 1–3 minutes the pancreas of the other dog began also, both continuing for some 15–20 minutes. This type of experiment can be criticized as unphysiological. Nevertheless, Matsuo felt justified in concluding that it was 'beyond doubt that the secretion of pancreatic juice is caused under physiological conditions by some chemical substance which is liberated by the injection of acid into the duodenum or jejunum, enters into the general circulation, and stimulates the cells of the pancreas'.

Another criticism was that the effect of the supposed hormone was not a specific one, produced by one particular secretion, but was due to the vasodepressor action of tissue extracts. This was the criticism that was also applied, as we have seen, to the gastrin theory of Edkins. Bayliss and Starling were very well aware that the injection of intestinal extracts gave a marked lowering of blood pressure, which is clearly seen in Figs 2.6(a) and (b), but they showed that this effect was much reduced if the extraction was carried out for twenty-four hours with absolute alcohol in a Soxhlet apparatus instead of with acid (Fig. 2.6(c)). They also found that the epithelial lining of the intestine was mostly shed if the dorsal aorta was temporarily occluded, and that extracts prepared from these desquamated cells still had a marked effect on pancreatic secretion, but only a negligible one on blood pressure.

Moreover, they were able to show that 'secretin' was specific in its site of origin within the body, for it was not present in extracts of a variety of other tissues and, most significantly, it could not be obtained from the mucosa of other parts of the alimentary canal (Fig. 2.6(d)). In fact, potent extracts could only be obtained from those parts, the duodenum and jejunum, which were normally acted upon by the acid gastric chyme. Thus the supposition that 'secretin' was no more than a generalized 'vasodilatin' was never very well founded.

2.4. Secretin and cholecystokinin/pancreozymin: physiology

We must now consider in more detail the physiological significance of 'secretin'. The initial complication is that the secretory activity of the pancreas is influenced by the vagus nerve as well as by hormonal action. Pavlov's technique for demonstrating this in dogs has already been mentioned, but it can also readily be shown in acute experiments of the type used by Bayliss and Starling. For this purpose the vagus is prepared for faradic stimulation and a cannula inserted into the pancreatic duct so that the drops of secretion can be counted and can also be collected for subsequent analysis, particularly for their protein (enzyme) content. Fixation of pieces of the pancreas at the beginning and end of the experiment makes it also possible to prepare sections showing whether or not there has been any discharge of secretory granules.

The main effect of vagal stimulation in these experiments is to bring about an extensive discharge of enzymes. This is indicated by their increased concentration in the pancreatic secretion, while examination of sections shows a marked reduction in the granule content of the cells. On the other hand, the effect upon the volume of secretion is very variable; an increased output in the dog was, as we have seen, clearly shown in Pavlov's experiments, but in the anaesthetized cat there may be little or no increase.

In contrast to this, the main effect of the injection of 'secretin' preparations into the blood stream is to promote a great increase in the volume of the secretion, while the juice so produced has at most only a low concentration of enzymes. Indeed, there was for many years disagreement as to whether 'secretin' had any effect at all upon the discharge of the latter. This disagreement, perplexing at the time, can now be seen as the result of the use of different technical procedures in different laboratories. Investigators in the United States were preparing their 'secretin' by saturating the initial acid extract with sodium chloride. This brought down the hormone in a so-called 'A precipitate', which was a putty-like substance, containing up to 72 per cent water and a considerable amount of impurities, but relatively free of vasodilator activity. Alcohol extraction of this salt cake, followed by evaporation and precipitation by trichloracetic acid, yielded a highly potent material known as 'SI', which proved an excellent starting-point for further purification. Those who used this preparation concluded that 'secretin' produced some discharges of enzymes as well as of fluid, although the enzyme output was slight in comparison with that evoked by vagal stimulation.

In England, however, J. Mellanby was exploiting another method of preparation, in which the intestinal mucosa was extracted with absolute alcohol and the active material precipitated in association with bile salts, to which it was adsorbed. A potent preparation of the hormone was then obtained by elution. Using this material, Mellanby was unable to obtain any evidence for discharge of enzymes. He thus concluded that enzyme output was entirely under the control of the vagus, and that the function of 'secretin' was to bring about secretion of the fluid in which the enzymes were transported. In arriving at this conclusion, he had moved a very long way indeed from the position taken up initially by Bayliss and Starling, who had at one time claimed that the hormonal method of control was 'the normal one', and that 'a concomitant nervous process . . . is superfluous and therefore improbable'.

Renewed investigation of these disagreements by Harper and Vass in 1941 showed that the entry of food material into the duodenum of the cat undoubtedly promoted an increased discharge of enzymes from the pancreas, even when all the nerves to the intestine had been severed. Mellanby's view, therefore, could not possibly be correct, yet they were able to confirm his finding that the hormone did not stimulate the discharge of enzymes *if it was prepared by his method*. From this, they went on to demonstrate the explanation of the disagreements, which is that two hormones are concerned, both of them being secreted by the duodenum, and that different extraction methods give different yields. One of these hormones, secretin *sensu stricto* (which we shall refer to without the use of inverted commas), is defined as the hormone, extractable from the mucosa of the small intestine, which stimulates fluid and bicarbonate secretion by the pancreas. The other, to which they gave the name pancreozymin, brings about the discharge of enzymes. With Mellanby's method of preparation the secretin is extracted with the bile salts, while the pancreozymin remains in solution and can then be obtained by precipitation with sodium chloride. This explains why his material

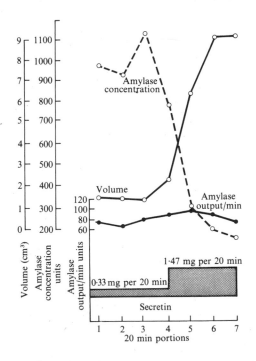

FIG. 2.7. Effect of increasing the rate of secretin administration on the volume and enzyme content of pancreatic juice in an unanaesthetized dog. (From Wang *et al.* (1948). *Am. J. Physiol.* **154**, 358–68.)

evoked no discharge of enzymes. The 'SI' prepara-tion, however, contains both hormones, so that those who used it were perfectly correct in claiming that their 'secretin' did evoke enzyme discharge. The two hormones can be separated from this material by making the final precipitation with bile salts and acetic acid instead of with trichloracetic acid; both come down in the precipitate and the secretin can be extracted from this with alcohol, the pan-creozymin remaining with the alcohol-insoluble residue. That pancreozymin is actually transmitted through the blood stream has been demonstrated in dogs prepared, in the manner outlined earlier, with a subcutaneously auto-transplanted pancreas;

the introduction of food substances into the duo-denum through a fistula evokes the discharge of pancreatic fluid and an increased output of enzymes and, in the absence of any nervous connections, the stimulus must be a hormonal one.

Data illustrating the contrasting effect of these two hormones are summarized in Figs 2.7 and 2.8(a) and (b). Fig. 2.7 presents data obtained from an experi-ment in which secretin was administered to an unan-aesthetized dog, initially at a rate of 0.33 mg per twenty minutes; the volume of secretion and its amylase concentration remain approximately constant and so also, in consequence, does the output of amylase per minute. When the rate of administration of secretin

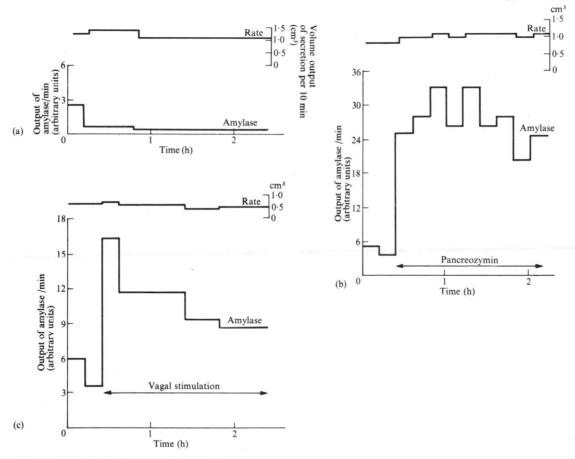

Fig. 2.8. Demonstration of hormonal and neural influences on pancreatic secretion in the cat.

(a) Secretin only injected, injections regularly repeated throughout resulting in a flow of juice of low enzyme content, with no alteration in the granule content of the zymogen cells (cf. Fig. 2.9).

(b) The flow of pancreatic juice was maintained by injections of secretin. In addition, during the period indicated by the arrows, 9 mg of a pancreozymin preparation was given every 12 min. This resulted in a sustained increase in the output of amylase and a depletion of the granule content of the zymogen cells (cf. Fig. 2.10).

(c) The flow of pancreatic juice was maintained by injections of secretin. In addition, during the period indicated by arrows, the dorsal vagus trunk was stimulated in the thorax. This resulted in an increase in the output of amylase and a depletion of the granule content of the zymogen cells. (From Harper and Mackay (1948). *J. Physiol.* **107**, 89–96.)

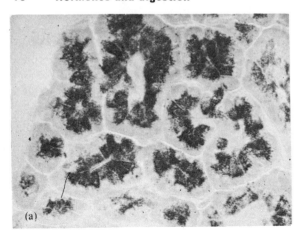
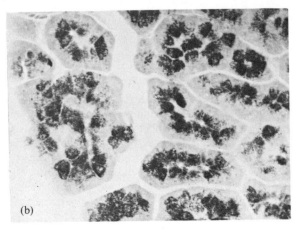

FIG. 2.9. Sections of pancreatic tissue of the cat removed (a) before and (b) after stimulation by secretin; there is no reduction in its content of zymogen granules (cf. Fig. 2.8(a)).

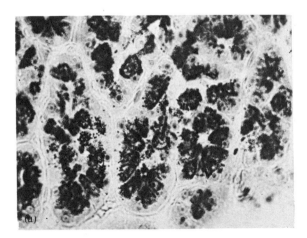
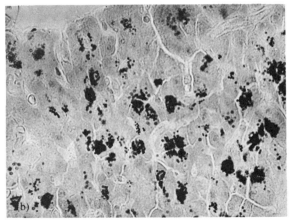

FIG. 2.10. Sections of pancreatic tissue of the cat removed (a) before and (b) after stimulation by secretin and pancreozymin; there is marked depletion of the zymogen granules (cf. Fig. 2.8(b)). (From Harper and Mackay (1948). *J. Physiol.* **107**, 89–96.)

is suddenly increased more than threefold, to 1·47 mg per twenty minutes, the volume of secretion and its amylase concentration remain approximately constant and so also, in consequence, does the output of amylase per minute. When the rate of administration of secretin is suddenly increased more than threefold, to 1·47 mg per twenty minutes, the volume of secretion immediately increases but there is a reciprocal fall in the concentration of the enzyme, so that the output of this per minute remains approximately constant. Thus the secretin is affecting the rate of output of the fluid but not the rate of output of the enzyme. Actually, there is often a temporary small rise in the latter when the rate of administration is in-

creased, but this is due to the washing-out of accumulated enzyme from the pancreatic alveoli, the small cavities into which the cells discharge. A similar effect is usually seen at the beginning of an experiment, when the secretin is administered for the first time; the early samples of juice carry a high enzyme content which is also a result of this washing-out.

The effects of secretin and of pancreozymin are contrasted in Fig. 2.8 (see also Figs 2.9 and 2.10). The injection of secretin at regular intervals into an anaesthetized cat produces a steady output of pancreatic juice with a low amylase content, and at the end of the experiment there has been no noticeable diminution of the zymogen content of the cells. If pancreozymin is injected in addition, however, there is no change in the volume output but a marked increase in the output of amylase, accompanied by a reduction of the zymogen granules. If, instead of the injection of pancreozymin, the stimulation of the vagus is superimposed upon the secretin treatment, the result is very similar; amylase output is increased (its subsequent decline being due to fatigue of the preparation) without any concomitant increase in the volume of the fluid secretion, while the cells again show a marked decrease in their zymogen content (Fig. 2.8(c)). In fact, the action of the vagus almost exactly parallels that of pancreozymin except for one difference. Atropine has no effect upon the action of the hormone, but it abolishes the secretomotor effect of the vagus as a result of its normal paralyzing influence upon the parasympathetic nerve endings.

These reactions can also be readily demonstrated *in vitro*, slices of the pancreas of the pigeon being particularly suitable for the purpose. If such slices are incubated in saline media in Warburg baths it is found that extrusion of preformed secretory granules will take place on the addition to the medium of either pancreozymin or acetylcholine. The latter mimics the effect of vagal stimulation since it is the normal chemical transmitter at parasympathetic nerve endings (p. 59), and its effect is therefore abolished if atropine is also added, since this prevents it from acting upon effector cells. The effect of pancreozymin, however, is uninfluenced by atropine, a clear demonstration of the distinction between the hormonal and the neurohumoral types of action which we shall be discussing later. Another distinction can equally clearly be made by the substitution of secretin for pancreozymin; this shows that the former has no influence upon discharge of the zymogen granules.

So far we have referred to the discharge of hormones by the duodenum as though hydrochloric acid were the only stimulating agent involved. This assumption is, in fact, often implicit in accounts of the process, but it is certainly not correct, for it is known that gastrectomy (removal of the stomach) and achlorhydria (reduction of gastric acidity) need not affect intestinal digestion. The evidence shows that only a part of the total response of the pancreas can be accounted for by the stimulating effect of the acid that enters the duodenum, and that in dogs the response of the gland to a meal of meat continues even if the duodenal contents are neutralized by the introduction of a solution of sodium bicarbonate. By using an animal with the auto-transplanted pancreas and duodenal loop described above, it has been

shown that acid in the latter is a powerful releaser of secretin but that its effect on pancreozymin is much weaker. Peptones and amino acids, on the other hand, are strong stimuli for the release of pancreozymin and are second only to acid in their effect on secretin. Fatty acids are also effective stimulants, but carbohydrates are not. That these substances act by releasing the relevant hormones, and not by direct stimulation of the pancreas, is shown by the fact that they have no effect upon that organ when they are injected into the blood stream. It is thus clear that the pancreatic hormonal mechanism does not rely only upon acid, but that it makes use also of the class of stimulants known as secretagogues; these may be defined as substances present in food, or produced by its digestion, which excite the production of digestive secretions either by local action, or by entering the blood, or by causing hormones to be released.

The disentangling of the actions of secretin and of pancreozymin upon the pancreas is not the end of the line of research established by Bayliss and Starling, for both of these hormones have actions also upon the liver. Bayliss and Starling themselves noted that their 'secretin' preparations strongly stimulated the flow of bile, but they did not establish whether one hormone only was involved. Later work with pure preparations has made it clear that secretin (*sensu stricto*) has a weak stimulating action upon the flow of bile, but that it does not promote the secretory activity of the hepatic cells. The action is adaptively meaningful, for it can be said that both actions of secretin encourage intestinal digestion by contributing to the neutralization of the gastric juice.

Secretin can also inhibit gastric motility and the secretion of acid. These effects, too, are adaptively meaningful, but this cannot be said of other reported activities, such as the promotion of pepsin secretion. It is possible that some of these other actions are pharmacological rather than physiological, or that they are artifacts resulting from modification of the hormone molecule during its purification. We shall return later to these overlapping actions.

2.5 Secretin and cholecystokinin/pancreozymin: chemistry

Evidence of hormonal regulation of contraction of the gall bladder in mammals first emerged in 1928, when Ivy and Oldberg gave the name cholecystokinin to a hormone that they believed to have this effect. Their proposition aroused little interest, but attention revived when, during Harper's work on pancreozymin, it became apparent that his material had a marked action on the gall bladder. At first this suggested that there was indeed another hormone secreted by the intestine. Later, however, it became clear that this was not quite so. Cholecystokinin certainly exists in one sense, but it and pancreozymin have proved to be one and the same hormone, which has been termed, somewhat inconveniently, cholecystokinin/pancreozymin, or, for short, CCK/PZ. However, it is likely that the more convenient term cholecystokinin will come into general use, since it can be justified on grounds of priority, although this will obscure the interesting story of the discovery and characterization of the hormone. The conclusion that only one hormone is involved follows decisively from chemical studies. These, aimed initially at the preparation of material in a form sufficiently pure for clinical use, have led to the determination of the amino-acid

Because of the potential medical importance of these two preparations, Mutt was asked by Swedish clinicians, after the Second World War, to restudy the problem of their purification. He has recorded how at first he hesitated to undertake the work, because the problem seemed to contain 'nothing of scientific interest'. Soon, however, he found that the earlier preparations had been far less pure than had been supposed; an understandable consequence of the lack in those earlier years of techniques suitable for the purification of labile peptides. By 1952 new methods involving ion exchangers were available, and these formed the basis for the new attack. As a result, Jorpes and Mutt were able to isolate the pure hormone, and to determine its amino-acid sequence along the lines laid down by the pioneer work of Sanger (p. 35).

Secretin (Fig. 2.11) is a single-chain polypeptide

Secretin	His	Ser	Asp	Gly	Thr	Phe	Thr	Ser	Glu	Leu	Ser	Arg	Leu	Arg	Asp	Ser	Ala
	1	2	3	4	5	6	7	8	9	10	11	12	13	14	15	16	17
	Arg	Leu	Gln	Arg	Leu	Leu	Gln	Gly	Leu	Val-NH$_2$							
	18	19	20	21	22	23	24	25	26	27							
Glucagon	His	Ser	Gln	Gly	Thr	Phe	Thr	Ser	Asp	Tyr	Ser	Lys	Trp	Leu	Asp	Ser	Arg
	1	2	3	4	5	6	7	8	9	10	11	12	13	14	15	16	17
	Arg	Ala	Gln	Asp	Phe	Val	Gln	Trp	Leu	Met	Asn	Thr					
	18	19	20	21	22	23	24	25	26	27	28	29					

FIG. 2.11. Primary structure of secretin and glucagon. Positions in which no substitutions have occurred are underlined.

sequences of cholecystokinin/pancreozymin and of secretin. The story goes back to 1933. At that time Swedish workers had obtained a preparation of 'secretin' in the form of a crystalline picrolonate, derived, after crystallization from pyridine, from a salicylate. This material proved of some value in clinical studies. By persuading a patient to swallow a lead ball, a silk cord, and a double stomach-and-duodenal tube, it was possible to aspirate the duodenal contents. Study of the composition of the pancreatic juice secreted in response to intravenous injections of the preparation made it possible to judge the functional condition of the pancreas.

In 1938, workers in the United States obtained another crystalline picrolonate, also by the use of pyridine, but the two substances were not identical. Chemical and X-ray diffraction studies indicated that they must be complexes of uncertain composition, although it seemed probable by now that the hormone itself was a polypeptide.

of low molecular weight, with 27 amino-acid residues, and bearing a strongly basic charge due to the arginine and histidine residues, and to the amidation of two of the glutamic acid ones. The cells that secrete it have been located in the mammalian intestine by immunohistochemistry. The whole molecule is needed for normal biological activity. Fragments obtained by degradation or synthesis show no more than a trace of this; for example, sequence 5–27 has no biological activity, 2–27 has only very slight activity, and 1–6 and 1–14 have little or none. The molecule provides another example of resemblances between the sequences of biologically active polypeptides, for there are considerable structural resemblances between secretin and glucagon. Indeed, the differences are little greater than those sometimes found between functionally similar polypeptide molecules from distantly related species (Fig. 2.11, and see p. 43).

Bayliss and Starling had suggested that secretin

was stored as a prosecretin that was in some way activated by hydrochloric acid. Jorpes points out that this view is in principle correct, if restated in different terms. Secretin, because it is strongly basic, is electrostatically bound to ionized carboxyl groups within the cell, and it cannot be easily extracted. The acid, when it enters the cell, can be supposed to neutralize the negative charge of the proteins and so to set the secretin free as a hydrochloride that can readily diffuse into the blood.

Purification of secretin involves its extraction into methanol. The methanol-insoluble residue contains material that acts both on the gall bladder and on the secretion of pancreatic enzymes; in other words, it contains both the cholecystokinin and the pancreozymin components. Subsequent purification of this

more active than the whole molecule, even on a molar basis. This octapeptide closely resembles the molecules of gastrin II and also of caerulein, which is a secretion of the skin of certain anuran amphibians, and, while of unknown function in those animals, shares the biological activities of the two hormones. The COOH-terminal pentapeptide sequence is identical in all three molecules, and they all contain a sulphated tyrosine residue. Further, the 16–25 sequence of CCK/PZ also has some resemblance to part of the calcitonin molecule (p. 154). These various structural resemblances account to some extent for the overlap of the actions of the gastro-intestinal hormones, but the resemblances have other implications as well, and these we shall discuss later (p. 101).

The dramatic circumstances connected with the

Human gastrin II	Glu	Gly	Pro	Try	Leu	Glu(5)	Ala	Tyr(SO$_3$H)	Gly	Try	Met	Asp	Phe-NH$_2$
	1	2	3	4	5	6–10	11	12	13	14	15	16	17
Caerulein				Glu	Gln	Asp	Tyr(SO$_3$H)	Thr	Gly	Try	Met	Asp	Phe-NH$_2$
				1	2	3	4	5	6	7	8	9	10
Porcine cholecystokinin/ pancreozymin				(1–25)		Asp	Tyr(SO$_3$H)	Met	Gly	Try	Met	Asp	Phe-NH$_2$
				1–25		26	27	28	29	30	31	32	33

FIG. 2.12. Primary structure of human gastrin II, cholecystokinin/pancreozymin, and caerulein.

material over ion exchangers results in a 10 000-fold increase in hormonal activity, but there is no change in the ratio of cholecystokinin to pancreozymin. This in itself is strong evidence that there is only one hormone exerting both types of effect, and this has been confirmed by determinations of the amino-acid sequence of the molecule, and by further studies of its properties.

Cholecystokinin/pancreozymin is a single-chain polypeptide with thirty-three amino acids (Fig. 2.12), and with a sulphated tyrosyl. As with gastrin and secretin, it has a number of actions additional to its primary ones upon the gall bladder and the secretion of pancreatic enzymes. It stimulates secretion of gastric acid and of the duodenal succus entericus, it inhibits gastric motility, and it increases duodenal motility. These actions largely depend on the COOH-terminal heptapeptide, the sulphated tyrosyl being also a necessary requirement. In these respects it contrasts with secretin, for which virtually the complete molecule is required for activity. Indeed, the COOH-terminal octapeptide 26–33 of CCK/PZ, obtained by degradation, is several times

discovery of 'secretin', and the importance which this assumed in the development of endocrinological principles, led to an overshadowing of the part played by the nervous system in pancreatic regulation in mammals. Neural regulation came to be regarded as redundant or, at best, baffling. However, in the light of our earlier summary of the regulation of gastric secretion by neural and endocrine interactions, it is possible to interpret pancreatic regulation along similar lines.

Here again we can distinguish first a cephalic phase, evoked in the same way as the cephalic phase of gastric digestion, and mediated by the vagus nerve. This can convey impulses directly to the gland, or can influence the pancreas indirectly by evoking the release of gastrin, which then, as we have seen, can exert some action upon the pancreas. The result in both cases is predominantly the release of pancreatic enzymes, but it is possible that the vagal impulses also adjust the pancreatic blood vessels to facilitate the prolonged secretory activity that will follow.

This cephalic phase is followed by a gastric phase, in which the vagus is again involved. Stimulation of the fundus of the stomach by the presence of food sets up impulses that are propagated by vago-vagal reflex pathways to the pancreas, while stimulation of the antrum liberates gastrin which acts again as a pancreatic stimulant. As with the cephalic phase, the main result of the gastric phase is the liberation of enzymes.

The major part of the regulatory mechanism, however, is a third phase, the intestinal phase, which is primarily under endocrine regulation by secretin and cholecystokinin/pancreozymin. Whether the nervous system is also involved in this phase is not clear, but there is some evidence that vagal stimulation increases the sensitivity of the pancreas to the two hormones. The main releasing agent in this phase is, of course, the acid of the gastric chyme, but fatty acids and amino acids also play a part, and it is possible that the bile does so as well.

2.6. Other intestinal polypeptides

Several other polypeptides besides secretin and cholecystokinin/pancreozymin have been extracted from the small intestine. Their physiological significance is not always clear, but there is evidence to justify regarding at least one of them as a hormone.

Bulbogastrone, which inhibits gastric acid secretion, is secreted in the upper duodenum (duodenal bulb). This substance is not yet chemically characterized, but the physiological evidence for its hormonal nature is good. It is released from the mucosa by the acid pH resulting from the entry of the acid chyme, this stimulus being a highly specific one; in particular, fats, which inhibit gastric activity, do not influence its release. That it is distinct from secretin and cholecystokinin/pancreozymin can be shown by perfusing the duodenal bulb with acid; this inhibits gastric secretion without affecting the output of either fluid or enzymes from the pancreas. Another inhibitor of gastric acid secretion is urogastrone, which is a polypeptide extracted from urine. It cannot on present evidence be regarded as an alimentary hormone, but it is at least possible that it may be a metabolite of one.

Gastric inhibitory polypeptide (GIP) is a well characterized product of the small intestine, inhibiting both gastric motility and gastric secretion. On the evidence of immunohistochemical studies, it is probably secreted by certain granular cells of the duodenal and jejunal glands. It has 43 amino acids, its sequence showing strong resemblances to secretin and glucagon (p. 18). Fifteen of the first 26 amino acid residues at the NH_2-terminal end are in the same position as in porcine glucagon, while 9 of the first 26 amino acids are in the same position as in secretin.

It has been suggested that this substance is identical with a supposed duodenal hormone, known since 1930 as enterogastrone, which has been thought to be released by the entry of fats and their digestive products into the duodenum, and thus to be responsible for the gastric inhibition produced by fats. Whether enterogastrone is indeed gastric inhibitory polypeptide is a little uncertain, since the chemical characterization of enterogastrone is not complete, while the normal physiological stimulus for the release of gastric inhibitory polypeptide remains unknown.

Another of these intestinal polypeptides is motilin, with 22 amino-acid residues, isolated from the intestinal mucosa of the pig. It is probably secreted by certain of the argentaffin enterochromaffin cells of the small intestine. Cells of this category are distributed throughout the gastro-intestinal mucosa, and are best known for their secretion of serotonin (5-hydroxytryptamine). Motilin, which has no sequence resemblance to any other of the gastro-intestinal polypeptides, stimulates gastric motor activity, but, as with gastric inhibitory polypeptide, it is uncertain what is the physiological stimulus for its release. Its hormonal significance thus remains in doubt.

Finally, vasoactive intestinal polypeptide, from the upper intestine of the pig, has 28 amino acids in a sequence which, like that of gastric inhibitory polypeptide, resembles that of secretin and glucagon. It relaxes smooth muscle, and, in consequence, increases splanchnic blood flow. Additionally, it has secretin-like effects on the pancreas, and produces hyperglycaemia (cf. glucagon, p. 43). Its hormonal status, like that of motilin, is uncertain, but even so, it is remarkable that the intestinal wall contains at least four biologically active polypeptides with related amino-acid sequences, and with some overlapping of actions. We shall discuss later the evolutionary implications of this situation (p. 105).

2.7. Some evolutionary considerations

A remarkable conclusion that emerges from the study of the regulation of digestion in mammals is the lack of precise demarcation between the actions of the nervous system and of the hormones, and between the multiple actions of the individual hormones themselves. What is the explanation of this? It is necessary first to bear in mind that the evidence is by no means straightforward to interpret. Only a very few species have been studied in this context, and, even so, there is much interspecific variability in response. It is necessary also to take account of the possibility that even preparations of a supposedly high level of purity may be contaminated with another hormone. For example, 100 units of one particular commercial preparation of secretin may

fortunately, little is known of the normal blood levels of these hormones; thus the decision that a particular effect is physiological and not pharmacological must be largely subjective.

However, having taken these difficulties into account, it can reasonably be assumed, as a basis for

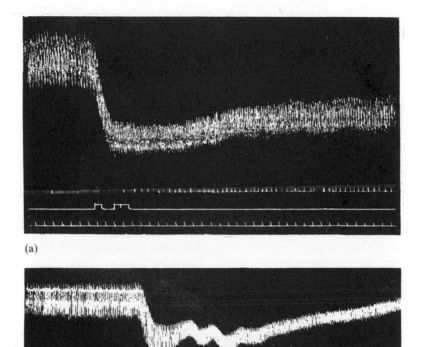

(a)

(b)

FIG. 2.13. Effect on pancreatic secretion in the dog of injecting intravenously (a) 15 ml of a 'secretin' solution prepared from the intestine of the fowl, and (b) 5 ml of a 'secretin' solution prepared from the intestine of a dogfish (cf. Fig. 2.6 for further explanation). (From Bayliss and Starling (1903). *J. Physiol.* **29**, 174–80.)

contain as much as 25 units of pancreozymin activity. The demonstration that a particular response, when such impurities have been allowed for, is truly physiological, rests in part upon formal definitions. One of these (and it is a rigorous one) is that an effect, to be regarded as physiological, must be produced by an amount of the hormone concerned that does not exceed the amount that would be released during normal digestion. Un-

argument, that some of the interactions and overlaps mentioned earlier are likely to be physiological ones. It has been suggested that they are characteristic of a primitive and imperfectly differentiated regulatory system. Conceivably, the alimentary system has remained at a primitive level of organization in this respect because it is a self-regulating system that is essentially independent of the rest of the endocrine system. Whether or not this is so,

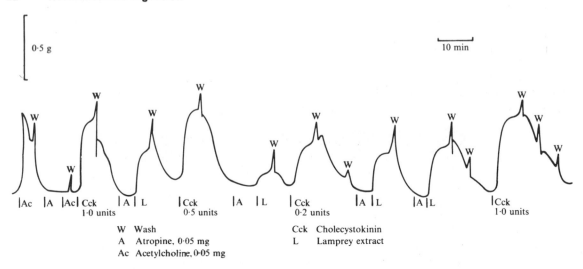

0·5 g

10 min

| Ac | A | Ac | Cck | A | L | Cck | A | L | Cck | A | L | A | L | Cck |
| --- | --- | --- | 1·0 units | --- | --- | 0·5 units | --- | --- | 0·2 units | --- | --- | --- | --- | 1·0 units |

W	Wash
A	Atropine, 0·05 mg
Ac	Acetylcholine, 0·05 mg

Cck	Cholecystokinin
L	Lamprey extract

FIG. 2.14. Trace showing the action of cholecystokinin (= cholecystokinin/pancreozymin, Boots Pure Drug Company) and extract of the intestine of the river lamprey (*Lampetra fluviatilis*) upon an *in vitro* preparation of the gall bladder of the rabbit. The contractions of the gall bladder were measured by a strain gauge (vertical scale) and recorded by a pen recorder. Both evoke similar contractions. (From an unpublished experiment of G. Dockray.)

however, is a question that cannot be answered until we know much more about digestive regulation in the lower vertebrates. It may well be found eventually that adaptation within the endocrine system of the alimentary tract is more subtle than we can at present appreciate. As regards neural regulation, however, there are certainly indications that the lower forms may be at a more primitive level of organization than are mammals. In the latter, the whole of the alimentary tract is under the dual and antagonistic regulation of the parasympathetic and sympathetic components of the autonomic nervous system. In fish, however, this system does not show such marked antagonism of the two components, nor do the two overlap so far in their distribution over the alimentary tract. For example, both vagal and sympathetic fibres evoke motor responses in parts of the musculature of the alimentary tract. There is no clear-cut antagonism of stimulation and inhibition of the gut musculature in fish, nor is it certain that the vagus extends further back than the pyloric region of the stomach.

As for the regulation of secretory activity in the alimentary tract, too little attention has been given to gastric digestion to permit useful conclusions, although there is some evidence that chemical influences play a part. For example, histamine stimulates gastric secretion in all the major groups, while mammalian gastrin stimulates the secretion of acid by the isolated gastric mucosa of the bullfrog. Generalization is not yet possible, although it seems

very likely, on general evolutionary grounds, that hormonal regulation will prove to be widely spread in the vertebrates. Some measure of nervous control certainly seems to be of general occurrence, sometimes mediated through vagal pathways, and sometimes through local reflexes stimulated by distension of the stomach wall.

The results of study of the pancreas are more positive, in that Bayliss and Starling showed that 'secretin' was widespread in vertebrates, for they were able to prepare active extracts from the intestine of the fowl, tortoise, frog, salmon, dogfish, and skate (Fig. 2.13). The information relating to these lower forms, however, remained incomplete, although it was later shown that secretion in rays could be increased by introducing acid into the intestine, and by intravenous injection of 'secretin' preparations.

More recently these studies have been carried further, owing to the development of improved extraction procedures, together with the use of acute preparations of the rat for the assay of small quantities of intestinal extracts. It has thus been shown that extracts of the intestine of cyclostomes and fish contain active material that influences the rate of output of fluid and enzyme from the pancreas of the rat. These extracts can thus be said to have both a secretin-like and a pancreozymin-like activity. Moreover, the use of an assay involving the isolated gall-bladder of the rabbit has shown that these extracts also have a cholecystokinin-like activity (Fig. 2.14). Secretin-like activity has also been identified in *Myxine* (representing the other main surviving group of cyclostomes) and in the chimaeroid *Hydrolagus* (a member of the ancient group of Holocephali, related probably to the elasmobranchs). These active factors have not been chemically characterized, but the evidence suggests at this stage that the production of substances capable of influencing pancreatic activity is an ancient property of the vertebrate alimentary tract. We shall consider later the wider implications of this conclusion (p. 105).

Whether the nervous system is involved in the regulation of pancreatic activity in the lower vertebrates is unknown. Some early experiments of Babkin suggested that there was no parasympathetic or sympathetic control of the secretory activity of the pancreas in these animals, for acetylcholine and adrenaline had no significant effect upon the volume of secretion discharged, but it is obviously impossible to generalize from such fragmentary information.

The whole field of alimentary regulation in the lower vertebrates is one in which there is need for much more work, and for the relating of the results to the physiological and ecological factors which influence feeding and digestion. In mammals the pancreas can be capable of spontaneous secretion, notably in the rabbit; in this animal it can continue to secrete after complete denervation of the organ, and even after decapitation and the removal of the whole of the alimentary tract with the exception of the liver and pancreas. It is possible (but this is only guesswork) that such a property, together with some degree of modulation by a simple hormonal mechanism, could meet the needs of the sluggish alimentary activity of fish, in which the digestion of a meal may take at least two days for completion. But feeding habits and digestive activities are highly variable, even in these lower groups, and undoubtedly present much scope for specialization in the details of their regulation.

3

Hormones and metabolism I

3.1. Diabetes mellitus and the pancreas

We shall now examine the effects of a hormone which, although it apparently originated within the alimentary tract, has come to form part of a physiological system very different from that of the digestive hormones. Diabetes mellitus (the 'pissing evil' of the seventeenth century) is a condition arising from profound disturbances of metabolism, the most obvious feature of which is a defective utilization of carbohydrate. This is reflected in an abnormally high concentration of glucose in the circulating blood (hyperglycaemia) and a reduction in the amount of glycogen stored in the liver and muscle. The affected individual passes a large quantity of urine (polyuria) which possesses a sweet taste as a result of the presence of excreted glucose. It is this taste that gives to the condition its name (*diabainein*, to pass through; *mellitus*, sweetened with honey). Not only the carbohydrates are affected, however, for protein and fats are called upon to supplement them as energy sources, and this leads to increased excretion of non-protein nitrogen, to wastage of the tissues despite high food intake, and to ketosis, which is the accumulation of ketone bodies (acetoacetic acid, acetone, and β-hydroxybutyric acid) in the blood and urine.

The cause of this condition remained unknown until recent times, despite its early recognition, and attempts to control it by regulation of the diet met with only limited success. A new phase, however, opened in 1889, in which year Minkowski, working under von Mering, undertook removal of the pancreas (pancreatectomy) from a dog as part of their study of digestive physiology. We have already seen that it is sometimes well not to be unduly inhibited by previous work. Von Mering doubted the practicability of the operation, but Minkowski was happily ignorant of Claude Bernard's statement that animals could not survive total pancreatectomy, and (as he subsequently confessed) was led by his youth to 'presumptuous overestimations of his capacities'. So

he carried out the operation, and found not only that it had been successful, but that it had been followed quite unexpectedly by the development of symptoms of diabetes mellitus. The recognition of this was a result of the dog persistently micturating in the laboratory, a lapse that led Minkowski to examine its urine and thus to find that it had a high glucose content. The discovery was of fundamental importance, for it showed that some disorder of the pancreas might be the origin of the diabetic condition, and also provided a technique for its experimental analysis. It could not, however, have been exploited so effectively had there not already existed some important information relating to the structure of the organ. We are dealing, in fact, with a striking example of the importance of linking experimental studies with histological observations, and it is the latter that we must first consider.

3.2. The islets of Langerhans

The digestive secretion of the pancreas arises within secretory alveoli or acini, which discharge into a branched system of ducts, but there is also an endocrine component present. The first step towards the recognition of this was taken when a twenty-two-year-old medical student, Paul Langerhans, published in 1869 a doctorate thesis in which he presented an account of the microscopical anatomy of the organ. He noted the zymogen granules, although since they were blackened by osmic acid he erroneously concluded that they were fat droplets, but he also found small groups of cells that lacked these granules, and which he thought might be associated in some way with the nervous system. The work was left incomplete, to his own regret, and he did not live to associate it with von Mering and Minkowski's discovery. By 1893, however, Laguesse had already realized the potential importance of these groups of cells and was referring to them as the islets of Langerhans, a name that they have retained ever since. This was a period in which observations on several organs, and particularly the thyroid gland and the gonads, were beginning to establish the foundations of endocrinology, although the time was not yet quite ripe for the synthesis of the scattered and sometimes confusing data. It was still being suggested that the relationship of the pancreas to the diabetic condition might result from that organ being concerned with the removal of some impurity from the body, but Laguesse was considering the possibility that the islets might be producing an internal secretion, and he seems to have been the first to use in this connection the terms endocrine and exocrine as descriptive of internally and externally secreting tissue.

The islets of Langerhans (Fig. 3.1) are scattered irregularly throughout the pancreas of mammals and vary greatly in size and number, even within the same species; in the guinea-pig there are from 15 000 to at least 40 000, while in the human pancreas counts ranging up to 2 300 000 have been recorded. They arise from the duct epithelium, and they often remain connected with the delicate extensions of this which pervade the whole organ. A feature related to their endocrine function is their very rich blood supply, with capillary vessels or sinusoids lying close against the irregular cords in which the islet cells come to be arranged. This provides for the removal of their secretion, and facilitates a direct response of the cells to the level of glucose in the blood, but the possibility that nervous reflexes may also be involved in islet activity is not entirely excluded.

An initial difficulty in relating pancreatic structure to the diabetic condition was that when the islets first came under detailed scrutiny it was impossible to say whether they were an independent tissue or whether they were stages in the development or degeneration of the zymogen cells. This problem was the focus of much of the early histological work. By the turn of the century, evidence had accumulated that the islet cells did show distinctive characteristics, and this view was supported by evidence of another type, which was later going to bear unexpected fruit. Schulze reported in 1900 that careful ligation of peripheral parts of the pancreas of the guinea-pig led to the degeneration of the zymogen tissue while the islets remained unaltered. From this he drew the conclusion that the latter must be independent structures, that they were vascular glands of the same type as the pituitary, and that they might well be involved in some way in the regulation of blood sugar.

Following upon these pioneer studies, particularly important advances were made by Lane, in 1907, and

Bensley, in 1911. The former introduced the use of so-called neutral stains such as neutral gentian, obtained as a precipitate by adding a solution of orange G to one of gentian violet. With such dyes, and by varying the fixative, he found evidence for the existence in the islet tissue of two distinctive cell types, the A (or alpha) and B (or beta) cells, distinguishable from each other and from the zymogen cells by the reactions of their granular contents. He recognized that these might be two different phases of the same fundamental cell, but rightly pointed out that even if this were so it would not exclude the possibility of the production of two different secretions. He concluded, in fact, that the islets were discharging into the blood stream 'a twofold substance' with an important effect upon metabolism. These observations were developed much more fully by Bensley, who, using a greater range of fixatives and stains, and studying the pancreas of the toad as well as the mammalian organ, firmly established the concept of the pancreas as an organ combining exocrine with endocrine functions. The award to him in 1952 of the Banting Medal of the American Diabetics Association was a well-merited tribute to the value of histological studies in the solution of endocrinological problems.

The neutral stains used so successfully by Lane and Bensley were found by later workers to be capricious in their effects, particularly when applied to other species. Much use was subsequently made of the Azan technique of Heidenhain, first introduced for this purpose by Bloom in 1931. In general, the granules of the A cells stain bright red with azocarmine, and those of the B cells orange-grey. Bloom was the first to identify also a third cell type, the D (or delta) cell, in which the granules stain bright blue. A fourth type is sometimes mentioned; this is the C cell, which, however, probably represents stages in the exhaustion or recovery of one or other of the other types.

The Azan technique and its later variations give beautiful results, but still suffer from the need to control most carefully all stages of the procedure. There is a markedly subjective element in deciding what constitutes a 'good' preparation, which may mean no more than a preparation demonstrating what the observer hopes to find. Moreover, the staining reactions are not specific for any particular cell component, so that identity of response, in comparing one species with another, must be analyzed by other procedures. A number of these are now available. They have given much greater certainty to interpretations of islet organization, especially since some of them can be used in series to stain the same section, thus making it possible to establish the properties of individual cells. Even so, however, they still have to be used with caution. For example, a method which is reliable histochemically, in the sense that it reveals a known chemical reaction, may be used to demonstrate the presence of a particular hormone, but need not be specific for that hormone alone. The undermentioned methods are thus of value when applied to material that is already known to be vertebrate pancreatic tissue, but their value

declines when they are applied to other tissues, including those of invertebrates, of which the hormonal content has still to be defined.

A wide range of evidence has now confirmed that mammalian islet tissue (Fig. 3.1) contains at least three types of cell, distinct in appearance and in function. They are referred to as A, B, and D cells, or alternatively as A_2 ($=A$), B, and A_1 ($=D$). We shall see in due course that the A_2 cells secrete the hormone glucagon; the B cells secrete the hormone insulin; and the A_1 cells possibly secrete gastrin.

Amongst the most useful of the newer staining methods are two procedures, introduced by Gomori, which also have found wide application in other fields of endocrinology. In one of these methods, the B granules are stained dark blue by chrome-alum–haematoxylin; in the other, they are stained violet magenta by aldehyde–fuchsin. The A granules are then counter-stained by acid dyes such as phloxin or ponceau de xylidine. Both methods require experience before reliable results can be obtained; careful attention needs to be given to the oxidation procedure, as well as to the age of the staining fluids and the methods of preparing them. Neither of them is specific for insulin. Nevertheless, the response of the B granules to aldehyde–fuchsin has some histochemical basis, in that it results from the production of SO_3 groups from the sulphydryl groups of the insulin molecule, after oxidation with permanganate, which splits the S—S bonds. Other cytochemical reagents and procedures are available, but again they are not specific for the islet hormones. One of these reagents is pseudoisocyanin, which yields metachromasia and fluorescence in the presence of SO_3 groups formed by performic acid or potassium permanganate oxidation (Fig. 3.2). The dihydroxy-

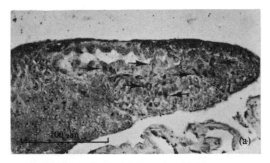

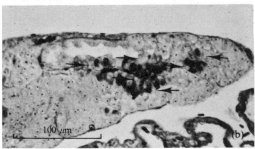

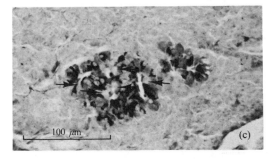

FIG. 3.1. Identification of A ($=A_2$), B, and D ($=A_1$) cells in sections of the pancreatic islets of a lizard, *Lygosoma laterale*. Fixation in Bouin's fluid. (a) Impregnated with silver; several argyrophil D cells are seen (arrows). (b) The same section, after removal of silver and staining with phosphotungstic acid–haematoxylin; the secretory granules of the A cells are black (arrows), but the argyrophil D cells are unstained. (c) Another section, stained with aldehyde fuchsin–trichrome. The A cells, stained by ponceau–acid fuchsin, are dark grey. The B cells, stained by aldehyde fuchsin, are black. The D cells, stained by light green, are light grey (arrows). (Photographs by courtesy of W. B. Rhoten.)

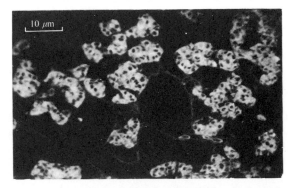

FIG. 3.2. Pseudoisocyanin reaction of the B cells of the adult river lamprey. They appear white by fluorescence microscopy. (There is no evidence that the other cells contain immunoreactive glucagon.) (From Ermisch (1966). *Zool. Jb.* (*Anat.*) **83**.)

dinaphthyldisulphide (DDD) procedure of Barrnett and Seligman, with appropriate blockage and reduction, identifies S—S and SH groups in insulin, while the dithizone method identifies zinc, which is associated with insulin secretion and storage, but which may also be present in A_2 and A_1 cells as well. A_2 cells can be identified by the dimethylaminobenzaldehyde-nitrite method; this reveals tryptophan, which is present in the glucagon secreted by these cells, but which is absent from insulin; B cells are therefore negative. Silver impregnation techniques are valuable, since both the A_1 and the A_2 cells are argyrophil, but the result depends upon the particular technique used. The procedure of Hellman and Hellerström impregnates only the A_1 cells, while that of Grimelius impregnates both types. Argyrophilia means that the cells can be impregnated with silver, but require light or a reducing agent to produce the black deposit of metallic silver. This is quite different from the argentaffin reaction; this depends on the reduction of silver salts in the dark, and without a reducing agent.

Finally, electron microscopy contributes a more precise image of the secretion granules of these cells. The A_1 granules are in general large, with moderate to low electron density, and with a surrounding membrane that is closely applied to the core. The A_2 granules are smaller, and electron dense, with a membrane that is less closely applied to the core. The B granules have cores which vary in density and shape, and which are often widely separated from their membranes. Electron microscopy reveals only occasional granules in the C cells, which confirms the view that these are immature or exhausted. They are more common in lower vertebrates, although they may be conspicuous in islet cell tumours of mammals, or during stages of regeneration.

These three main types of cells (A_1, B, and A_2) seem to be universally present in mammals, varying only in the details of their arrangement. Sometimes they are mixed together indiscriminately, as in the guinea-pig; sometimes they show a degree of segregation, as in the rat and rabbit, where the A_2 cells tend to occupy the periphery of the islets. The association of these three cell types, however, is by no means a purely mammalian situation. Comparative studies show that the pattern is a long-established feature of vertebrate organization, for an essentially similar arrangement is found throughout the gnathostomes.

In the Agnatha a simpler pattern is present, and it is, of course, in this group that we might expect to find some clues to the evolutionary history of the islets. Conditions in the ammocoete larva of the lamprey are of particular interest. At the interior end of the intestine, and in close association with the bile duct, cells grow out from the intestinal epithelium and become arranged in the submucosa in groups that have been called the follicles of Langerhans (Figs 3.3 and 3.4). There is no

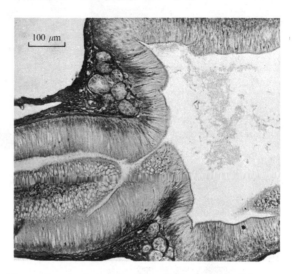

FIG. 3.3 Longitudinal section through the junction of the oesophagus (left) and the anterior intestine (right) of a larval lamprey to show the follicles of Langerhans embedded in the submucosa in the angle between the intestine and the oesophagus. (From Morris and Islam (1969). *Gen. comp. Endocrin.* **12**.)

morphologically differentiated pancreas in these larvae, but cells corresponding with the exocrine pancreatic cells of higher forms are found in the intestinal epithelium; these cells are concentrated at the anterior end of the intestine, so that they are in close relationship with the follicle cells. At metamorphosis, the follicles give rise to a compact gland-like tissue; this interdigitates with a blind caecum of the intestine, containing many exocrine cells, to form a compound structure which is visible on the surface of the intestine at its anterior end, and may be called the cranial pancreas (Fig. 3.5). The bile duct, which degenerates at this stage of the life-cycle, gives rise to additional follicle cells which largely become embedded in the liver; they may be called the caudal pancreas. Scattered groups of follicle cells are also found between the cranial and caudal concentrations.

The follicle cells of the larva, and the corresponding cells of the cranial and caudal pancreas of the adult, are undoubtedly homologous with the B cells of gnathostomes. This is shown by their light- and

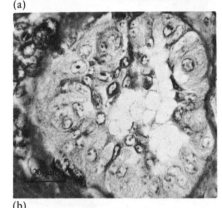

(a)

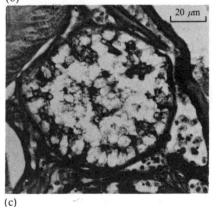

(b)

(c)

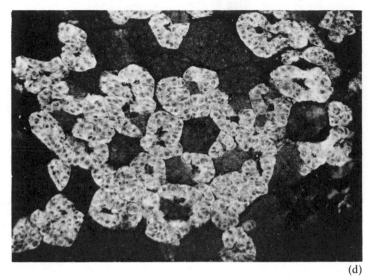

(d)

Fig. 3.4. Follicles of Langerhans of larval lampreys. (a) Follicles developing at the base of the oesophageal epithelium and passing into the submucosa (cf. Fig. 3.2). (b) A vacuolated follicle from a larval lamprey that had been injected with glucose. (c) Cellular breakdown in a follicle of a larval lamprey that had been injected with alloxan, at 200 mg kg⁻¹. (From Morris and Islam (1969). *Gen. comp. Endocrin.* **12**.) (d) Section of islet tissue of adult lamprey showing immunofluorescent staining of B cells with antiserum to mammalian insulin. (There is no evidence that the other cells contain immunoreactive glucagon.) (cf. Fig. 3.2). (From van Noorden *et al.* (1974). *Gen. comp. Endocrin.* **23**, 311–24.)

electron-microscopical features. Moreover, they can be destroyed selectively by alloxan (Fig. 3.4(c)), like B cells (p. 31); they become degranulated and vacuolated (Fig. 3.4(b)) when the animals are subjected to a glucose load (p. 31); and insulin can be demonstrated in them by immunohistochemistry (Fig. 3.4(d), and see p. 9). On present evidence they are the only cell type; neither A_1 nor A_2 cells have yet been identified. It is apparent, therefore, that in all respects, both anatomical and cytological, the conditions in larval and adult lampreys are highly suggestive of a primitive stage in the evolution of a true pancreas, with a simple form of islet tissue

becoming associated with an outgrowth of exocrine tissue.

Conditions in the myxinoids (*Myxine, Polistotrema*) are similar in principle, except that their islet tissue is concentrated in a compact organ; this is easily visible to the naked eye, close to the bile duct where this enters the intestine. Here again, only B cells have so far been found.

These facts indicate that islet tissue in a simple form arose very early in vertebrate evolution, and that it must have originated within the alimentary tract, as, indeed, is implied by its mode of development in the higher vertebrates. From this point of

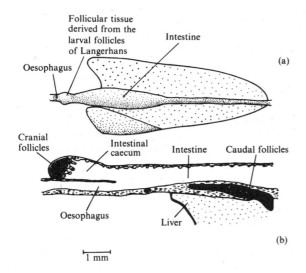

Follicular tissue derived from the larval follicles of Langerhans

Oesophagus

Intestine

(a)

Cranial follicles

Intestinal caecum

Intestine

Caudal follicles

Oesophagus

Liver

(b)

1 mm

FIG. 3.5. (a) Dorsal view of the liver and the associated region of the alimentary canal of the adult lamprey, *Lampetra fluviatilis*. (b) Vertical longitudinal section of the same. (From Barrington (1945). *Q. J. microsp. Sci.* 85, 391–417.)

view, its endocrine secretions should be classed with the digestive hormones that we have considered in the previous chapter. The important difference is that these latter hormones are concerned with the food before it has been absorbed, whereas the islet secretions have become involved in the regulation of the subsequent metabolism of the digestive products. It is doubtless because of this that the islet hormones have become involved in complex interactions with other endocrine secretions, as we shall see.

The islet tissue of the lower gnathostomes is more complex than that of agnathans, showing, in general, a fundamental similarity to that of mammals, with A_1, A_2, and B cells usually identifiable. These three types are identifiable in elasmobranchs, together with amphiphils, so called because they show features of both A and B cells. Such cells, of intermediate type, have been reported in other lower vertebrates as well; their significance is not clear, but they perhaps indicate that one cell type can transform into another under appropriate stimulation. There is variation in the anatomical arrangement of islet cells in elasmobranchs. Typical islets occur, but often the endocrine cells may additionally be found in the pancreatic ducts, arranged as an outer layer of the duct epithelium. It is not clear whether this represents a primitive condition.

The Holocephali are probably related to the elasmobranchs, but must have separated from them

at a very early stage, for the group is already well defined in the Devonian period. It is perhaps in keeping with this long history of independence that, in addition to A_1, A_2, and B cells, *Hydrolagus* has a unique cell type, provisionally termed the X cell, constituting up to 50 per cent of the islet cells: its function is unknown.

The pancreas of teleost fish is usually a diffuse organ, scattered around the intestine and spleen, and often extending into the liver. It is thus difficult to see with the unaided eye, but this is not so of the endocrine component, which, in addition to forming scattered islets, is often concentrated as well into one or two large bodies, called the principal islets or Brockmann bodies. The usual three cell types are present.

The situation in tetrapods calls for little further comment, for in general the pancreas is a compact organ containing scattered islets that include the expected three cell types. There is variation in detail, the most noteworthy being in birds. These animals have a high percentage of A cells, with A_1 cells constituting at least 30 per cent of the total cell count in the pigeon. Moreover, the islets tend to be differentiated into three types: mixed islets, with the three cell types; dark islets, with A cells predominating; and light islets, composed chiefly of B cells. This situation obviously lends itself to experimental exploitation.

The general uniformity of pancreatic islet tissue throughout the gnathostomes, and its greater simplicity in agnathans, is not unexpected. It is in line with what emerges from the comparative study of other aspects of the vertebrate endocrine system. What is remarkable, and too often taken for granted, is that this endocrine tissue should be commonly present as scattered islets. That islet tissue and zymogen tissue should be associated in the same organ can perhaps be seen as a consequence of their closely related origin, as revealed in lampreys, but even this must presumably have some functional explanation. Perhaps it signifies that islet cells originated from alimentary epithelial cells that monitored the passage of nutrients across the epithelium into the blood stream. Later the metabolic products of these cells may have evolved into endocrine secretions; a concept that is hypothetical, but yet logical.

What is not so easy to understand is why the endocrine tissue remained fragmented into islets, and why those of man, for example, are of the same order of size as in the rat; their mean dimension is 100–200 μm, although there is, of course, variation in size and number, even within one species. The explanation of the fragmentation may lie in the large surface area that is thereby created between the endocrine and zymogen tissue, for this suggests that there must be some important metabolic relationship between them. What this might be we can only guess. Conceivably, insulin and/or glucagon facilitate in some way the synthetic activity of the zymogen cells; insulin, for example, might promote incorporation of amino acids into their protein secretion. The problem, a much neglected one, merits further study. Relevant to it is the suggestion that the association of adrenocortical and chromaffin tissue in the adrenal gland of the higher vertebrates (another puzzling feature of their endocrine organization) may be associated with a metabolic relationship between the two. In this instance it has been shown that a high concentration of glucocorticoid secretion is essential for the activity of the enzyme phenylethanolamine-N-methyl transferase, which is involved in the formation of adrenaline from noradrenaline (p. 191).

3.3. The discovery of insulin

We have seen how the trend of thought at the end of the nineteenth century was leading to the view that some secretion of pancreatic islet tissue might be related to diabetes mellitus. The results of transplantation experiments were lending support to this, for it had been shown in 1892 that a diabetic condition caused by removal of the pancreas could be reduced or abolished by transplanting a portion of the organ under the skin and allowing it to remain there after it had established vascular connections. If, however, the transplant was then removed, the typical symptoms of diabetes reappeared.

During the early years of the present century many investigators, encouraged by the successes that had been achieved in the preparation of active extracts from the thyroid and adrenal glands and from the 'posterior lobe' of the pituitary, were endeavouring to prepare from the pancreas some extract that would alleviate the symptoms of diabetes mellitus. So convinced were they that the islets were secreting a hormone, that in 1909 it was designated insuline (*insula*, island), well in advance of its actual discovery. Even with this unusual abandonment of caution, however, success continued to elude these investigators, although it seems probable that some came very close to it. It is likely that extracts prepared by Zuelzer in 1908 did contain the hormone, but their use was abandoned because of alarming clinical results; a striking warning of the importance of testing new preparations in carefully planned experiments upon animals.

It was not until 1920 that Banting initiated a renewed and intensive attack upon the problem and, in collaboration with Best, finally prepared the long-awaited extract and thereby demonstrated the existence of an islet hormone for which the name insulin, a modification of the earlier suggestion, was immediately adopted. Banting had just settled down to a career of general practice in London, Ontario, but had in addition taken up an appointment as instructor in the Medical School. Those who hold that it is no disadvantage for a member of a university to undertake a modicum of teaching will take encouragement from the fact that the germ of his idea is said to have come to him at 2 a.m. on the morning of 1 November 1920, when he was preparing a lecture on pancreatic function. He was struck by the account of experiments, similar in principle to those of Schulze mentioned above, in which ligation of the ducts had destroyed the zymogen tissue but had left the islets substantially intact. Banting saw that by preparing extracts from such an organ, it would be possible to avoid the risk of the supposed hormone being destroyed by pancreatic digestion, an occurrence which might well account for previous failures in extraction.

His idea was inscribed in his notebook in the succinct words 'Tie off pancreas duct of dogs. Wait six or eight weeks. Remove and extract.' He was not, in fact, the first to have had this particular idea, nor is it uncommon for investigators to be pursuing the same project quite independently of each other. In 1912 a similar experiment had been started, but the worker concerned seems to have abandoned it owing to the great technical difficulties involved. These were, of course, also encountered by Banting and Best, but in this case they were overcome. After months of concentrated work during the summer of 1921, taking turns at watching and sleeping in order to keep their experimental dogs under continuous observation, they finally obtained extracts that lowered the elevated blood sugar of dogs that had been made diabetic by removal of the pancreas (Fig. 3.6). The importance of ensuring that the hormone was not destroyed by the digestive secretion during extraction was shown by incubating the active extract with pancreatic juice; after such treatment it was found to have lost its anti-diabetic effect. On 11 January 1922, pancreatic extracts were successfully administered to diabetic patients in the Toronto General Hospital. They had been developed just in time to benefit George R. Minot who, five years later, was to repay the debt by playing a leading part in the discovery of the erythrocyte-maturing

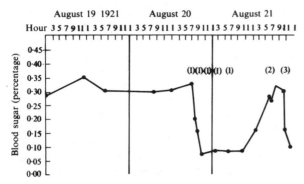

FIG. 3.6. The effect of insulin on the blood sugar of a de-pancreatized dog. (1) Injection of extract of ligated and degener-ated pancreas; (2) injection of extract after incubation with pan-creatic juice; (3) injection of extract incubated without pancreatic juice. (From Best and Taylor (1940). *Physiological basis of medical practice.* Williams and Wilkins, London.)

factor of liver, which provided a treatment for pernicious anaemia.

As to the source of the hormone, it is certain that it is secreted by the B cells of the islets. This can be shown by immunohistochemistry (p. 9; Fig. 3.4(d), p. 28), and there is also experimental evidence. For example, if the major part of the pancreas is removed from cats or dogs, the B cells in the small portion remaining become degranulated and then vacuolated and finally may degenerate, a consequence of the excessive demands made upon them for the protection of insulin. A similar demand, with similar results, can be established by the prolonged admini-stration of glucose into a normal and intact animal, for the consequent rise in blood sugar again stimu-lates an increased output of the hormone.

Another procedure, which has useful application in experimental studies, is the administration of

alloxan, the ureide of mesoxalic acid. This substance has a destructive action upon the B cells, which may show signs of degranulation within five minutes of the intravenous injection of a suitable dose. Ultimately it may bring about complete destruction of these cells, while the A cells and the zymogen tissue are virtually unaffected. The result is the establishment of a typical diabetic condition known as alloxan diabetes; direct assay of the damaged pancreas will then confirm its lack of the hormone.

The demonstration that insulin is actually present in the circulating blood (which we have seen to be an essential condition for confirming hormonal activity) depends in part upon the fact that plasma from normal animals will lower the blood-sugar levels of normal or diabetic ones. The most con-vincing evidence, however, rests upon radio-immuno-assay (p. 51), which makes possible the measure-ment of the circulating levels.

3.4. The effects of insulin

We have seen that insulin has a readily demonstrable effect upon the blood-sugar level. This level, in an animal that is not absorbing glucose from its intest-ine, is normally an expression of an equilibrium between the utilization of glucose as an energy source and its replenishment by the breaking down of glycogen stores. Additional elements in the equilib-rium, when the animal is feeding, are the absorption of glucose into the blood stream, and its uptake and subsequent metabolism by the tissues. To under-stand how the endocrine regulation of this equilibrium is achieved in mammals, it is necessary first to review in general terms the metabolic pathways that are involved in the storage and release of energy in these animals (Fig. 3.7).

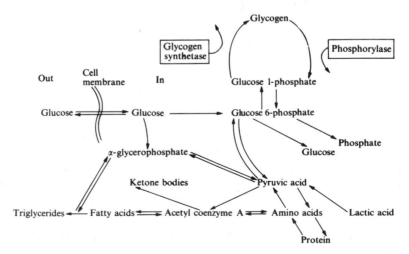

FIG. 3.7. Diagram of metabolic pathways.

Glucose absorbed from the intestine passes first via the hepatic portal system to the liver. Some of it enters the hepatic cells, but much passes through the liver and enters the muscle cells. These two tissues have certain metabolic pathways in common. In both of them the glucose is phosphorylated to glucose 6-phosphate, some of which is then converted into stored glycogen (glycogenesis) by the glycogen synthetase pathway. Part of the glucose 6-phosphate, however, is broken down with the release of energy for the immediate needs of the liver and muscle cells. An additional source of glucose 6-phosphate for this purpose is the stored glycogen. This is broken down first to glucose 1-phosphate by the mediation of phosphorylase, along a pathway which is different, therefore, from that leading to the synthesis of glycogen. Release of energy from the glucose takes place in two stages, after the isomerization of glucose 1-phosphate to glucose 6-phosphate The first stage (glycolysis) is the anaerobic breakdown of glucose 6-phosphate to pyruvate, which is then converted into either lactate or acetyl coenzyme A. The second stage is the aerobic (oxidative) breakdown of the acetyl group through the citric acid cycle, leading to the formation of carbon dioxide and water.

In addition to these pathways, there are two others which are found in liver but not in muscle, and which enable the liver to contribute to the energy resources of the whole body. First, it contributes to the homeostasis of blood sugar by releasing glucose that is formed by the breakdown of glycogen (glycogenolysis). This process depends upon the enzyme glucose 6-phosphatase, which is present in liver but not in muscle. Its absence from muscle cells makes it impossible for them to release glucose for use elsewhere; their function is to use it to bring about muscular contraction, not to maintain blood-glucose levels.

The second of these two hepatic pathways provides for the formation of carbohydrate from non-carbohydrate sources (gluconeogenesis). This is needed because the supply of glucose by glycogenolysis yields only a short-term reserve of energy. Longer-term needs, such as might arise during starvation, are met by calling upon other sources. These are primarily amino acids, including alanine, cysteine, glycine, and serine, which are glucogenic amino acids. They are degraded by transamination to pyruvate, which can then either be oxidized through the citric acid cycle, or transformed into stored glycogen. It is the formation of carbohydrate from these precursors which is sometimes regarded as

gluconeogenesis in the strict sense. However, pyruvate and lactate, formed in muscle and passed to the liver, can also serve as sources of carbohydrate, following the same pathways, and this source is often included within the term. The process of gluconeogenesis depends upon the enzyme fructose 1,6-diphosphatase. This enzyme is present in liver, but not in muscle, which is why muscle cannot carry out this process. Liver, by contrast, has a remarkable capacity for absorbing amino acids from the blood stream and has the prime responsibility for maintaining homeostasis of blood sugar during starvation.

Adipose tissue, although primarily a centre for the deposition and mobilization of fat, also plays an important part in carbohydrate metabolism. Fatty acids are taken up by adipose cells, and so is glucose. The latter is converted to fatty acids, via acetyl coenzyme A, and to α-glycerophosphate, with which the acids are esterified to form triglycerides (lipogenesis). These triglycerides are the main storage form of fat. They can subsequently be broken down to glycerol and fatty acids (lipolysis), which are then released into the blood to provide a further source of energy. These pathways are not peculiar to adipose tissue; both lipogenesis and lipolysis occur in the liver as well.

The regulatory action of insulin upon this very complex metabolic system is demonstrated by the routine clinical test of glucose tolerance. Blood-sugar levels are determined before the drinking of glucose solution, and for a period of two hours afterwards (Figs 3.8 and 3.9). The rapid absorption of the

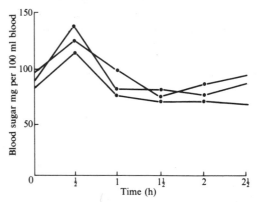

FIG. 3.8. Glucose tolerance test. Blood-sugar curves from three normal human subjects after the ingestion of 50 g glucose.

glucose results in the level rising to a peak in about 30–45 minutes; after this, the level falls again, and, in normal subjects, returns to a normal value within

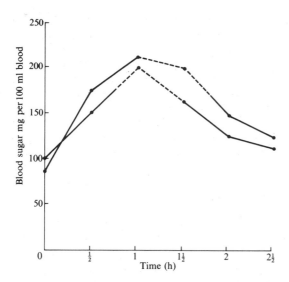

FIG. 3.9. Glucose tolerance test. Blood-sugar curves from two mildly diabetic patients. The fasting blood sugar is nearly normal but the response is abnormal, the broken lines indicating glycosuria. (Figs 8 and 9 from Bell *et al.* (1959). *Textbook of physiology and biochemistry*. Livingstone, Edinburgh.)

$1-1\frac{1}{2}$ hours. The fall is a result of insulin being released from the B cells, which are directly stimulated by the increased glucose level in the blood that is reaching them. The effectiveness of this signal can be demonstrated by perfusing pancreas slices *in vitro*; insulin is released from these if the glucose content of the perfusing fluid is raised. Nevertheless, this direct signal is not the only factor involved. Nervous reflexes may possibly play a part, while in normal feeding the passage of glucose into the intestine can also evoke the release of insulin. In this instance the signal may be the release of entero-glucagon (p. 45), which is able to evoke the release of insulin from the B cells.

The insulin so released facilitates the peripheral utilization of glucose in three main ways, along the pathways just outlined. First, it acts upon muscle to promote carbohydrate metabolism and the storage of glycogen. It was at one time suggested that the hormone did this by stimulating the activity of hexokinase, which mediates the phosphorylation of glucose, but this view is no longer held. It is now believed that the effect actually results from insulin influencing the cell membrane of muscle cells so as to facilitate the transfer of glucose from the extracellular fluid into the cell. A gradient of free glucose is maintained between the external medium and the interior of the cell, because the glucose is immediately phosphorylated; this gradient encourages further

entry. The enzymes required for the subsequent metabolism of glucose 6-phosphate are present in muscle cells in quantities sufficiently large to make the entry of glucose the main rate-limiting factor, and it is doubtful whether they are affected by insulin. Nevertheless, it is likely that insulin influences muscular tissue in other ways as well. Probably it favours glycogenesis by increasing glycogen synthetase activity, while it also favours the deflection of more glucose into the glycolytic pathway.

The second important field of action of insulin is the liver. Here, in contrast to its action upon muscle, it does not affect the cell membrane, for hepatic cells are always freely permeable to glucose. What the hormone probably does is to favour glycogenesis and glycolysis, while it also decreases hepatic gluconeogenesis, favours the uptake of fatty acids, and increases lipogenesis.

Thirdly, insulin acts upon adipose tissue, its effect here being in some respects similar to its effect upon muscle. In particular, it enhances the membrane transfer of glucose, which may then be stored as glycogen, or used immediately as an energy source. It also enhances the uptake of fatty acids by adipose tissue, promotes lipogenesis, and decreases lipolysis.

Finally, insulin stimulates, in all of these three tissues, the uptake of amino acids and their incorporation into tissue protein. It also facilitates the oxidation of glucose in most peripheral tissues; the exceptions to this are the brain and the retina, which, although obligatory users of glucose, do not require insulin for this purpose.

These various actions of insulin, all of which interact to promote a fall in blood sugar, can be demonstrated more directly by observing the result of injecting the hormone into normal individuals that have been on a controlled diet for several weeks (Fig. 3.10), as well as into hyperglycaemic ones. There is an initial fall, for the reasons already stated, but this fall is followed by a recovery phase. This is due to the release of carbohydrate from the liver, primarily through the action of hormones which maintain equilibrium by antagonizing the effect of insulin, and which we shall be considering below.

The facts outlined above make it possible to understand the nature of the diabetic syndrome. Insulin lack decreases the capacity of muscle to utilize glucose, both by oxidation and by glycogenesis. The effect of this is seen in the glucose tolerance test (Figs 3.8 and 3.9). If the supply of insulin in the subject is defective, the blood-sugar level rises to an abnormally high level and falls more slowly. This results in the level exceeding the renal

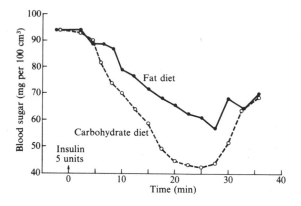

FIG. 3.10. The effect of the injection of insulin upon the blood sugar of a normal human subject after he had been on controlled diets for some weeks. A high-fat diet results in a decreased sensitivity to the action of insulin. (From Winton and Bayliss (1937). *Human physiology* (2nd edn). Blakiston, Philadelphia.)

threshold, which is the level at which the kidney tubules can reabsorb all of the glucose in the glomerular filtrate. Sugar therefore appears in the urine (glycosuria) to an extent that will depend upon the severity of the diabetic condition. This accounts for the polyuria, since the passage of the glucose demands an increased output of fluid in order to maintain it in solution. If the condition is untreated, the persistence of these symptoms leads along a potentially deadly chain to loss of water and electrolytes, dehydration, haemoconcentration, and circulatory failure.

Fat metabolism is also affected by insulin lack, for lipogenesis is impeded both in the liver and the adipose tissue, while fat stores are mobilized as an adaptation for securing an alternative source of energy. This leads to the production of considerable quantities of acetyl coenzyme A. Normally this should combine with oxaloacetate and then be metabolized by the citric acid cycle, but in the diabetic condition a block develops, possibly because the defective carbohydrate metabolism leads to an inadequate provision of oxaloacetic acid. Whatever the reason, however, the accumulating acetyl coenzyme A condenses to form acetoacetate within the liver, and from this arise the other ketone bodies. Further, a diabetic animal is unable in the absence of insulin to convert carbohydrate into fat, whereas in a normal rat, for example, as much as 35 per cent of ingested carbohydrate can be used in that way.

Finally, we have seen that the diabetic condition is accompanied by a loss of protein. This is due to increased gluconeogenesis, the decreased availability of energy from carbohydrate resulting in protein being called upon, like fat, to make up the deficiency. The causal chain, however, is complex. As we have already noted, insulin promotes the incorporation of amino acids into peripheral tissues. In this way it counterbalances the deaminating action of the glucocorticoids (p. 55) upon protein metabolism. The absence of its influence in the diabetic condition contributes to the characteristic increase in nitrogen excretion. Evidently, therefore, the metabolic effects of insulin cannot be adequately evaluated without taking into account the effects upon these processes of certain other hormones. These we shall be considering shortly.

In the meantime, however, we may summarize the effects of insulin as an enhancement of the use of glucose as an energy source, and of the storage of surplus glucose as glycogen or as fat; increased storage of fat and a reduction in its use as an energy source; and enhancement of protein anabolism and inhibition of the use of protein as an energy source. To say, then, that insulin lowers blood-sugar levels, while correct as far as it goes, is to conceal a very broad spectrum of enzyme-mediated actions, which in some cases at least may depend on mRNA synthesis as a basis for enzyme synthesis. How this diversity of action is brought about by one hormone is not yet understood. One suggestion is that, since insulin influences the surface membrane of the muscle cell, it may also act upon other cell membranes, including those of the endoplasmic reticulum and the nuclei. It is possible also that cyclic AMP (p. 46) may be an intermediary, but to say this is obviously not to explain the diversity of responses which must depend upon intracellular specialization. No doubt the complexity of the data relating to insulin action is a measure of the intensive research to which this hormone has been subjected because of its immense clinical importance. It may be expected, therefore, that advancing knowledge will show the actions of other hormones to be no less complex.

3.5. The chemistry of insulin

The great clinical importance of insulin has caused much attention to be given to its purification and to the elucidation of its chemical structure. The results have been remarkably successful, and have had far-reaching consequences. Insulin was isolated in crystalline form in 1926. Later it was found that this crystallization requires the presence of zinc ions (p. 27), but that cadmium, cobalt, iron, or nickel can be substituted. X-ray diffraction photographs of its rhombohedral crystals were obtained in 1935. Later, between 1945 and 1955, Sanger elucidated at Cambridge the primary structure of the molecule, a brilliant pioneer achievement which earned for him the Nobel Prize for Chemistry for 1958, and which paved the way for the determination of the peptide sequences of many other polypeptide and protein hormones. Some of these we have already mentioned; others will be encountered later. Insulin was thus shown to be a protein of relatively small size (molecular weight of about 6000), composed of two polypeptide chains, a shorter A-chain of twenty-one residues and a longer B-chain of thirty (Fig. 3.11).

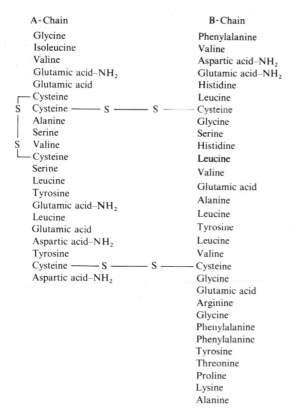

FIG. 3.11. Amino-acid sequences of the insulin molecule of cattle. (After Sanger (1960). *Br. med. Bull.* **16**, 183–8.)

The two chains are connected by two disulphide (—S—S—) linkages, while a third such linkage forms an intra-chain bridge in the A-chain. These disulphide bridges, which contribute to the tertiary structure of the molecule, are essential for its biological activity. Insulin particles, detectable within the B granules by electron microscopy, are now thought to be hexamers, with six molecules arranged around two zinc ions. The hormone circulates in the blood stream, however, as a mixture of monomers and dimers.

Bovine insulin was synthesized *de novo* in 1963, and then, in 1965 and 1966, human insulin was synthesized, this being the first human protein to be prepared in the laboratory. At first it was thought that the biosynthesis of the hormone was effected, like its laboratory synthesis, by the formation of separate A- and B-chains, followed by their linkage, but this is now known not to be so. Insulin is, in fact, synthesized as a single-chain precursor, called pro-insulin, in which the future A- and B-chains are linked end to end by a peptide strand, before being joined by their —S—S— bonds. It is supposed that this arrangement facilitates biosynthesis, enabling it to be completed as a monomolecular reaction instead of a bimolecular one.

The importance of these molecular studies, quite apart from the hope which they hold out of eventually achieving laboratory synthesis in amounts adequate for clinical use, is that they should lead to the identification of those structural features that are responsible for the biological activities of the molecule. However, determination of primary structure takes us only a short way towards this goal, for insulin has a secondary and tertiary structure which are of critical importance in its functioning. Fortunately, the relatively small size of the molecule has permitted remarkably successful studies of its three-dimensional structure (Fig. 3.12). Not all of the amino acids are of equal importance in determining the activities of so complex an organization. The identification of the more important ones is, however, greatly aided by studies of variations in the peptide sequences of the naturally occurring hormones,

TABLE 3.1

Variations in the amino-acid sequence of mammalian insulins (Data collected from various authors by Young (1962). *Proc. R. Soc.* B**157**.)

	A-chain				B-chain		
	4	8	9	10	3	29	30
Ox	Glu	Ala	Ser	Val	Asn	Lys	Ala
Sheep	Glu	Ala	Gly	Val	Asn	Lys	Ala
Horse	Glu	Thr	Gly	Ile	Asn	Lys	Ala
Sei whale	Glu	Ala	Ser	Thr	Asn	Lys	Ala
Pig	Glu	Thr	Ser	Ile	Asn	Lys	Ala
Sperm whale	Glu	Thr	Ser	Ile	Asn	Lys	Ala
Dog	Glu	Thr	Ser	Ile	Asn	Lys	Ala
Human	Glu	Thr	Ser	Ile	Asn	Lys	Thr
Rabbit	Glu	Thr	Ser	Ile	Asn	Lys	Ser
Rat 1	Asp	Thr	Ser	Ile	Lys	Lys	Ser
Rat 2	Asp	Thr	Ser	Ile	Lys	Met	Ser

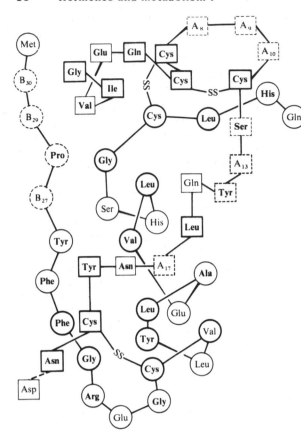

FIG. 3.12. Much simplified diagram (after Hodgkin) of the amino-acid composition and the interrelationship between the A-chain (squares) and the B-chain (circles) of a monomer of pig insulin. The A-chain consists of three parts: an initial α-helix from the NH$_2$-terminal, opening out at A$_9$–A$_{11}$; a brief straight region; and a second helical structure of non-α type, starting at A$_{13}$. The B-chain also consists of three parts: an initial octapeptide from the NH$_2$-terminal; an α-helix between B$_9$ and B$_{19}$; and the sharp U turn at B$_{20}$ and B$_{23}$ with the COOH-terminal residues B$_{24}$–B$_{30}$ folded back against the body of the molecule. The A-chain lies in a pocket formed by the three parts of the B-chain and the monomer is stabilized by several invariant covalent and hydrogen bonds, the **three cystine bridges between A$_6$–A$_{11}$, A$_7$–B$_7$, and A$_{20}$–B$_{19}$ forming** the backbone of the molecule.

Invariant amino-acid residues are indicated by heavy squares and circles. Residues that are highly variable among insulins from other mammals, and from birds and teleost fish, are drawn with interrupted lines. Symbols lightly drawn with uninterrupted lines show residues that are conservative (i.e. only rarely substituted, and, when so, usually by an amino-acid residue belonging to the same type (acid, basic, ambivalent, or hydrophobic). The residues A$_{22}$, B$_0$, and B$_{31}$ do not occur in pig insulin and are found only exceptionally.

Residues designated by letters in bold type are common to pig and hagfish insulin. All invariant residues are the same, except at B$_{18}$; 9 out of 16 conservative residues are the same, and so are 3 highly variable ones. This indicates remarkable constancy in the basic structure of the insulin molecule. (From Falkmer *et al.* (1975). *Am. Zool.* **15**, suppl.)

together with studies of the properties of synthetic molecules, or of those which have been structurally modified by some form of chemical action.

The extent of the variations found in naturally occurring insulins may be judged from Tables 3.1 and 3.2. Those in mammals are few, affecting positions 4, 8, 9, and 10 in the A-chain, and positions 3, 29, and 30 in the B-chain. Evidently, therefore, there is some species specificity of structure, but no obvious phylogenetic pattern emerges from it. Indeed, certain species that are clearly not closely related may share identical sequences. One remarkable exception to this general stability in mammals

is provided by the guinea-pig, which has replacements at no less than seventeen positions.

Other vertebrates that have been studied from this point of view include the fowl, which has replacements at six sites, and some species of teleost, which have replacements comparable in number with those of the guinea-pig. Altogether, the substitutions so far recorded in these groups have occurred at 29 of the 51 available sites; they are summarized in Table 3.2. An additional feature in fish insulins is that there may be an extra residue at the end of the B-chain (methionine in the toadfish, *Opsanus tau*, for example, and valine in the angler fish (goose fish), *Lophius*

TABLE 3.2

Accumulated variations in insulin A-chain and B-chain sequences in mammals, chicken and fishes. Invariant residues are circled. The sequences are divided into three groups; unless an entry is included, the residue is the same as in the sequence of pig insulin given in the top line. Deletions are indicated by a dash (—). (From Blundell et al. 1971.)

Insulin A-chain sequences

	①	②	3	4	⑤	⑥	⑦	8	9	10	⑪	12	13	14	15	⑯	17	18	⑲	⑳	㉑
Chicken + mammals except guinea-pig	Gly	Ile	Val	Glu / Asp	Gln	Cys	Cys	Thr / Ala / His	Ser	Ile / Thr / Val	Cys	Ser	Leu	Tyr	Gln	Leu	Glu	Asn	Tyr	Cys	Asn
Fishes			Leu					His	His / Lys / Arg	Pro		Asn / Asp	Lys / Ile	Phe	Asp		Gln / Glu	Ser / Asn			
Guinea-pig				Asp				Ala	Gly	Thr		Thr	Arg	His							

Insulin B-chain sequences

	−1	1	2	3	④	⑤	⑥	⑦	⑧	9	10	⑪	12	13	14	15	⑯	17	⑱	⑲	⑳	21	22	㉓	㉔	㉕	㉖	27	28	29	30
Mammals (except guinea-pig and chicken)		Phe	Val	Asn / Lys	Gln	His	Leu	Cys	Gly	Ser	His	Leu	Val	Glu	Ala	Leu	Tyr	Leu	Val	Cys	Gly	Glu	Arg	Gly	Phe	Phe	Tyr	Thr	Pro	Lys	Ala
Fishes	Met / Ala / Val	Ala / Pro	Ala / Pro											Asp														Asn	Pro	Lys	Ser / —
Guinea-pig		Phe		Ser / Arg							Asn			Glu	Thr			Ser				Glu	Asp				Ile			Lys	Asp

piscatorius), while residue 30 is missing in all of those investigated. Thus the B-chain of teleosts may contain less than 30 residues.

Mention of these substitutions, however, must not be allowed to obscure the strong conservative element in the evolutionary history of the insulin molecule. Especially remarkable is the fact that of the 21 invariant residues in the molecules of the gnathostomes so far studied, no less than 20 are also invariant in *Myxine*, the exception being the substitution of alanine for valine at position B-18 (Fig. 3.12).

One feature of particular interest from the standpoint of molecular evolution is that the rat has two insulins, one of which has lysine at position 29 of the B-chain (resembling the insulins of other species in this respect) while the other has methionine substituted there. Two insulins are also secreted in certain species of teleosts: the bonito (*Katsuwonus* sp.), the flounder (*Pleuronectes flesus*), and *Lophius*. In these cases it is not known whether each individual secretes both forms of the hormone, but both of the rat insulins have been found in each individual rat that has been studied. We shall consider later, and in a broader context, the genetic implications and the evolutionary significance of the occurrence of two forms of a hormone within a species, and the importance of establishing whether or not each individual carries the two forms (p. 100).

Amino-acid substitutions in polypeptide molecules may be expected to affect the properties of the molecules. Actually, the effects upon the insulin molecule are less than might at first be expected, but they are nevertheless shown in both its immunological activities and in its biological properties.

Insulin, like other proteins, can act as an antigen and evoke the production of antibodies in the blood of animals that are not adapted to the particular form in which it is presented to them. Fortunately for clinical practice, insulin is a weak antigen, although insulin-binding antibodies do occur in the serum of patients who have received large doses of the hormone. Insulin antibodies, however, are readily raised in guinea-pigs, which are particularly sensitive to the bovine hormone, and their action can be demonstrated in the laboratory. Ox serum, for example, will normally, by virtue of its insulin content, promote the uptake of glucose by isolated rat diaphragm, but this effect can be completely abolished by the addition of the guinea-pig antiserum to the medium.

Insulin-binding and insulin-neutralizing antibodies show little specificity. Bovine and pig antibodies will react with many other insulins, including those of the mouse, whale, sheep, and man; yet quantitative differences in reaction do exist, and seem to be associated with degrees of difference in the primary structure of the molecules. Thus the reaction of bovine insulin with anti-bovine-insulin serum is stronger than the reaction of either bonito or cod insulin. The antigenicity of the molecule undoubtedly depends upon tertiary structure, for it largely disappears when the A- and B-chains are separated. We have noted the variations at sites 8, 9, and 10 in the mammalian A-chain. It has been suggested that these changes, which seem likely to influence the surface properties of the molecule, may play some part in specific recognition of the molecule. It is noticeable, from this point of view, that the invariant residues of the molecule are clustered in its core, rather than at its surface. On the other hand, the positions of the invariant residues suggest that many of them are concerned with the relative arrangement of the two chains, while others are involved in establishing the contacts needed for the formation of the dimer.

Table 3.3 shows the amounts of guinea-pig antiserum to ox-insulin, and guinea-pig antiserum to cod-insulin needed to inhibit activity of insulins from various species. All the insulins can be inhibited provided enough of the antisera are available, but the amounts of antisera required vary a great deal. For example, fish insulins require a high level of ox-antiserum, indicating that these insulins are immunologically very different from that of the ox. Within the fish group, however, the antisera requirements bear no relationship to phylogenetic relationships of the various fish species. Indeed, the remarkable case of the guinea-pig, which requires more than a 250-fold excess of anti-ox-insulin, shows how unreliable these results can be as an index of relationships. Peptide sequences of insulin molecules of fish are known for only a few species, as we have already seen. Even so, it is apparent that the marked structural differences between fish insulins and the insulins of the fowl and of mammals are in broad agreement with the immunological data.

Insulin antibodies are a valuable experimental tool, for they provide a precise demonstration of the presence of the hormone in the blood, or in tissue extracts. This precision may at times have important practical applications, as is illustrated by a case of the death of a healthy young woman in her bath. The immediate cause of death was drowning, but the absence of any signs of struggle suggested that she was unconscious prior to this, while there were also indications that

TABLE 3.3

(*Immunological behaviour of insulins extracted from various species* (From Falkmer and Wilson (1967). *Diabetologia* 3.)

Group of animals	Source of insulin	Species	Amount of antiserum which neutralizes 1 mU insulin activity in mouse diaphragm test	
			Ox-insulin antiserum (m/units)	Cod-insulin antiserum (m/units)
Mammals	Ox	(*Bos taurus*)	1	60
	Guinea-pig	(*Cavia porcellus*)	> 250	
Birds	Chicken	(*Gallus domesticus*)	1	1–2
Amphibians	Bullfrog	(*Rana catesbeiana*)	0·26	1–2
Bony fish	Sculpin	(*Cottus scorpius*)	4	1–2
	Tunny	(*Thunnus thynnus*)	27	9
	Bonito	(*Katsuwonus pelamis*)	9	3
	Cod	(*Gadus callarias*)	30	1
	Bowfin	(*Amia calva*)		
Cartilaginous fish	Dogfish	(*Squalus acanthias*)	20	30
Cyclostomes	Hagfish	(*Myxine glutinosa*)	50	30

she had been hypoglycaemic. Since there were no signs of disease, this suggested that she might have been poisoned by insulin, and a careful search of the body surface did, indeed, disclose four marks of hypodermic injections on her buttocks. Extracts were accordingly made of the tissues surrounding these marks. The proof that insulin was present in them had to depend upon biological tests, for the hormone could not be identified by chemical means in a crude protein mixture. The extracts were shown to have a hypoglycaemic action on injection into mice and guinea-pigs, but the evidence that did most to convict her murderer was that they also stimulated glucose consumption by the isolated rat diaphragm (p. 55), and that this effect was abolished by guinea-pig-insulin antiserum.

The fact that there are some differences in immunological properties of insulin molecules raises the question whether there are corresponding differences in their biological activities. The answer is that differences in the peptide sequences of the naturally-occurring hormones have little effect upon activity, as judged from the results of interspecific injections. Indeed, there is little change in activity even with differences of up to 23 of the 51 amino acids; the specific activities of fish insulins, when tested in mammals, are quite comparable with those of the mammalian insulins themselves. Differences are not, of course, entirely absent. For example, there are differences in biological activity between the populations of cod (*Gadus callarias*) from North American waters and those from European waters, and chemical studies show that there are also differences in the primary structure of the insulin molecules of these populations. This is an instructive example of a population difference of the same nature as the interspecific differences that we have already noted. It is a situation to be expected in the light of current evolutionary theory, in which differences between species arise initially as differences between populations.

Nevertheless, the underlying resemblances in biological properties of the variant insulin molecules shows that early hopes of identifying an 'active core', where biological activities would be localized, were based upon an oversimplification. No doubt retention of the three-dimensional shape of the molecule is essential for activity. Those substitutions, therefore, that do not affect the stabilizing interactions within the molecule will not greatly influence activity, whereas significant reduction or loss of activity would be expected to result from substitutions that bring about conformational changes. Such substitutions would inevitably be rejected by natural selection.

3.6. Insulin and blood sugar in the lower vertebrates

The remarkable refinement of control which we have just been reviewing is one aspect of the physiological mechanisms which ensure the constancy of the internal environment of mammals. This constancy, or homeostasis, is, in the well-known aphorism of Claude Bernard, an essential condition for the maintenance of their independent life. Probably the control of homeostasis is less precise in the lower vertebrates, but the essential foundations for it are certainly present, as is apparent from the wide distribution of the hormones that we have been considering. Moreover, regulation of the disposal of nutrients into tissue stores, and of the levels of fuels circulating in the blood, is a widespread feature of vertebrate organization, and it is likely that the endocrine mechanisms involved are similar in principle to those found in mammals. There are, however,

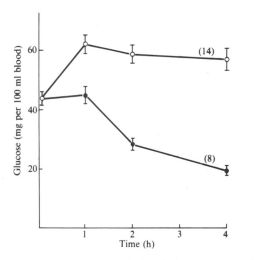

FIG. 3.13. Effects of insulin on the blood glucose concentration of the lamprey. ●——● 1 unit of insulin per animal injected intraperitoneally (8 animals). ○——○ controls injected with 0.9% NaCl solution (14 animals). The vertical bars represent the standard errors. (From Bentley and Follett (1965). *J. Endocrin.* **31**, 127–37.)

many differences in detail; some of these may reflect differences in the properties of those hormones, while others may be a consequence of the diversification of modes of life in the lower groups, and of the influence upon them of seasonal factors.

In general, mammalian insulin causes a decrease of blood-sugar levels in cyclostomes (Fig. 3.13) and fish (Fig. 3.14), with an eventual return to normal levels, but with great variation in the duration of the hypoglycaemia. Examples are the holocephalan fish *Hydrolagus colliei*, the ratfish, with a normal blood-glucose level of 60 mg per 100 ml, and an elasmobranch one (*Squalus acanthias*), with a level of 50 mg per 100 ml. Bovine insulin, or extracts containing the insulins of these fish, are hypoglycaemic in both species, the maxima after bovine insulin being reached within 24–48 hours (Fig. 3.14). The level of blood glucose in *Squalus* which have received injections of their own insulin returns to normal after 3 days, indicating that this animal has an endogenous mechanism for controlling hypoglycaemia. Whether the same can be said of *Hydrolagus* is less clear from the data available. In any case the situation is not simple to interpret, for dogfish insulin seems to have no effect on the levels of glycogen in the liver and muscle of either *Squalus* or *Hydrolagus*.

One factor that may be relevant here (and one

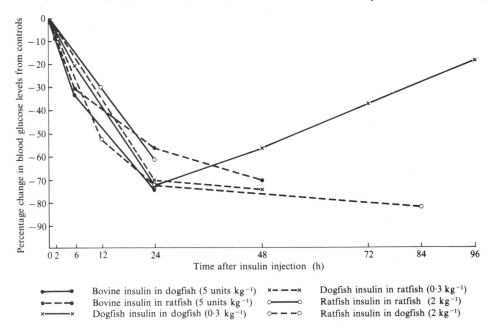

FIG. 3.14. Effects of bovine or chondrichthyan insulins upon blood-glucose levels in dogfish and ratfish. Results are expressed as percentage change in blood-glucose levels when compared with controls. Dosages are given in parentheses. All insulins tested are potent hypoglycaemic agents in these fishes. (From Patent (1970). *Gen. comp. Endocrin.* **14**, 215–42.)

which certainly has shown the importance of taking into consideration the general biology of experimental animals) is the presence of very large amounts of lipid in the livers of these fish (70 per cent of the wet weight in dogfish, and 80 per cent in *Hydrolagus*). This material, because of the large size of the organ in chondrichthyans, has an important effect in lowering the sinking factor, thereby increasing the efficiency of swimming. To this extent it presents some functional analogy with the gas in the swim bladder of a teleost fish, although at a lower level of effectiveness. It could be, therefore, that insulin in these animals is more important for the regulation of lipid than of carbohydrate metabolism.

Finally, some brief reference to the lower tetrapods, where also, however, information is exceedingly fragmentary, and where, as so often with poikilotherms, the results vary with the season. Insulin certainly reduces blood-glucose levels in *Rana temporaria* and *Xenopus laevis*, but, at least in the frog, it has little or no effect on levels of liver and muscle glycogen. Frogs are slow to recover, and may die 24 hours after an injection. As we shall see (p. 54), pancreatectomy of the toad *Bufo arenarum* produces marked hyperglycaemia; survival after this operation averages only 9 days.

A few other examples must serve, this time from reptiles. Pancreatectomy of the snake *Xenodon merremi*, and of the lizard *Tupinambis* spp., produces hyperglycaemia, after an initial hypoglycaemia. Total pancreatectomy in *Alligator mississipiensis* also produces hyperglycaemia (Fig. 3.15), in this instance without an initial hypoglycaemia (Fig. 16). Blood-glucose levels in *Alligator*, starting at 73 mg per 100 ml, show progressive increase to 606 mg after 16 weeks, with death, accompanied by pronounced

ketosis, ensuing after 2–4 months. The effects, however, can be alleviated by insulin injections (Fig. 3.16). Conditions in this species are clearly very

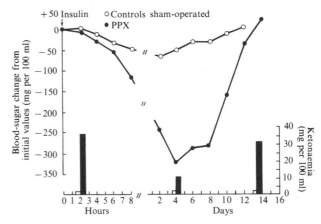

FIG. 3.16. Changes in blood-sugar and ketone-body levels of control sham-operated or pancreatectomized (PPX) alligators given insulin intraperitoneally (0.25 units per kg body weight). (From Penhos *et al.* (1967). *Gen. comp. Endocrin.* 8, 37–43.)

much in line with the mammalian type of response to pancreatectomy.

It is hardly necessary to emphasize that a great concentration of effort upon the lower vertebrates is essential before any approach can be made to an understanding of the biology of insulin in vertebrates as a whole. And this is true also of the other hormones that we shall see to be so closely involved with insulin in metabolic regulation.

3.7. Insulin and the invertebrates

The presence of insulin throughout the vertebrates is not surprising; it is to be expected from the uniformity of the islet tissue of these animals. What is less expected is evidence that insulin-like material is present in various invertebrates. Of course, this conclusion demands rigorous proof, by well-established procedures. One requirement is that the material, after adequate purification, should enhance the uptake of glucose and the resulting synthesis of glycogen in the isolated mouse diaphragm. This, as we shall see, is a standard bioassay for insulin. Further, it is necessary to show that this response can be inhibited by antisera to various known vertebrate insulins. Another test is to treat the material with mercaptoethanol; this destroys the disulphide bridges of the insulin molecule, and should therefore destroy any biological activity which is due to insulin. Immunological cross-reactions with known mammalian insulins can also be investigated.

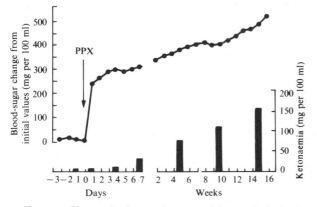

FIG. 3.15. Changes in the blood-sugar and keytone-body levels of alligators after pancreatectomy (PPX). (From Penhos *et al.* (1967). *Gen. comp. Endocrin.* 8, 37–43.)

By these methods, in conjunction with histochemical procedures, it has been shown that insulin is secreted throughout the vertebrates. Applied to invertebrate material, these methods have given evidence of insulin-like substances in the pyloric caeca of the starfish, *Pisaster ochraceus*, and in various parts of the alimentary tract of *Ciona intestinalis*, *Buccinum undatum*, and *Eledone cirrosa*, and perhaps in the digestive gland of the crab *Carcinus maenas*. On the other hand, there is no trace of such material in cnidarian coelenterates. At present the biological significance of these findings is unknown; the functions of the material are unexplained, while the cells secreting it have not been satisfactorily identified.

However, these results, although they need much further exploration, have already suggested a line of thought regarding the origin of the insulin molecule. It seems possible that hormones may often have arisen from some chance association between a metabolite and some process that it proved able to influence. As we have suggested earlier, the position of the B cells within the intestinal wall of the lamprey larva suggests that they might initially have been cells that monitored the passage of glucose through the intestinal epithelium into the blood stream. If we pursue this argument further, it is conceivable that a pro-insulin-like protein may initially have served as a digestive enzyme. This might itself have been partly broken down during digestion, with the release of an insulin-like protein which was then taken up into the blood. Later in evolution it might have been secreted directly into the blood without passing into the intestine. It is been suggested that two factors favour this view, which is, of course, entirely hypothetical. One is that insulin can be absorbed from the intestine into the blood stream. The other is that the B cells release insulin in response to stimulation by several of the digestive hormones that primarily regulate digestive processes.

4

Hormones and metabolism II

4.1. Glucagon

It was noted when insulin was discovered, and was observed by Banting and Best, that the hypoglycaemic effect of pancreatic extracts was preceded by a transitory hyperglycaemic one. This effect, readily seen after intravenous injection of insulin (Fig. 4.1), was at first attributed to the liberation

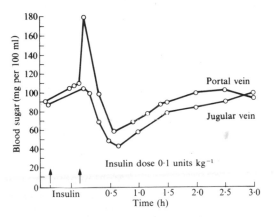

FIG. 4.1. Blood-sugar changes in mammal after intravenous injection of insulin. (From Foa (1964). In *The hormones*, Vol. 4 (eds G. Pincus, K. V. Thimann and E. B. Astwood). Academic Press, New York.)

of adrenaline, but by 1923 it was already being suggested that it was due to a distinct substance which was capable of mobilizing glucose, and for which the name glucagon was proposed. The existence of this hyperglycaemic substance, and its secretion by the A_2 cells, is now fully substantiated, but the history of glucagon research nevertheless presents an extraordinary contrast with that of insulin. The existence of insulin had been forecast confidently well in advance of its actual discovery. The existence of glucagon, secreted by immediately adjacent cells in the pancreatic islets, was doubted for many years, and its study attracted little attention. This neglect was partly due to variability in commercial methods of manufacturing insulin, and the

consequent difficulty of establishing uniformity in the hyperglycaemic action of the glucagon which was present as a fluctuating impurity. A further difficulty was the lack of suitable methods for handling a substance that is present in most mammals in only very small quantities, amounting to less than 10 ng per g pancreatic tissue. Such are the chances upon which depend advances in biology and medicine.

The glucagon of the pig was isolated and crystallized in 1953, and its primary structure (confirmed by synthesis) determined in 1957. It is a single-chain polypeptide with twenty-nine amino acids, and with a molecular weight of 3485 (Fig. 2.11, p. 18). Bovine glucagon is identical and probably human is as well, while that of the bird is at least closely similar. Complete integrity of the molecule is required for its immunological and biological activities. A remarkable feature of the structure is that the amino-acid sequence closely resembles that of secretin (p. 18). Glucagon has 29 amino acids and secretin 27; of these, 14 are common to the two molecules and are located at identical sites. We shall return to this feature in a later discussion (p. 105).

Knowledge of the composition of glucagon has made possible the accurate identification of the A_2 cells as being the cells that secrete it. As we have seen already, the A_2 cells react positively to the histochemical test for indoles because of the relatively high tryptophan content of glucagon, while the presence of the molecule within the cells has been directly demonstrated by its immunoreactivity in tissue sections. There is, unfortunately, no satisfactory cytotoxic substance as specific for the A_2 cells as is alloxan for the B cells. Cobalt chloride and synthalin have been used for this purpose, but the results of their action have been difficult to interpret.

Even after the synthesis of glucagon, and the identification of its source, it remained uncertain whether or not it could be regarded as a hormone, released into the blood in physiological conditions. However, cross-circulation experiments with dogs had shown that the release of glucagon was suppressed by a rise in blood-sugar levels and promoted by a fall. Conclusive evidence resulted from the later use of radioimmunoassay, which clearly established the presence of glucagon in the blood, and made it possible to study the conditions that influence its secretion. As a result of all this, it is now clear that glucagon is indeed a hormone involved in the regulation of carbohydrate metabolism.

A clue to its function is that it passes first to the liver in the portal circulation, its level here being higher than in the peripheral blood. Evidently the liver is its first target, and probably its main one, but some glucagon passes on and is able to influence other targets. The same, of course, is true of insulin; it has been said rightly that it can be no accident of evolution that the islet cells lie just upstream of the liver. What glucagon does is to promote hepatic glycogenolysis and inhibit glycogenesis; as a result, it increases, within a matter of seconds, the output of glucose from the hepatic cells, producing a hyperglycaemic effect which provides an immediate defence against hypoglycaemia.

This defensive action seems to be one of its major functions, but it is also an important regulator of amino-acid metabolism. It activates gluconeogenesis and, given sufficient time, promotes adaptive synthesis of enzymes within the hepatic cells. These latter actions enable the hormone to provide long-term protection against hypoglycaemia. This is why in birds and lizards, where A_2 cells make up a large proportion of the islets, pancreatectomy of fasted animals results in severe hypoglycaemia. The effect is less easy to demonstrate in other groups, where the A_2 cells are less concentrated, because (as already mentioned) there are no specific cytotoxic substances with which to destroy these cells.

The relation between insulin and glucagon, while easy to visualize in these simple terms, is not easy to formulate in a deeper analysis. One suggestion is that the A_2 and B cells are a single functional unit, controlling the movement of nutrients into and out of certain cells in accordance with the needs of the animal and the availability of the nutrients. On this view, insulin promotes the entry of exogenous nutrients into liver, muscle, and fat cells, while glucagon promotes the release of stored nutrients and their distribution to tissues that require fuel. It is thus suggested that when, for example, hyperglycaemia results from ingestion of a meal (Fig. 4.2), the combination of a negative feedback response of the A_2 cell, and of a positive feedback response of the B cell, ensures optimal hepatic storage without the

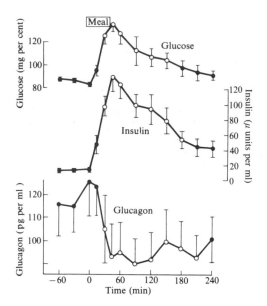

FIG. 4.2. Effect of a large carbohydrate meal upon the plasma concentration of pancreatic glucagon, insulin, and glucose in eleven normal human volunteers. (From Lefebvre and Unger (1972). In *Glucagon* (eds P. J. Lefebvre and R. H. Unger). Pergamon Press, Oxford.)

large increase in the secretion of insulin that would be needed if this were the only hormone involved. The dual action would also help in ensuring survival during hunger. Glucagon could then promote the distribution of nutrients, and the production of new glucose from non-carbohydrate sources, while reduction of insulin secretion could minimize glucose uptake by muscle and so ensure that glucose uptake is concentrated in the insulin-independent tissue of the brain. The influence of blood-glucose levels upon glucagon secretion can be demonstrated in both man and the dog. In the dog, an increased level of blood glucagon is found when the blood-glucose level falls below 50 mg per 100 ml, and a decreased level of the hormone when blood glucose rises above 160 mg per ml. Similarly in man (Fig. 4.1), the infusion of glucose results in a fall in blood glucagon as the level of blood glucose rises above 150 mg per ml. Apparently, then, the secretory responses of the A_2 cells are adjusted to ensure that blood-glucose levels remain within the normal range.

There is, however, an alternative view of the regulating mechanism. According to this, the levels of nutrient metabolites in the blood are regulated not by two separate servo systems, but through a single insulin–glucagon negative feedback system. This view derives from evidence that glucagon can directly stimulate the release of insulin from the B cells. Infusion of glucagon thus promotes an increased secretion of insulin in advance of the rise in the level of blood glucose which eventually results from the infusion. It is thus proposed that the function of glucagon, at least in man, is to sense and amplify those stimuli that act to increase the secretion of insulin. This would explain why nutrient levels in the blood change little during ingestion of a meal, whereas the insulin secretion increases very greatly. In other words, there is a device ensuring a very sensitive homeostatic control of nutrient levels; this, it is supposed, is a consequence of the involvement of the A_2 cells.

It remains uncertain what is the correct explanation of the mechanism, but it is evident that insulin and glucagon provide an excellent illustration of hormonal interaction, other examples of which we shall encounter later (see, for example, p. 54). It is equally uncertain at what evolutionary stage these two hormones became functionally associated. However, glucagon is present in the lower gnathostomes, as might be expected from their possession of A_2 islet cells; and its hyperglycaemic action, antagonistic to the action of insulin, has been demonstrated in certain species (Fig. 4.3).

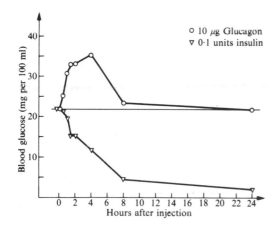

FIG. 4.3. Concentration of blood glucose in *Rana temporaria* after a single injection of insulin or glucagon (experiment done in March). (From Hanke and Neumann (1972). *Gen. comp. Endocrin*, Suppl. 3 (eds W. S. Hoar and H. A. Bern.))

Another fact which may be significant from this point of view is that a widely distributed glucagon-like substance, identifiable by its glucagon-like immunoreactivity, is present in intestinal extracts of many vertebrates, including man and other mammals, the tortoise, frog, axolotl, goldfish, and eel. Cells binding fluorescent glucagon antibody have

been identified in the stomach of the dog, and in various parts of the intestine, and are likely to be the source of this substance. Intestinal glucagon (alternatively called enteroglucagon) differs from pancreatic glucagon both chemically and immunochemically. For example, it exists in the dog in two molecular weights (6000–10 000 and about 3000) and in the duck it has a molecular weight of 6000. Moreover, the plasma levels of pancreatic and intestinal glucagon are inversely related during the absorption of glucose. The physiological significance of this intestinal component is uncertain. It seems, however, that it is released in response to ingestion of a high glucose load, and it has therefore been suggested that its function is to provide an early stimulus for increased release of insulin from the pancreatic islets.

The potential evolutionary interest of the existence of two forms of glucagon has been increased by the identification of radioimmunoassayable glucagon in the digestive glands of a crab, *Cancer pagurus*, a limpet, *Patella caerulae*, and a snail, *Helix pomatia*. It has also been found in whole extracts of a tunicate, *Cynthia papillosa*, and in amphioxus (*Branchiostoma*). The cells producing this material have not yet been identified, nor is it known what action, if any, it has in these various species. Here again, however, there is evidence that a hormone previously regarded as a vertebrate one, and (in the case of glucagon) only recently characterized for certainty in that group, may be widespread in the animal kingdom. Does this imply that the regulation of carbohydrate metabolism in invertebrates is along lines similar to those found in mammals? Only further research will show.

Much, therefore, remains to be learned about glucagon and related problems of pancreatic islet tissue, but the study of this particular hormone has already led to one very striking advance, the importance of which reaches beyond that of the hormone itself. This advance, which concerns the mode of action of glucagon, arose from studies of the mechanism by which glucagon and adrenaline (p. 55) produce their hyperglycaemic effects. Phosphorylase, which is the principle rate-limiting factor in hepatic glycogenolysis, exists in two forms; one of these, the active form (phosphorylase a), is phosphorylated, and the other, the inactive form (phosphorylase b), is dephosphorylated. Glucagon and adrenaline both increase the amount of the active form, the activation being associated with the transfer of phosphate to the enzyme from ATP. Study of liver homogenates showed that the activation could take place when the hormones were added to the homogenates in the presence of ATP and Mg^{++}, but that it could not take place if the homogenates were first centrifuged. This led to the discovery that activation was produced by the interaction of either hormone with the particulate fraction, and that this interaction resulted in the formation of a heat-stable factor which was then identified as cyclic AMP (adenosine $3',5'$-monophosphate). Cyclic AMP (Fig. 4.4(a)) is formed

identifiable in bacteria as well as in metazoans. Evidently it is a feature of living organisms that must have arisen very early in evolutionary history. Its importance in endocrine processes is that it serves as a 'second messenger', by no means confined to the action of glucagon and adrenaline. These hormones, and many other as well, including vasopressin, parathyroid hormone, and corticotropin, produce

Fɪɢ. 4.4. (a) Chemical structure of cyclic AMP. (b) Formation of prostaglandins PGE_1, PGF_{1a}, and PGA_1 by cyclization of a long-chain polyenoic acid. (From Ramwell and Shaw (1970). *Rec. Prog. Hormone Res.* **26**.)

from ATP through the action of an enzyme, adenylate cyclase (formerly called adenyl cyclase). This enzyme is located within the cell membrane, supposedly in an inhibited state; what the two hormones do is to remove the inhibition, or at least to activate the enzyme in some way. The result is to catalyze the formation of cyclic AMP and increase its intracellular level; the level is then rapidly lowered because of metabolism of the enzyme. (It is believed that the symptoms of cholera are traceable to a loss of the ability to maintain low levels of the enzyme substance in the epithelial cells of the intestine.)

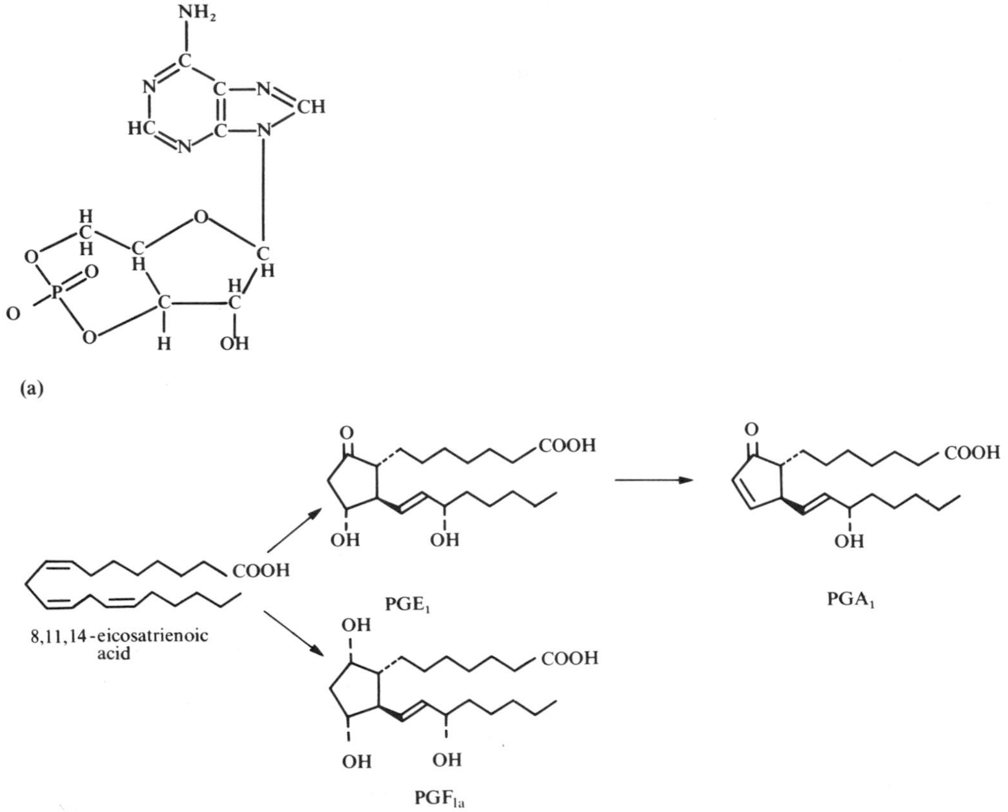

Cyclic AMP is a widespread regulatory agent,

their effects by interacting with specific receptors that are probably located on the outer surfaces of the cell membranes of their targets. This reaction increases in some way the activity of adenylate cyclase, which then builds up the intracellular levels of the second messenger.

In general, cyclic AMP increases protein kinase activity, but the precise effect of this in any particular target must depend upon the specialisation, or programming, of the cells concerned. For example, phosphorylase kinase is involved in the response to glucagon. Cyclic AMP, in the presence of ATP and Mg^{++}, converts inactive (dephosphorylated) phosphorylase kinase to the active (phosphorylated) form. This, in the presence of calcium, then converts phosphorylase from the less active to the more active form.

It is possible that the action of cyclic AMP may be associated with the enigmatic compounds called prostaglandins, which have been described, a little optimistically, as hormones in search of a function. Prostaglandins, formed by enzymic conversion from long-chain polyenoic acids (Fig. 4.4(b)), were first found in seminal fluid, but are now known to be present in most, and perhaps all, mammalian tissues. They have a wide range of pharmacological activity, sometimes at a very high level, upon many effectors, including smooth muscle, peripheral vessels, gastric glands, and various hormonal targets. Probably they are important in maintaining renal blood flow, and in facilitating expulsion of the uterine contents at birth.

In many tissues there is some correlation between their action and the activation of adenylate cyclase. One suggested explanation of this is that adenylate cyclase activity depends upon the availability of membrane calcium, which is displaced by prostaglandins. If this suggestion is well founded, it follows that hormonal responses of target tissues may be regulated to some degree by the production of prostaglandins within those tissues. Less conventional is the suggestion that vaginal absorption of prostaglandins from seminal fluid would permit a secretion of one individual to act as a circulating hormone in another. At present, however, the function of these substances remains obscure, and it is impossible to judge whether or not they are indeed hormones, either local or circulatory. However, the discovery that aspirin and similar compounds inhibit the biosynthesis of prostaglandins is likely to enlarge an understanding of their significance.

The action of cyclic AMP, although attracting much attention in its endocrine context, is not confined to endocrine tissues (so much is clearly implied by its presence in bacteria), and a great deal remains to be learned regarding its regulatory functions. However, its importance is already sufficiently evident for its discoverer, E. W. Sutherland, to have been awarded a Nobel prize.

4.2. Somatotropin (pituitary growth hormone)

Direct demonstration of the existence of a growth hormone, secreted by the pars distalis of the pituitary gland, dates from 1921, when Evans and Long showed that saline extracts of the 'anterior lobe' of the gland of cattle could accelerate growth in rats. Later,

it was shown by Smith that such extracts could restore the growth of hypophysectomized animals, and in due course it became apparent that a pituitary growth hormone (now named somatotropin) was secreted throughout the gnathostome vertebrates. It is possible that it is also secreted in cyclostomes, but this is less certain.

Well-defined symptoms result in man from disturbances in the secretion of this hormone. Gigantism, due to over-production of the hormone, is a rare condition which begins in childhood, and which is often associated with a tumour (adenoma) of the acidophil cells of the pars distalis. It is characterized by an abnormally high growth rate, which leads in males (more commonly affected than females) to a body height of between seven and eight feet, largely resulting from the excessive growth of the legs. Acromegaly, first associated with pituitary malfunction in 1886, is due to hypersecretion of the hormone which sets in during the adult stage, after the fusion of the epiphyses. As a result, it is impossible for gigantism to develop, but there is an enlargement of the head and extremities and a thickening of the skin and subcutaneous tissue, with protrusion of the lower jaw. Hyposecretion of the hormone during childhood results in the slowing or cessation of growth and an arrest of sexual development. The affected individuals become short or dwarfed, but they differ from hypothyroid dwarfs in lacking the cretinous appearance of the latter, being in fact well formed, with normal proportions and a youthful appearance.

Somatropin is not, of course, the only factor that determines growth in man; genetic and nutritional factors are also involved. For example, short stature in children may be due to a genetic restriction that cannot be overcome by any hormonal treatment, or it may be due to a slow rate of development, which will be corrected by the passage of time. Other and less obvious factors are intra-uterine growth disturbances, or psycho-social causes, including disturbed family relationships, which may influence a child to eat less and therefore grow less. These considerations are important, for, owing to the species specificity of growth hormone, to be discussed later, treatment of human patients rests at present upon the limited supply of human hormone that can be obtained from human pituitaries, and it is important none is wasted by applying it where it is not required. The hormone is obtained by removing pituitaries at autopsy and preserving them in acetone. About 60 000 glands are collected each year in the United Kingdom, a quantity which is impressive, but which

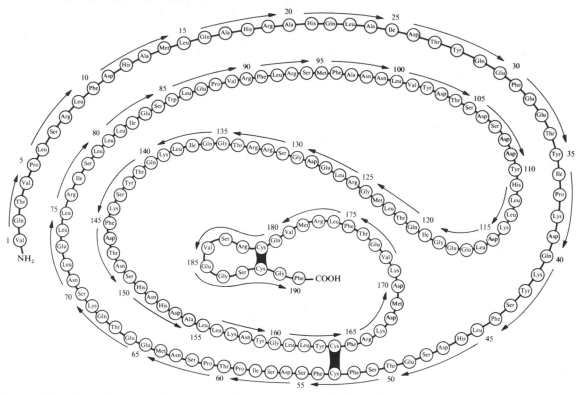

FIG. 4.5. The amino-acid sequence of human growth hormone (somatotropin). (From Li (1972.) In *Growth and growth hormone* (eds A. Pecile and E. E. Müller). Excerpta Medica, Amsterdam.)

still imposes a need for restraint in their clinical use. However, if appropriate hyposomatropic patients (i.e. with growth-hormone deficiency) are treated with somatotropin until the end of the growth period, with supplements of gonadotropin (p. 119) at adolescence if necessary, they can be brought to within normal height limits. Increases in height of about 10–12 cm in girls and 15–18 cm in boys can be expected; decisive contributions to happily fulfilled lives.

With somatotropin, as with insulin, clinical importance has been the spur to remarkable chemical achievements in chemical investigation, culminating in the determination of the primary structure of the human hormone (Fig. 4.5). This hormone, with 190 amino acids and two disulphide linkages, closely resembles in structure another pituitary hormone, prolactin (p. 122), and also a third hormone, human placental lactogen (p. 123), with properties similar to those of prolactin. We shall discuss later the functional and evolutionary implications of these resemblances. Bovine growth hormone had already been isolated in 1944 as a highly purified protein. The homogeneity of the preparation was established by appropriate methods, including solubility studies, zone electrophoresis, and counter-current distribution, yet hopes that it would be of therapeutic value in man were

TABLE 4.1

Some physicochemical properties of growth hormones (From Li (1968). *Persp. Biol. Med.* 11.)

	Human	Monkey	Bovine	Sheep	Pig	Whale
Molecular weight	21 500	23 000	45 000	47 800	41 600	39 900
Isoelectric point (pH)	4·9	5·5	6·8	6·8	6·3	6·2
Sedimentation coefficient	2·18	1·88	3·19	2·76	3·02	2·84
Diffusion coefficient	8·88	7·20	7·23	5·25	6·54	6·56
Disulphide linkages	2	4	4	5	3	3

disappointed. The preparation was inactive in human patients, and by 1954 this inactivity was described as presenting a 'frustrating dilemma'. A few years later the explanation of the frustration became clear when it was shown that preparations of the growth hormone of teleost fish were inactive in the rat and also differed chemically from the bovine hormone; yet the sheep and bovine hormones were active in the hypophysectomized teleost *Fundulus*. Further, the Rhesus monkey, like man, failed to respond to the hormones of other mammals, but both man and the monkey responded to human and to monkey hormones. In short, somatotropin is markedly species specific in its action, although, since 25 per cent of the molecule can be digested away without any decline in potency, only part of it can be concerned with its growth-promoting action.

Nevertheless, this specificity is correlated with differences in molecular structure, for differences in physicochemical properties, shown in Table 4.1, are reflected in the immunological as well as the biological activities of the various preparations. As regards immunological activity, antibodies to somatotropin can be raised in mammals, and their properties demonstrated by the double diffusion technique of Ouchterlony. The antiserum is placed in a central well of an agar plate, and the preparations to be tested are placed in wells surrounding the central one (Fig. 4.6). The appearance of localized precipitin lines between the central well and the peripheral ones is an indication of antigen–antibody reactions between the diffusing materials.

For example, it can be shown that rabbit anti-bovine serum reacts with the bovine and sheep hormones, but not with others, so that these two must be closely related antigenically. Similarly, rabbit anti-human serum reacts with human and monkey hormones, but not with others, so that these two must also be closely related. As with insulin, the antiserum will neutralize the biological activity of its specific antigen. For example, the injection into hypophysectomized rats of bovine growth hormone together with normal rabbit serum results in a gain in weight of 18 g per rat in ten days, whereas the simultaneous injection of the hormone with its rabbit antiserum gives virtually no gain at all.

These reactions can be analyzed further with the more sensitive procedure of quantitative micro-complement fixation. This procedure shows that degrees of immunological relatedness correspond very well with phylogenetic relationships established by other evidence. Thus the chimpanzee and orangutan cross-react strongly with the human hormone,

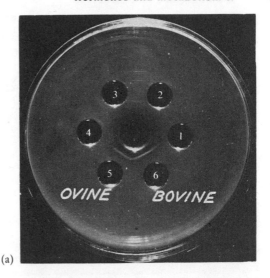

(a)

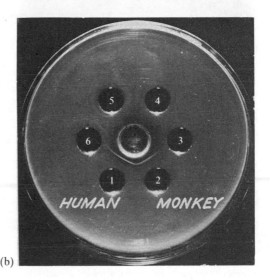

(b)

Fig. 4.6. (a) The interaction of rabbit antiserum to bovine growth hormone (centre well) with purified growth hormones (1, human; 2, monkey; 3, pig; 4, whale; 5, sheep; 6, bovine). Precipitation lines have developed between the centre well and wells 5 and 6, indicating close antigenic relationship between the sheep and bovine hormones. (b) The interaction of rabbit antiserum to human growth hormone (centre well) with purified growth hormones arranged as before. Precipitation lines between the centre well and wells 1 and 2 indicate close antigenic relationship between human and monkey hormones. (From Hayashida and Li (1959). *Endocrin.* **65**, 944–56.)

the Rhesus monkey less strongly, and the squirrel monkey still less. Further, the growth hormones of the pig, cattle, and sheep also cross-react with the antiserum to human growth hormones. Their reactions are much weaker than the primate ones, but

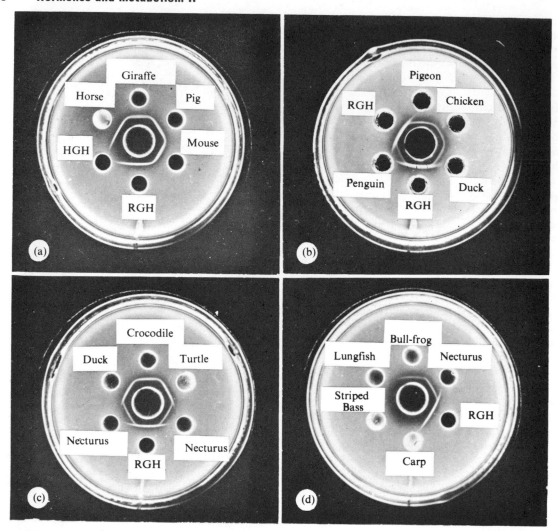

FIG. 4.7. The interaction of monkey antiserum to rat growth hormone (RGH; centre well) with growth hormone in extracts of pituitaries from various vertebrates. In (a) note reactions of qualitative identity, except that human growth hormone (HGH) gives no precipitin reaction. In (b) note that extracts of pigeon, chicken, duck, and penguin give reactions of only partial identity with rat growth hormone (indicated by the formation of spurs), but show reactions of identity with each other (including the penguin, on the basis of a separate test not shown here). In (c) note that the duck gives a reaction of qualitative identity with the crocodile and turtle; the amphibian *Necturus* gives reactions of only partial identity with the duck, turtle, and rat. In (d) note that the bull-frog gives a reaction of almost complete identity with *Necturus*, while the lung-fish (*Protopterus*) and two teleosts (striped bass and carp) give no reactions with rat growth hormone. (From Hayashida (1970). *Gen. comp. Endocrin.* **15**.)

their existence implies that there must be some similarities of structure between all of these hormones.

Immunological relations within the vertebrates have been explored over a wider spectrum of groups (Fig. 4.7) by using the double-diffusion procedure to test a range of purified preparations against monkey antiserum to rat somatotropin. The following are amongst the results of this examination. A

number of mammalian orders gave reactions that were qualitatively identical, with the exception of human somatotropin; this, as expected, was negative. Extracts from four orders of birds gave qualitatively identical results, but showed only partial identity with respect to rat somatotropin. Crocodile and turtle extracts were qualitatively identical with each other and with the duck. These results indicate that avian and mammal hormones share some immunological determinants, but that rat somatotropin has additional determinants that are not found in birds. All of these conclusions, together with the identity in reaction of birds and the two reptiles, are obviously in line with the known phylogenetic relationships of the groups concerned. It will be recalled that birds and mammals are independent offshoots of a reptilian ancestry, and that birds are more closely linked with surviving reptiles than are mammals.

Studies with other vertebrate groups are generally in line with this argument, although there are matters of detail that would not always be predictable from known phylogenetic relationships. For example, teleosts (striped bass and carp) are negative to the monkey antiserum, whereas chondrosteans (sturgeon, *Polyodon*) and holosteans (*Amia*, *Lepisosteus*) are clearly positive. This suggests that teleosts have moved further from the common ancestry of osteichthyans and tetrapods than have the more primitive members of the actinopterygian line. Amphibians show partial identity with mammals and birds, whereas *Protopterus*, despite the close relationship of lung-fish to the tetrapod line, is negative. This could doubtless be interpreted as indicative of the isolated position of the modern dipnoans, which are highly specialized derivatives of that line. Finally, sharks (*Squalus acanthias* and *Mustelus canis*) have partial identity with mammals, as also has the skate, *Raja eglanteria*, but less so.

The results obtained in double-diffusion studies are confirmed by radio-immunoassay, which is a special case of a type of a procedure called competitive protein-binding analysis. This depends upon the availability of a protein with specific binding sites for the hormone under investigation, and upon the availability also of an isotopic form of the hormone, which can be readily assayed by radioactive counting. Suppose that both the unlabelled and the labelled forms of the hormone are mixed with the binding protein, that the binding sites are saturated, and that association and dissociation occur spontaneously. If more of the unlabelled form is added, the two forms will compete for the binding sites in proportion to their concentrations, according to the law of mass action. Further addition of unlabelled hormone will therefore reduce the percentage of bound labelled hormone in the system, so that determination of this percentage provides a very sensitive measure of the amount of unlabelled hormone present (cf. Fig. 4.8). Proteins with binding sites for such small molecules as thyroxine and steroids may be obtainable direct from the plasma, where they may be serving under physiological conditions as specific carrier proteins

for the hormones. This may also apply for large hormonal molecules, such as insulin, but in assaying these molecules it is usual to prepare specific binding proteins in the form of antibodies, raised by the administration of the hormone from another species, acting therefore as a foreign antigen. This is the basis of radio-immunoassay.

Immunological procedures, because of their sensitivity and specificity, are of great value in studies of protein hormones, and in this book we refer to them in various contexts. It is important, however, to remember that the use of these procedures is an exploitation of the precise specificity of reaction between antigen and antibody, and not of the biological activity of the hormone concerned. It is thus essential to be able to show that the immunological and biological properties under investigation are associated in the same molecule.

Radio-immunoassay requires a system comprising pure preparations of the hormone and of its antibody, together with a sample of the hormone which has been labelled with radioactive iodine (^{131}I). The antibody will bind a certain percentage of the amount of labelled hormone which is presented to it. Addition of increasing amounts of the unlabelled hormone to the system will then progressively reduce this percentage by competitive binding at the reactive sites. In other words, the ratio of bound labelled hormone to free labelled hormone falls in proportion to the increase in concentration of the unlabelled hormone, and it is this ratio that has to be determined. To do this, it is necessary first to separate the bound labelled hormone from the free labelled hormone, for this separation does not take place in the system owing to the low concentrations of reactants preventing spontaneous precipitation of the labelled antigen–antibody complex. Given a satisfactory procedure for this separation, together with purity of labelled antigen and specificity of antibody, radio-immunoassay (Fig. 4.8) provides a level of sensitivity which is usually far in advance of that which could be obtained with any other form of assay.

A summary of a widely used procedure for human growth hormone will illustrate the handling of the technique. Rabbit antiserum to human growth hormone (antigen) is prepared, and also a small amount of labelled antigen. The amount of antibody required to give 50–70 per cent binding of the labelled antigen is then determined. The labelled antigen is then incubated for 7 days with a predetermined amount of antiserum, together with the unknown, which will usually be a sample of plasma. At the end of incubation, the free antigen and the antigen bound to the

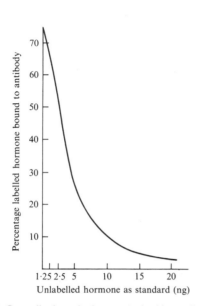

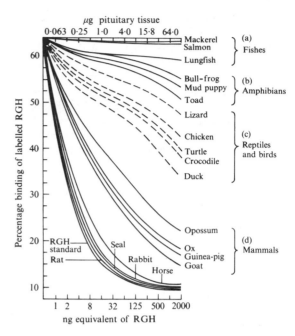

FIG. 4.8. Generalized standard curve obtained in a radio-immuno-assay. The dilution of antiserum chosen will bind only 76 per cent of the fixed amount of labelled hormone added. (From Greenwood (1967). In *Modern trends in endocrinology*, p. 3 (ed. H. Gardiner-Hill). Butterworth, London.)

FIG. 4.9. Composite diagram showing immunochemical related-ness of growth hormone in pituitary extracts from representatives of various vertebrate classes based on radio-immunoassay with monkey antiserum to rat growth hormone. (From Hayashida (1970). *Gen. comp. Endocrin.* 15.)

antiserum are separated, and the ^{131}I content of each is determined. The amount of unlabelled antigen in the test sample can then be calculated by reference to a standard curve. Various methods are available for the separation, including, for example, electro-phoresis on cellulose acetate, ion exchange chroma-tography, and adsorption on charcoal. The lower limits of sensitivity are estimated to be 0·07 ng/ml for purified human growth hormone, and 0·22 ng/ml for plasma samples.

Using this method, the immunological relation-ships of various somatotropin preparations can be compared by measuring the extent to which they com-pete with a standard (e.g. rat growth hormone) for binding with the antibody to the standard. Results for a number of species are shown in Fig. 4.9. It will be seen that a marsupial (opossum) gives the lowest degree of cross-reaction amongst the mammalian species studied; the other species conform to the results of double-diffusion studies. We may conclude that, in general, the sharing of antigenic determin-ants increases with decreasing phylogenetic distance, but it is equally clear that, with increasing distance, the immunological behaviour of the hormone be-comes increasingly unreliable for defining the details of phylogenetic history. Nevertheless, the isolation

of the teleosts conforms with the high degree of independent specialization of this group, which is apparent also in other features of their endocrine system.

The biological activity of somatotropin prepara-tions is determined by a bioassay that is usually carried out on hypophysectomized rats. Radio-immunoassay is now more sensitive and rapid than this procedure, but (as indicated above) the bioassay remains essential for confirming that the immuno-logically active material is actually capable of promoting growth, and that the results are not arti-facts of reaction. The bioassay involves measurement of the gain in weight or in width of the cartilage separating the epiphysis of the tibia from the shaft. Daily injections of appropriate strength give a gain that is proportional to the logarithm of the dose, provided that the test is not prolonged for more than eight days; thereafter, the response is diminished as a result of the formation of antibodies. Degrees of response are broadly similar to the corresponding immunological activity, but do not agree so closely in detail with the known phylogenetic relationships. For example, all mammalian extracts tested are more active than those of almost any other vertebrate group, one surprising exception being amphibians (bull-frog and toad), which show activities within the normal mammalian range. At the opposite extreme, teleostean extracts (striped bass, salmon, mackerel) are completely negative, whereas more primitive bony fish (*Polypterus*, the sturgeon, *Polyodon*, *Amia*, *Lepisosteus*) are positive. *Squalus*, *Mustelus*, and *Raja* are positive, their activities being inhibited by antiserum to rat somatotropin. These results suggest that the molecular determinants of the immunochemical activities of the somatotropin molecule are different from the determinants of its biological activities, as expressed in the tibia growth response.

Skeletal growth involves the uptake of sulphate, which passes into the chondrocytes of developing cartilage and is incorporated by them into the chondroitin sulphate which constitutes the mucopolysaccharide moiety of the cartilage matrix. One index of growth-hormone action is, therefore, an increase in this sulphate uptake, which can be demonstrated both *in vivo* and *in vitro*. But there is a complication in the study of this apparently simple parameter. This emerged when it was found that the addition of growth hormone to pieces of mammalian cartilage *in vitro* failed to stimulate sulphate uptake if the cartilages had been removed from hypophysectomized rats. On the other hand, serum from normal rats could induce this stimulation without any addition of the hormone at all, whereas serum from hypophysectomized animals failed to do so.

From these and other experiments it has been concluded that the action of growth hormone on skeletal chondroitin-sulphate synthesis is mediated in mammals by a non-dialysable component (probably a peptide) of the serum; this component, called sulphation factor (or somatomedin), is supposedly formed by the liver under the influence of growth hormone, and is released from this organ into the blood. The factor is therefore absent from the serum of hypophysectomized rats, but it can be restored to the serum of these animals if they are treated with growth hormone, which stimulates the production of the factor by the liver. Similarly, its serum level increases when human patients with pituitary dwarfism are treated with growth hormone (Fig. 4.10).

Sulphate uptake is not the only index of the presence of sulphation factor, for this substance affects many aspects of cell anabolism and cell replication. For example, it stimulates the incorporation of leucine into chondromucoprotein, of uridine into RNA, and of thymidine into DNA. Indeed, it is even possible that the sulphation effect is primarily the result of the stimulation of the synthesis of the

protein moiety of protein–polysaccharide complexes of skeletal matrix. In any case, however, there is good reason for regarding somatomedin as a second hormone, mediating the action of somatotropin upon skeletal tissue.

Not surprisingly, in view of the complexity of the growth process, somatotropin has other parameters of activity additional to its influence on skeletal growth. One is an effect upon nitrogen balance. Injections of the hormone cause nitrogen retention, with a marked decline in urinary nitrogen, while a fall in blood urea indicates that amino acids are being used in protein synthesis rather than for fuel. There is also retention of potassium and phosphorus (probably due to increase of cell mass) and of sodium and calcium. The calcium retention occurs during the treatment of hypopituitary dwarfs, despite an increased output of urinary calcium which is a particularly characteristic result of the treatment.

The nitrogen retention reflects, of course, an increase in protein synthesis, which is apparent in experimental animals, and also in hypopituitary children who are receiving somatotropin therapy. Since much of the body's protein is contained in the muscle, this effect can be demonstrated by measuring protein and DNA in samples of muscle obtained by biopsy. Increase in cell size and number is found, together with increase in DNA, which reflects cell hyperplasia. It is worth noting, however, that muscle growth is not totally dependent upon somatotropin, for it can take place as a result of prolonged exercise even in the absence of the hormone.

Another metabolic effect of the hormone, particularly evident after long-term treatment, is a modification of fat metabolism. An initial fall in free fatty-acid

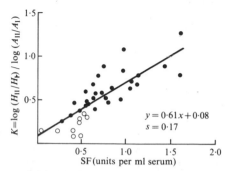

FIG. 4.10. Sulphation factor activity (abscissae) in serum, and corresponding growth rate (ordinates), in patients with pituitary dwarfism before (○) and during (●) treatment with human growth hormone. K is an expression relating height (H) to age (A). The line represents the regression equation. (From Hall and Uthne (1972). In *Growth and growth hormone* (eds A. Pecile and E. E. Müller). Excerpta Medica, Amsterdam.)

levels is followed by a rise which results from fat mobilization; this is shown in increased lipolysis in adipose tissue and in an increase in the uptake of fatty acids by muscular tissue. The significance of this for growth is not clear; it has therefore been suggested that somatotropin may be of importance in metabolism generally, by facilitating a supply of energy during periods in between meals when the body is more dependent upon fatty acids for energy supplies.

Growth hormone also has profound effects upon carbohydrate metabolism. As with free fatty-acid levels, there is an initial period of lowered blood-glucose levels, but prolonged treatment with the hormone leads to increased output of glucose from the liver, as a result of increased gluconeogenesis, accompanied by an increase in glucose 6-phosphatase. There is also a marked impairment of glucose tolerance (i.e. the rate of disappearance of intravenously injected glucose is decreased). This results from a reduced transport of glucose into muscle and adipose tissue, and from a reduction in phosphorylation of the glucose that does enter the muscle. The consequence of this is marked hyperglycaemia. This, however, may be only a transient effect, since the normal reaction to this is an increased output of insulin, partly in response to the rise in blood sugar, and partly in direct response to the somatotropin itself. There is an element of paradox in all of this, for somatotropin is stimulating the secretion of insulin, and at the same time antagonizing the normal action of this hormone upon the promotion of glucose utilization. Because of this, somatotropin has a diabetogenic effect. If it is given to dogs for sufficient time, and in sufficient quantities, the B cells are severely and even irreparably damaged, because they are impelled by somatotropin to an excessive output of insulin. Persistent diabetes may result, accompanied by ketosis.

4.3. Hormonal interactions in growth and metabolism

Appreciation of this influence of growth hormone derives from the studies of Houssay, initiated on the toad, *Bufo arenarum* (Table 4.2). Pancreatectomy in this animal results in hyperglycaemia, just as in a mammal, and Houssay showed that this effect could be diminished by removal of the whole pituitary gland or of the pars distalis, while implantation of the latter re-established the condition, or even intensified it. The special importance of the pars distalis was shown by the fact that the neuro-intermediate lobe had little or no effect. These studies

TABLE 4.2

Effect of various combinations of treatment upon the blood sugar of the toad, Bufo arenarum (Fröm Houssay (1949). *Quart. Rev. Biol.* **24**.)

	Normal	Hypophys-ectomized	Pars distalis removed
With pancreas	64	51	56
Implantation of pars distalis	68	58	69
Pancreatectomy	199	94	94
Pancreatectomy plus implantation of pars distalis	256	228	214
Pancreatectomy plus implantation of neuro-intermediate lobe	199	110	116

were extended to mammals, and it was shown that if hypophysectomy was carried out on a pancreatectomized dog, showing the usual symptoms of diabetes mellitus, these symptoms were markedly reduced. So striking is the effect that such a doubly operated dog can survive for many months without the insulin treatment which is essential for the survival of a depancreatized animal with its pituitary intact. It follows that the pars distalis must be secreting a factor which augments the diabetic disturbances associated with insulin deprivation, and which, therefore, must normally be antagonizing the effects of that hormone. The conclusion seemed so surprising when it was first announced that one distinguished physiologist is said to have declared that it must be wrong, because metabolic control was known to be primarily the function of the 'posterior lobe' of the gland! As events turned out, however, this discovery helped to gain for Houssay a Nobel Prize.

There is also a well-documented interaction of growth hormone and the thyroid hormones. Thyroidectomy results in the decrease in number of the acidophil cells of the pars distalis of the rat, which are known to secrete growth hormone (p. 68), while the number can be restored by supplying to the animals a minimal dose of thyroxine. In this respect, thyroid hormones are growth-promoting agents because their presence is required for the endogenous production of growth hormone.

But the action of the thyroid goes further than this. Very high doses of thyroxine are required to restore normal growth rates in thyroidectomized rats, whereas smaller doses of growth hormone are adequate if they are administered in combination with thyroxine. Evidently, therefore, the effective action of growth hormone depends upon the presence of thyroxine; but the opposite also applies, for thyroxine, while certainly a growth-promoting agent in mammals, can only act in this way in the presence of growth hormone. For this reason, treating hypopituitary dwarfs with thyroxine will not bring the patients to normal growth rates. The growth-promoting influence of the thyroid hormones will be discussed further in a later chapter (p. 175). It will be sufficient to add now that this hormonal inter-relationship is not confined to the mammals. Thyroid treatment of normal and intact teleost fish may improve their growth rate, but will not restore normal growth in hypophysectomized fish.

The interaction of hormones in metabolic regulation is further exemplified by the glucocorticoid hormones of the adrenocortical tissue, with which we deal in more detail later. We can note here that they influence carbohydrate metabolism, in part by inhibiting the peripheral utilization of glucose, and in part by promoting the deamination of amino acids and hence the formation of glucose from protein sources in the liver. In general, therefore, they are part of the system which opposes the effects of insulin, tending to produce an increase in nitrogen excretion and a rise in blood sugar. Prolonged administration of them may, in fact, establish a diabetic condition; this results from damage to the B cells, in consequence of the increased demand for the secretion of insulin to antagonize their action.

Hyperglycaemia is also evoked by adrenaline, and, to a less extent, by noradrenaline (p. 191). These hormones, like glucagon, act upon phosphorylase to stimulate hepatic glycogenolysis. Unlike glucagon, however, which acts primarily on the liver, they also act upon muscle phosphorylases to promote the glycolytic breakdown of glycogen, with a consequent increase in the lactic acid level of the blood. These responses to adrenaline and noradrenaline are essentially emergency responses, which are regulated by the nervous system, and which facilitate the extra activity required when an animal is responding to some stressful stimulus (p. 193). One such circumstance would be a development of hypoglycaemia, such as might result in man or in experimental animals from an overdose of insulin. However, adrenaline can only produce a rise in blood sugar if there are adequate reserves of hepatic glycogen; since these might well be lacking during hypoglycaemia, a direct supply of sugar would be a more certain remedy.

Precision has been given to this and other aspects of hormonal interaction in the regulation of carbohydrate metabolism by the use of the isolated diaphragm of the rat. This can be incubated *in vitro* in the presence of suitable reagents, and it is then possible to measure its uptake of glucose from the medium, and the extent to which it is synthesizing new protein as reflected in its uptake of amino acids labelled with radioactive carbon (Fig. 4.11). These

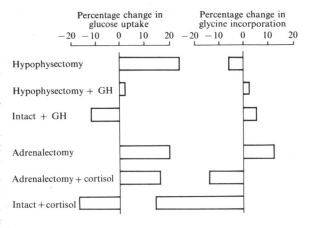

FIG. 4.11. Summary of the effects of hypophysectomy adrenalectomy, and treatment with growth hormone (GH) or with cortisol, on uptake of glucose and incorporation of [^{14}C]glycine into the protein of isolated rat diaphragm. Results are expressed as the percentage change induced by a particular treatment; comparisons are not quantitatively accurate but illustrate general trends. (From Manchester *et al.* (1959). *J. Endocrin.* **18**.)

activities will be influenced by the presence of insulin and other hormones in the incubation medium. Thus, for example, it is possible to make direct measurements of the relative insulin content of different types of plasma by comparing the activity of the diaphragm in these with its activity in a suitable control medium.

Some results of such hormonal interactions, as exemplified in reactions of the isolated diaphragm of the rat, are illustrated in Fig. 4.11 Growth hormone depresses the uptake of glucose and thus, by restraining carbohydrate metabolism, has an influence opposed to that of insulin; at the same time it increases the incorporation of amino acid into the protein of the diaphragm, as we would expect. Such nitrogen retention can, in fact, be demonstrated in intact experimental animals during a period of administration of growth hormone. Fig. 4.11 also shows that cortisol (p. 200) resembles growth hormone in restraining carbohydrate metabolism, but differs from it in decreasing nitrogen uptake. It is believed, however, that this is a consequence of its stimulation of gluconeogenesis in the liver, for associated with this is the transfer of protein to the latter organ from the other tissues. Thus the increased wastage of nitrogen in the diabetic animal may be ascribed at least in part to the action of the glucocorticoid hormones.

It will be apparent, even from this selective survey, that the hormonal control of metabolism in mammals is extraordinarily complex. The essential subtlety of the regulatory mechanisms can be sensed by considering what probably happens when insulin is injected into a normal mammal. We have seen that the level of blood sugar is first lowered and then restored (Fig. 4.1), and that the latter phase is attributed mainly to the action of agents that antagonize the effect of the insulin. We can now define these agents in more precise terms by noting that the hypoglycaemia will evoke the secretion of gluco-corticoids, which, by restraining the peripheral utilization of carbohydrates, will tend to counterbalance the stimulating influence of the insulin upon carbohydrate metabolism, while they will also stimulate gluconeogenesis and thereby favour a rise in blood sugar. Meanwhile, somatotropin will join in restraining the use of carbohydrates (Fig. 4.11) and, by encouraging nitrogen retention, will tend to counterbalance the influence of the glucocorticoids upon the amino acid metabolism of the non-hepatic tissues. Finally, the hypoglycaemia will also cause an increased output of adrenaline from the chromaffin tissue and this will promote a rise in blood sugar by stimulating glycogenolysis, provided that there are adequate reserves of glycogen in the liver.

5

Organization and evolution of the pituitary gland

5.1. Neurosecretion

The pituitary gland is a dual organ, formed of an ectodermal component, the adenohypophysis, and a neural one, the neurohypophysis. The explanation of this duality is that the gland is adapted to secure functional interrelationship of the nervous and endocrine systems. We have noted already that each of these systems has its own special characteristics; the nervous system being concerned with responses that are localized in space and time, while the endocrine system is concerned with diffuse and prolonged reactions. Effective regulation of the body depends upon co-ordinated action of the two, ensuring that afferent signals from the environment, both internal and external, are transmitted to the endocrine glands.

It might seem that the simplest way to bring about this co-ordination would be for endocrine cells to be innervated by conventional nerve cells (the *neurones banales* of French writers) through nerve fibres that are in direct synaptic connection with the cells at secretomotor junctions. This is certainly possible, yet such junctions are the exception rather than the rule. They have been identified most clearly in the pineal gland and in the adrenal medulla, but these are special cases, for the secretory cells concerned are themselves of neural derivation. It is clear, from the difficulty that has been found in identifying such connections elsewhere, that they are not a common feature of the vertebrate endocrine system.

Further reflection will in any case show that direct and conventional innervation of endocrine cells must necessarily be of only limited effectiveness in endocrine regulation, simply because of the fundamental difference in mode of operation of the two regulatory systems. It is essential, to ensure the effective discharge of hormones, that many of the cells of an endocrine gland should be brought into action simultaneously, and that the secretory activity of these cells shall be of long duration. These require-

ments run counter to the localization in space and time, characteristic of conventional innervation. It is undoubtedly for this reason that another type of neural control has evolved, mediated by specialized nerve cells called neurosecretory cells. This type of control is so fundamental to the regulation of animal activity that it is found throughout the animal kingdom, from coelenterates to mammals.

Neurosecretory cells (Fig. 5.1) have large cell bodies, and contain stainable granules or droplets, both in their cytoplasm (perikaryon) and in their axons. They were first reported by Speidel, who in 1919, following earlier observations of Dahlgren, described granules in cell bodies of the spinal cord of fish (p. 266). The nature of these Dahlgren cells remained unknown, and it was not until 1928 that E. Scharrer drew attention to similar appearances in the cells of the supraoptic and paraventricular nuclei, and of the preoptic nuclei which are their homologues in the lower vertebrates (Figs 5.17, 5.18, and 5.19).

It was his view that these cells might be concerned in secretion, and the eventual justification of this belief shows how the development of a new biological principle may have to wait upon the availability of suitable techniques. Trichrome stains will demonstrate inclusions in these cells (Fig. 5.1(c)), but it was the introduction into this field by Bargmann in 1949 of a modification of the chrome-alum–haematoxylin procedure of Gomori (p. 26) which opened up a phase of intense investigation of the problem. With this method, the granular contents of the cells are stained blue–black, and identical material can be seen in their axons and in the neural lobe itself (Fig. 5.1(a)). Within the axons it forms concentrations which are responsible for the varicosities that are characteristic of them, and that had led to the belief that they might be undergoing degeneration. When appropriately stained, however, the

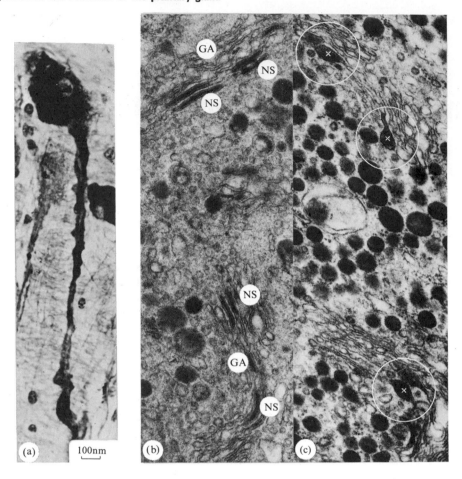

FIG. 5.1. (a) Neurosecretory cell from the nucleus supraopticus of a dog. Bouin's fixative, chrome-alum–haematoxylin and phloxin. (From Scharrer and Scharrer (1954). In von Moellendorff's *Handbuch der mikroskopische Anatomie des Menschen*, Vol. II, 5, pp. 953–1066.) (b) and (c) Electron micrographs of neurosecretory cells in the supra-oesophageal ganglion of an earthworm. Note in (b) neurosecretory material (NS) within cisternae of the Golgi complex (GA). Note in (c) neurosecretory granules developing in the Golgi complex, indicated by circles. (From Scharrer and Brown (1961). *Z. Zellforsch. mikrosk. Anat.* **54**, 530–40.)

material is clearly visible within the fibres, often looking like a string of beads. Larger accumulations of this material form conspicuous masses that used to be called Herring bodies, before their true nature was understood.

Other staining procedures are also useful for revealing the same features. A commonly used one is the aldehyde–fuchsin technique of Gomori, which, as we have seen earlier (p. 26), reveals sulphydryl groups. Both methods of Gomori can be used for bulk staining, making it possible to show the course of the fibres and to demonstrate the anatomy of the fibre tracts in whole preparations. Other methods are the thioglycollate–ferric ferricyanide technique of Adams, and the performic acid–Alcian blue tech-

nique of Adams and Sloper. These selectively demonstrate a high concentration of cystine in the material, the former method by reducing this amino acid to cysteine, and the latter one by oxidizing it to cysteic acid.

Light microscopy, however, gives only a partial view. Electron microscopy (Figs 5.1 and 5.2) reveals that the secretory products of these cells are highly characteristic electron-dense granules, bounded by single membranes, and derived from the Golgi cisternae; there is ample experimental evidence, to be discussed later, that the neurohypophysial hormones are contained within them. These granules appear in several size categories, but are commonly about 100–300 nm in diameter. It is accumulation of these gran-

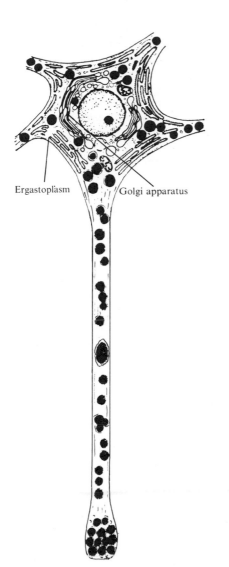

Ergastoplasm   Golgi apparatus

FIG. 5.2. Diagram of neurosecretory neurone showing organelles involved in the production of neurosecretory material. (From B. Scharrer (1970). *The neurosciences: second study programme* (ed. F. O. Schmitt) Rockfeller University Press, New York.)

or from a neuron to an effector cell, depends upon the production and, to some extent, the axonal flow, of chemical mediators. Typically in vertebrates these are either acetylcholine or noradrenaline. They are stored in the preterminal areas of the synapses, and are released into the synaptic clefts at cholinergic or adrenergic endings respectively.

Electron microscopy shows that cholinergic endings have accumulations of membrane-bound synaptic vesicles, electron-lucent, and within a size range of 20–50 nm. These are quantal units of acetylcholine, perhaps formed partly in the perikaryon (cell body) and also along the axon or at its ending. They are not visible by light microscopy. Noradrenaline is similarly represented by accumulations of granules, in this case electron-dense, and with a size of about 60 nm. Discharge of these chemical mediators or neurotransmitters takes place through openings formed by fusion of the synaptic vesicles with the cell membrane at the active sites, a mode of release termed exocytosis. The effect of the discharge is highly localized and transient, for acetylcholine is rapidly destroyed, while noradrenaline is probably taken up again into the axon. Because the action of these substances is so sharply localized, both in space and in time, and because they are not transmitted through the blood stream, they cannot be brought within the classical definition of hormones. They are termed neurohumours.

This, however, is not the only illustration of the secretory activity of the conventional neurone. Another is the dependence of receptors (taste-buds, for example) and muscle fibres for their differentiation upon some morphogenetic influence exerted upon them by the nerve endings that become associated with them. This effect is attributed to the production within the neurones of secretions which pass proximo-distally down the axon fibres, perhaps enclosed within dense-core vesicles similar to those just mentioned.

The secretory activity of neurosecretory cells, and the axonal flow which we shall see to be associated with it, is thus not without parallel in the conventional nerve cells. However, neurosecretory cells differ from these in certain respects, although they have the same fundamental morphological features of a perikaryon, axon, and dendrites. The ergastoplasm is extensively developed, as in all protein-secreting cells, but in contrast to the Nissl substance of the **conventional neuron (with which it corresponds),** **it tends to be found as a compact mass of lamellae** at one pole of the cell. Mitochondria and Golgi substance are also conspicuous.

ules, perhaps in association with carrier protein, that provides the so-called 'Gomori-positive material' of light microscopy.

A satisfactory evaluation of this concept of neurosecretion (which, in the light of later discussion (p. 61) we shall refer to as the classical concept) demands consideration of the properties of the conventional neuron. This is responsible for the propagation of nerve impulses, a process that involves electrical activity and ionic fluxes. These cells, however, are also involved in secretion, for the transmission of the impulse from one neuron to the next,

The secretion is thought to arise within the cisternae of the puromycin-sensitive ribosomal system of the ergastoplasm, but is first clearly visible as dense material within the Golgi cisternae and vesicles, from which it separates as the membrane-bound granules (elementary granules) which provide for its storage (Fig. 5.2).

After release from the Golgi region, the elementary granules accumulate between the ergastoplasmic cisternae, so that the ergastoplasm itself becomes broken up. The Golgi region becomes quiescent, as the perikaryon becomes filled with secretion; this forms the concentrations that are so conspicuous in the perikarya by light microscopy. These concentrations are not normally released from the perikaryon to the outside of the cell, although this possibility is not entirely excluded in some neurosecretory systems. They pass down the axon of the cell, to be released at distinctive points that are mainly located at or near the axon terminations in the neural lobe. These points of discharge have clusters of small vesicles like synaptic vesicles. In some systems they may also have thickened electron-dense membranes, termed synaptoid configurations. These may be defined as ultrastructural specializations which resemble those of synapses, but are not necessarily involved in synaptic transmission.

The secretion, having passed into the axons, may be temporarily stored within them, but eventually it is discharged from the nerve endings, and sometimes from other parts of the axons as well. Discharge takes place in structures called neurohaemal organs, where the neurosecretory endings are in close contact with blood vessels (Fig. 5.3), by which the secretion is distributed, ultimately to reach its target cells.

How the secretion is discharged from the axon is uncertain. Only rarely have intact membrane-bound granules been reported outside the axon. Ultrastructural studies suggest that sometimes the granules may fragment, this being followed by extrusion of their secretory contents. Omega-shaped bodies in contact with the axon membrane suggest that release may also take place by exocytosis, just as we have described for the synaptic vesicles carrying the neurohumours. This mode of discharge is undoubtedly advantageous. It avoids the passage of the secretion across membranes, and prevents its dispersion through the cytoplasm, with consequent dilution and risk of enzymic destruction. It may well be the main reason for the evidently common tendency for neuronal secretions to be enclosed in membrane-bound granules. Some of the synaptic-type vesicles may well arise as fragmentation pro-

ducts, but, if this is so, it is not clear whether their electronlucent contents are the secretory product, or whether this is represented by electron-dense material which is often seen lying against the axon membrane at sites of discharge. It may, of course, be that this material is carrier protein from which the active secretion has already separated, or will eventually separate. Clearly there is still much to learn about this process.

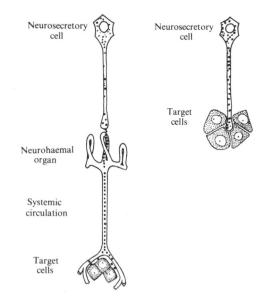

FIG. 5.3. (*Left*) Diagram of neurosecretory axon ending, with neurohaemal organ. (After B. Scharrer.)

FIG. 5.4. (*Right*) Diagram of neurosecretory axon ending, forming direct neurosecretomotor junction. (After B. Scharrer.)

Equally uncertain is the mechanism that brings about discharge at any particular time. There is direct evidence, from recordings made from neurosecretory cells in the spinal cord of teleosts (p. 266), that neurosecretory cells can propagate nerve impulses, characterized by action potentials of longer duration than those of conventional neurons. It is thus attractive to suppose that release is brought about by neural signals transmitted down the neurosecretory fibres, perhaps with synaptic-like vesicles releasing a neurohumour. On the other hand, axons lacking neurosecretory contents run with tracts of axons containing neurosecretion. This suggests that neurosecretory release may be regulated by neurons of conventional type, but of course it may be that axons lacking neurosecretion belong to neurosecretory cells that are temporarily denuded of their secretory product.

The nomenclature attached to this aspect of endocrinology needs careful definition. It is misleading to use the term neurosecretory material or neurosecretion for any material secreted by neurones, and visible with the light microscope after appropriate fixation and staining, and this remains so even if such material reacts positively to the chrome-alum–haematoxylin or aldehyde–fuchsin procedures. These methods are not specific, and it must be emphasized that the mere presence of some stainable material in neurones does not in itself establish the secretion of hormones. Physiological studies are essential for this, although the presence of membrane-bound granules of appropriate size in electron micrographs, and the association of the axons with neurohaemal organs, would be important contributory evidence.

When physiological investigation, combined with cytological and ultrastructural study, has established the probability that a particular group of neurones is secreting a neurosecretory material with hormonal activity, that material may be referred to as neuroendocrine material. In practice, however, the description of material as a neurosecretion commonly carries the implication that it is hormonally active, although the visible material may be a carrier substance and not the hormone itself. To the latter we apply the term neurohormone or neurosecretory hormone.

The concept so far outlined may be described as the classical concept of neurosecretion. Essential elements of it are that the secretion is a peptide (e.g. the neurohypophysial hormones), so that the cells are called peptidergic (or type A) cells. Another is that discharge of the hormone takes place into the blood stream at a neurohaemal organ. Advances in knowledge, however, have shown that neurosecretion is a much more diversified phenomenon than was at first appreciated. In particular, there is a wide spectrum of relationship between the nervous and the endocrine systems, and the dividing line between conventional and neurosecretory neurones is no longer as clearly defined as it formerly seemed to be. Thus, as so often with the growth of biological knowledge, we have to take account of borderline cases that are difficult to classify.

One respect in which the concept of neurosecretion has had to be broadened concerns the secretion. This need not necessarily be peptide material, for neurosecretory axons may also discharge biogenic amines. Those that do so are called aminergic (or type B) fibres. Clearly these fibres have much in common with those of conventional neurones, but they are not identical. That they produce biogenic amines can be demonstrated by the formaldehyde condensation technique which produces a fluorescence highly specific for this class of compound (p. 189), but it does not follow that the secretion is adrenaline or noradrenaline. Electron microscopy shows that the amines are associated with electron-dense and membrane-bound granules, of 500–1400 Å in size. They are smaller than the granules of peptidergic fibres, yet larger than typical synaptic vesicles of adrenergic nerve endings. Moreover, the axons differ from conventional adrenergic fibres in other respects as well. Their synaptic-type vesicles are found in all parts of the neurone, and not merely at the nerve ending, while the fibres often end in neurohaemal centres.

The other respect in which the concept has been broadened relates to the way in which signals are transferred from both type A and type B nerve endings to their targets. It is no longer justifiable to insist, as an essential criterion for neurosecretion, that the product should be discharged into the blood at neurohaemal organs. One possibility is for both type A and type B fibres to make direct contact with effector cells (Fig. 5.4), which may be either endocrine or neural, or perhaps neither. Such junctional sites can be termed neurosecretomotor junctions when endocrine cells are being innervated.

A second possibility is that the fibres may terminate very close to a group of effector cells, at a distance of perhaps only a few thousand ångström units; they may end in pericapillary spaces, for example, or against basement membranes. In such instances the space between nerve terminal and effector cell may sometimes be occupied by electron-dense material; the nature of this is not clear, but it has been suggested that it might serve as a temporary reservoir of discharged secretion, perhaps slowing down its propagation and permitting a more prolonged response to it.

Junctional sites of the two types outlined are difficult to classify in conventional nomenclature. The transmission of the neurosecretory signal does not involve the blood stream, so that the secretions cannot strictly be termed hormones. On the other hand, to call them neurohumours would be to conceal ignorance, for we cannot suppose that they are always identical with the established transmitter substances of conventional neurons, nor do we understand how they are released or how they function. Difficulties of interpretation may diminish with further research. For the present, it is enough to grasp the principle that communication between the nervous system and the endocrine system follows more than one route, involving the despatch of both local and distance signals. As has been well said, the vocabulary of neuroendocrine communication is richer than was earlier appreciated.

5.2. General organization of the pituitary gland in mammals

The name of the pituitary gland (from *pituita*, phlegm) derives from a misconception of the early anatomists, who believed that it was concerned with the evacuation of phlegm or mucus from the cavities of the brain. Vesalius supposed that this material was conducted into the infundibulum and that it trickled down from there into the pituitary gland (Fig. 5.5) below, so eventually reaching the palate

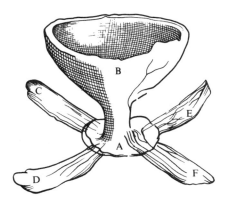

FIG. 5.5. Vesalius's interpretation of the pituitary gland. A, pituitary gland; B, infundibulum; C, D, E, and F, non-existent ducts supposedly leading to the palate and nasal cavities. (From Singer (1952). *Vesalius on the human brain.* Oxford University Press, London.)

and nasal cavities through four ducts. This sixteenth-century interpretation may seem to strain credulity. It is, however, no more remarkable than the one which has emerged from the results of twentieth-century research, and which, curiously enough, is also based upon the conception of a flow of secretion from the brain.

We have already seen that the gland is formed of two distinct components, known as the adeno-hypophysis and the neurohypophysis. The adeno-hypophysis arises in the embryo (Fig. 5.6) as Rathke's pouch, an outgrowth of the ectodermal lining of the stomodaeal ectoderm, while the neurohypophysis develops as the infundibular recess, a backwardly-directed outgrowth of the floor of the diencephalon. Rathke's pouch, which is hollow in most vertebrate groups, early differentiates into an oral and aboral lobe, separated by a constriction. The aboral lobe

comes into contact with the developing infundibular recess, this contact, as we shall see, having an important influence on the subsequent development of the adenohypophysis. Commonly a pair of lateral lobes grow out from the constriction separating the oral and aboral lobes, while a median anterior process also develops. This association of epithelial and neural components is of fundamental importance for the functioning not only of the pituitary gland, but also of the whole of the vertebrate endocrine system; growth in our understanding of it has illuminated our interpretation of endocrine systems throughout the animal kingdom. There could be no better demonstration of the importance of comparative studies in shedding light over areas much wider than those that are under immediate investigation.

The nomenclature of the pituitary gland has been confused in the past by the fact that in certain mammals it can readily be separated into two portions which have been termed the 'anterior lobe' and the 'posterior lobe'; from these, as we shall see (p. 90), correspondingly named commercial preparations have been prepared. This terminology is misleading, however, and it has been replaced by one that defines more satisfactorily both the mode of development of the gland and also its functional differentiation.

According to this terminology (Fig. 5.7), the adenohypophysis is composed of three regions: the pars distalis, the pars intermedia, and the pars tuberalis. The pars distalis and pars intermedia contain typical epithelial secretory cells, secreting a number of hormones. Those of the pars intermedia secrete at least one melanocyte-stimulating hormone. Those of the pars distalis secrete somatotropin, corticotropin, thyrotropin, prolactin, and two gonadotropins. We shall see later that each of these hormones is produced within a characteristic cell type. An important feature of the pars distalis is that in no group (with the exception of teleost fish, p. 77) do the secretory cells have a direct secretomotor innervation. Those nerve fibres that are present are vasomotor fibres related to the blood vessels.

The pars intermedia develops from the tip of Rathke's pouch, where this is in contact with the developing neurohypophysis. Contact is essential for the differentiation of this region of the pituitary. In birds, for example, the aboral lobe is eventually separated from the neurohypophysis by a layer of connective tissue, and in this group no pars intermedia develops. The same is true of whales and elephants, but this situation is to be distinguished

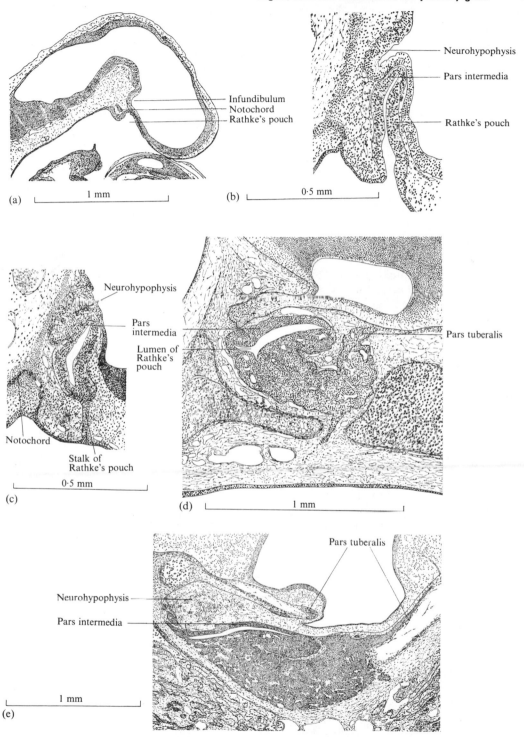

FIG. 5.6. Development of the pituitary gland of the rabbit, *Oryctolagus cuniculus*. Sagittal sections of (a), the head end of a ten-day embryo; (b) the pituitary region of a 13-day embryo, nasal end to the right; (c) a 15-day embryo; (d) a 20-day embryo; (e) a 30-day embryo (at term). (From Atwell (1918). *Am. J. Anat.* **24**.)

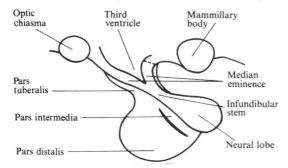

FIG. 5.7. Diagram to illustrate the nomenclature of the parts of the mammalian pituitary gland. (From Green and Harris (1947). *J. Endocrin.* **5**.)

from that in certain other mammals, including man, in which the pars intermedia undergoes reduction after being conspicuous at first in the embryo. In adult humans it constitutes only about 0·5–0·8 per cent of the gland, although the actual amount of intermedia tissue is actually greater than this because it invades the neurohypophysis. The pars intermedia of mammals always has a simpler cytological organization than the pars distalis, for the latter secretes six hormones, whereas the pars intermedia secretes only melanophore-(or melanocyte-) stimulating hormones (MSH), which may, however, be produced in more than one molecular form. The pars intermedia differs also in that its cells receive a secretomotor innervation, whereas those of the pars distalis do not (but see p. 62).

The pars tuberalis, which develops from the lateral lobes of Rathke's pouch, is characterized anatomically by its close contact with the median eminence. It provides a vascular bed for the hypophysial portal system (see later), but appears to have no secretory function.

The neurohypophysis also differentiates into three regions: the median eminence (of the tuber cinereum), lying in the floor of the diencephalon; the infundibular stem (which, with the pars tuberalis, forms the pituitary or hypophysial stalk); and the infundibular process, from which develops the neural lobe. The 'posterior lobe' of the old terminology, which is formed by the infundibular process and the pars intermedia, is sometimes separated from the 'anterior lobe' by a cavity which is the remains of the original lumen of Rathke's pouch.

The whole of the neurohypophysis has an essentially neural structure. A substantial part of the neural lobe is formed of non-myelinated nerve fibres (100 000 are said to enter it in man), but many cells are also present. Some of these are glial cells, similar

to those of brain tissue; many others are of a characteristic type, with short branching processes. The latter cells, known as pituicytes, were long regarded as the source of the hormones that are readily extractable from the neural lobe (p. 90), but this view has been abandoned. As we shall see later, the hormones are neurosecretions of the hypothalamus, which pass to the neural lobe along tracts of neurosecretory axons (Fig. 5.8(b)). However, the possibility that

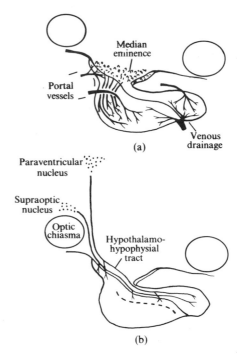

FIG. 5.8. Diagrams to show some features of (a), the blood supply and (b), the innervation of the mammalian pituitary gland. cf. Fig. 5.13. (From Harris (1955). *Neural control of the pituitary gland.* Edward Arnold, London.)

pituicytes have some secretory function cannot be wholly excluded. Clearly, however, these peculiarities of the neural lobe are not easy to reconcile with the expected organization of an endocrine gland. Their significance, however, is now well understood, the explanation of it having brought to light some important principles of endocrine function.

The dual organization of the pituitary gland, epithelial and neural, is reflected in its blood supply (Fig. 5.8(a)). That of the pars distalis is received from the internal carotid arteries along two paths. Part of this blood travels by a direct route, varying in its details, and sometimes negligible or absent, as it is, for example, in the rat. Most of the blood, however, follows an indirect route, constituted by the hypophysial portal system. This blood passes first into the pars tuberalis, the function of which is to provide a vascular bed. Here it enters a vascular plexus, the primary plexus of the portal system, from which capillary loops extend into the median eminence. This plexus drains into portal vessels, which run down the ventral surface of the pituitary stalk to enter the pars distalis. Here they break up into sinusoids and thereby form the secondary plexus of the portal system. We shall see that this hypophysial portal system is crucial in the control of endocrine regulation in mammals, and, indeed, in other vertebrate groups as well.

The blood supply of the neural lobe is very different from that of the pars distalis. It, too, is vascularized from the internal carotid arteries, but this blood supply is completely independent of that of the pars distalis, and is not derived from the hypophysial portal system (although in some species there may be a very small vascular connection leading from the adenohypophysis into the neurohypophysis.

5.3. Histology of the pars distalis in mammals

The mammalian pars distalis secretes six hormones. Four of these are tropic (or trophic) hormones, involved in regulating the output of other glands with which they are linked by negative feedback loops. These glands may conveniently be thought of as the target glands of the tropic hormones, although the relationship is necessarily a two-way one, with the target glands feeding back signals to the pituitary. Of the four hormones concerned, thyrotropin (thyroid-stimulating hormone; TSH) is related to the thyroid gland, corticotropin (adrenocorticotropic hormone; ACTH) to the adrenocortical tissue of the adrenal gland, and two gonadotropins (follicle-stimulating hormone, FSH; luteinizing hormone, LH) to the gonads. These relationships will be discussed in detail in later chapters. It will be sufficient now to say that, in principle, a fall in circulating level of a target hormone evokes an increased output of the corresponding tropic hormone, while a rise in level evokes a decreased output of the tropic hormone. Such changes can be brought about experimentally, and may then be reflected in visible changes in the cells secreting the tropic hormones.

The remaining two hormones are growth hormone (somatotropin) and prolactin; these are not involved in feedback relationships. All six hormones are polypeptides of varying molecular size. Thyrotropin and the gonadotropins are distinguished from the remaining three, however, by being glycoproteins, with a carbohydrate moiety included in their molecules. This distinction provides a valuable clue in interpreting the histochemical reactions of the cells of the pars distalis.

Understanding of the mode of functioning of the pars distalis requires a precise identification of the source of these several hormones. For this reason, a great deal of attention has been focused upon its cytological organization, interest in this having long antedated the chemical characterization of the hormones.

Earlier studies, up to the 1930s, were based upon the use of such staining mixtures as Mann's methyl blue–eosin, or the methylene blue and eosin mixtures of Giemsa and of Romanowsky. It had long been customary to classify the cells into those with a stainable cytoplasm (chromophils) and those with a non-staining one (chromophobes), and with these mixtures it was possible to differentiate the chromophils into basophils and acidophils, according to their affinity for basic and acidic dyes. Later, it became apparent that the basophilia largely resulted from the presence of ribonucleic acid, and could be removed by treatment of the sections with ribonuclease. As a result, these terms fell increasingly into disuse, to be replaced by a new terminology arising from the use of the Azan technique of Heidenhain. This stains acidophils either with orange G or with azocarmine, and the basophils with aniline blue, so that it is possible to refer to orangeophils, carminophils, and cyanophils.

With studies of the pituitary hormones making it increasingly likely that the cyanophils were secreting more than one hormone, attempts were made to subdivide this category. Some success was achieved in 1940 by Romeis, who distinguished in the human pars distalis five types of cell which he named with Greek letters. These were the α-cells (the classical acidophils), β-cells (basophils), γ-cells (chromophobes), δ-cells (a second category of basophils), ε-cells (orangeophils), and η-cells (found in pregnant women). This classification, however, was not entirely satisfactory. It was not concerned with function, the procedure proved difficult to repeat with other pituitaries, and, where it was repeatable, the issue was confused by investigators who applied the same Greek letters to cells that were not, in fact, similar in function.

Time has shown that there is only one satisfactory approach to this problem, and that is to establish the function of each cell type, and then to name it in terms of the function. The procedure required for this is not to be lightly undertaken. Staining techniques are required that are internationally acceptable, and that can be repeated in other laboratories. It is necessary to include cytochemical procedures, in which known chemical reactions are used to evoke some form of colour change or precipitation which can be interpreted in precise chemical terms. Immunohistochemical procedures are also of the utmost value in revealing the intracellular location of specific hormones, but of course they depend upon the availability of hormonal preparations that are sufficiently pure to yield specific antibodies. Electron microscopy is also obligatory, for this can reveal diagnostic features that are not apparent with light microscopy.

These techniques, however, are only a beginning, for descriptive studies must be integrated with physiological ones. The animal can be observed under natural conditions, so that changes in pituitary cytology can be correlated with cyclical changes in such physiological parameters as growth and reproduction. Interpretation of such changes must be confirmed by assay of the hormonal content of the pituitary, and here it is particularly advantageous if the species concerned has some regional localization of the several cell types. These observations need to by supplemented by experimental studies. Such studies might involve interference with pituitary feed-back, which can be achieved by removal or immobilization of its endocrine target glands, or by injection or ingestion of their hormones. Another field of study depends upon removal of the pituitary from its attachment to the brain. In ectopic transplanting, the gland is removed to another site (beneath the kidney capsule, for example, or into the orbit). Consequential changes in the cytology of the graft can then be correlated with physiological effects in the operated animal. *In vitro* studies provide another important approach. Here the gland is maintained in organ culture conditions, and its output of hormones correlated with its cytology.

For few species have these requirements been satisfied, either partially or entirely. But this does not mean that we cannot generalize from the very limited information that is at present available. The pituitary gland shows features of organization that are common to a wide range of vertebrate groups, and this fundamental uniformity justifies cautious extrapolation from what is known to what may reasonably be inferred. We can now consider some examples of these procedures, and judge of their wider applicability.

The periodic acid/Schiff (PAS) reaction has proved invaluable for pituitary research. This reaction is a specific test for 1,2-glycol groups (CHOH-CHOH), which are converted into dialdehydes (CHO-CHO) as a result of the oxidation of the C—C bonds by the periodic acid. Owing to the fact that this substance, unlike some other oxidizing agents, does not carry the oxidation any further, these dialdehydes can be identified by the use of Schiff's reagent, which reacts with them to give a compound with a magenta–red colour. The method is fully reviewed in current textbooks of histochemistry and will not be discussed further here beyond pointing out that it reveals three main types of biologically important materials: (a) glycogen; (b) mucoproteins, glycoproteins, and neutral mucopolysaccharides; and (c) various lipids, including sphingomyelin and certain glycolipids. Contrary to earlier views, it does not stain acid mucopolysaccharides. These, however, can be identified by staining them with Alcian blue, and by the reddish response (gamma metachromasia) which they give when stained with toluidine blue.

The cyanophilia of certain cells of the pars distalis is a property of their cell granules. These give a positive PAS response, which indicates (in conjunction with appropriate controls) that they secrete the glycoprotein hormones (FSH, LH, and thyrotropin). By itself this evidence would not be conclusive, but it can be strengthened by certain experimental procedures, which are devised to correlate cytological changes with changes in hormonal content. The results show that some cells secrete thyrotropin (thyrotropic cells) and that others secrete gonadotropins (gonadotropic cells). The two types can be distinguished by their form and position in the pars distalis of the rat (Figs 5.9 and 5.10). The gonadotropic cells are rounded in shape, with large granules, and are situated predominantly in a ventral zone and also in a narrow zone dorsally; they tend to be clustered closely around the larger portal vessels. The thyrotropic cells are somewhat larger, polygonal in shape, with fine granules, and are situated more centrally, where they show no particular relationship with the large vessels. The experimental evidence for their identification rests upon the following procedures (Figs 5.9, 5.10).

First, castration of either male or female rats results within one or two days in a marked increase in the size and number of the gonadotropic cells, with many mitotic stages, beginning in the ventral zone. After several weeks, many of these cells contain a hyaline vacuole, which is coloured a faint pink by the PAS reaction, and which is surrounded by deeply stained

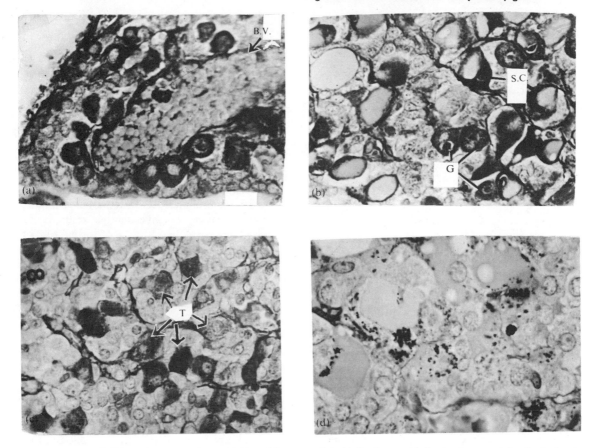

FIG. 5.9. Cytology of the pars distalis of the rat (PAS and haematoxylin). (a) At the anterior border in a normal animal, showing round or oval gonadotropic cells, with PAS-positive granules, surrounding a blood vessel (B.V.); (b) a similar region in a male rat, 15 months after castration. The majority of the gonadotropic cells (G) have been converted into signet-ring cells (S.C.), with vacuoles containing a hyaline substance, which stains a faint pink; (c) in the ventral region in a normal animal, showing polygonal thyrotropic cells (T) with PAS-positive granules; (d) a similar region in a male 66 days after thyroidectomy; the thyrotropic cells have an extensive accumulation of hyaline substance which contains vacuoles. (From Purves and Griesbach (1951). *Endocrin.* **49**.)

granules, giving a characteristic appearance known as the 'signet-ring stage'. This reaction, which can be correlated by bioassay with an increased gonadotropin content of the gland, is the result of the disturbance of the feedback balance by the withdrawal of the gonadal steroids. Conversely, the injection of oestrogen into the male will produce degranulation of the gonadotropic cells, leading sometimes to their degeneration.

Secondly, surgical thyroidectomy or goitrogen treatment causes the appearance of large numbers of 'thyroidectomy cells' (Fig. 5.9), originating in the thyrotropic region and again accompanied by many mitoses. These cells later develop hyaline vacuoles, which give a stronger PAS response than the vacuoles of the castration cells; later still, there may be an

extensive accumulation of hyaline material, perhaps containing vacuoles and granules of a peculiar character. Despite this increase in cell number, the thyrotropin content of the gland is found by bioassay to be low, and this is reflected in the fact that the fine granulation of the cells responds only faintly to the PAS test. This means that the disturbance of the feedback balance has resulted in an increased production of thyrotropin, which, however, is discharged so vigorously that the hormonal content of the gland is actually lower than under normal working conditions. This, incidentally, illustrates the difficulty of interpreting secretory status, for it shows how the condition of the cells depends upon the balance between synthesis and discharge. Cells with conspicuous stores of secretion may be relatively in-

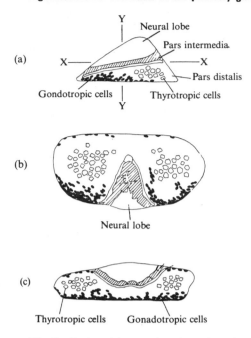

(a)

Y

Neural lobe

Pars intermedia

X——X

——X

Pars distalis

Gondotropic cells

Thyrotropic cells

Y

(b)

Neural lobe

(c)

Thyrotropic cells   Gonadotropic cells

FIG. 5.10. The distribution of thyrotropic and gonadotropic cells in the pars distalis of the male rat (cf. Fig. 5.9). (a) Sagittal section of the pituitary gland; (b) horizontal section in the plane marked X——X in (a); (c) transverse section in the plane marked Y——Y in (a). (From Purves and Griesbach (1951). *Endocrin.* **49**.)

active, while those with sparse contents may be highly active, but may be losing their product as quickly as they make it.

The difficulty is well exemplified by comparing the rat with the guinea-pig. In this species it has proved difficult to distinguish more than one type of PAS-positive cell. Moreover, prolonged goitrogen treatment of the guinea-pig actually raises the level of thyrotropin in its pituitary gland. This rise is paralleled by enlargement and multiplication of the thyrotropin cells, and an increase in their granulation and in their intensity of staining; but vacuolation is rare, and thyroidectomy cells do not appear. A likely explanation of the difference is that thyroid activity is low in the normal guinea-pig, and that hypothyroidism raises thyrotropin secretion only to a level approximating to that of a normal euthyroid rat. On this view, thyroidectomy cells in the rat represent a peak of thyrotropin secretion that is not attained in the hypothyroid guinea-pig.

The above analysis does not make any distinction between FSH-secreting and LH-secreting cells. However, it has been suggested that in the rat FSH is secreted in more peripherally situated gonadotropic cells, with coarse granules, and LH in cells which are centrally situated and which possess finer granulation. It has also been suggested that in other species the FSH-secreting cells tend to be the less acidophil of the two, so that a distinction can be made by counterstaining with orange G after using the PAS procedure. Functional analysis, as usual, is more convincing, and is exemplified in the bat *Myotis myotis*, which has a single and sharply defined reproductive period following the spring awakening. Activity of the LH-secreting cells is closely correlated in this species with the presence of corpora lutea (p. 110). These cells progressively differentiate during gestation, and undergo rapid involution after parturition, simultaneously with the disappearance of the corpora lutea. To give another example, LH-secreting cells are highly active during the brief rutting phase of the male mole, when the testes and the secondary sexual organs are very markedly enlarged.

The secretion of thyrotropin and of the gonadotropins has thus been convincingly attributed in certain mammals to PAS-positive cells with distinctive characteristics. They are the basophil cells of earlier terminology. The acidophil cells have been equally well studied, and they, too have been shown to include more than one functional type.

The classical acidophils of early descriptions (the α-cells of Romeis) are very strongly acidophilic, staining readily with eosin, acid fuchsin, orange G, and light green, to name some of the commonly used stains. Electron microscopy reveals a rich concentration of large granules (350–500 mm), electron-dense and membrane-bound, while histochemical evidence shows the granules to have a high concentration of cysteine and probably to contain lipoprotein. There is convincing and long-standing evidence for these cells being the source of somatotropin. Acromegaly has long been known to be associated with adenoma of the acidophil cells. Further, in the bovine pituitary these cells are mainly concentrated laterally, and extracts of the regions concerned have a strongly growth-promoting action, shown, for example, when applied to hypophysectomized tadpoles. Additional evidence is that these cells are lacking in a genetically determined strain of dwarf laboratory mouse. A confusing point is that the granules of these cells disappear in many species (but not in the guinea-pig) in conditions of thyroid deficiency, which might seem to suggest that they secrete thyrotropin. This, however, is not so. The reason for the disappearance of the granules is that a very low level of circulating thyroid hormone is needed for the synthesis of growth hormone by these cells. Thus the granules can be made to reappear in thyroidectomized mice by administering a dose of the hormone which, while large enough to permit the production of somatotropin, is still too small to meet the total demands of the body. The thyroidectomy cells, however, persist, which shows that they alone are the source of thyrotropin.

A second type of acidophil cell produces prolactin. The cells concerned (the η-cells of Romeis) are not easily distinguished from the somatotropin cells (they have, for example, a high cysteine content), but by judicious choice of fixation and staining procedures (the method of Cleveland and Wolfe, for example) the prolactin cells stain with erythrosin and contrast with the orange-G staining of the somatotropin cells. Electron microscopy can also be helpful, for the granules may be larger and of irregular outline. Immunohistochemistry, however, is decisive (p. 9), in conjunction with functional observations.

In the cat, where these cells are strongly carminophilic, they are plentiful during pregnancy and early lactation. Even more convincing, a high concentration of prolactin develops in lactating rats that are separated from their young, and this is paralleled by a storage of granules in the prolactin cells. Restoration of the young to the mother, and the consequent resumption of lactation, results in a very rapid decline in prolactin level in the pars distalis, and a parallel reduction in granulation. Ectopic grafts and *in vitro* cultures are also very illuminating. The pituitary of the rat, removed from its attachment to the brain and transplanted under the capsule of the kidney, or transferred to culture medium, is unable to secrete any of its hormones except prolactin. Cytological study shows that it is composed almost entirely of prolactin cells, the others having dedifferentiated or vanished. However, transfer of the grafts back to the region of the median eminence results in restoration of their cellular differentiation, and of their hormonal secretion. From this and other evidence, it is concluded that the brain exerts an inhibitory action on the prolactin cells, and that their secretory activity is promoted by removal of the gland from the brain. Clearly, however, connection with the brain is necessary for the production of the other hormones of the pars distalis. This is a fundamentally important conclusion, some implications of which will be seen in later chapters.

It remains to identify the cells that secrete corticotropin in mammals. This has long proved difficult, since the hormone is not stored in granules that are readily detectable by the usual staining methods, although faintly acidophil ones can be found. Lead haematoxylin sometimes (particularly in teleosts) reveals these cells as a distinct type, colouring intensely with this stain. The clearest evidence, however, comes from disturbance of the feedback relationship with the adrenal cortex. This is achieved by treating animals with metopirone (metyrapone), which inhibits corticosteroid production, and leads to hypertrophy and hyperplasia of the corticotropin cells. Conversely, cortisone treatment leads to their involution. The cells concerned are thus shown to correspond with the ε-cells of Romeis.

5.4. Neurosecretion and the neural lobe

The correlation of the hormonal activity of the neural lobe with its histological structure long presented problems quite different from those involved in the analysis of the pars distalis. This is because its structure is essentially neural in character. The nerve fibres found in it originate in part from the tuber cinereum, passing down the more dorsal region of the pituitary stalk as the tubero-hypophysial tract. The majority, however, arise in paired centres in the hypothalamus as the supraoptic and paraventricular nuclei (Fig. 5.8(b)). These fibres run down the more ventral region of the stalk as the supraopticohypophysial tract, passing close to the median eminence on the way. The interpretation of the neural lobe was clarified as soon as it was recognized that the cell bodies of these fibres were neurosecretory cells, responsible for the production of the polypeptide neurohypophysial hormones (oxytocin and vasopressin in mammals), which are passed down their axons into the neural lobe. It is probable, too, that some secretion (but not necessarily the same) is discharged into the median eminence. The absence from the neural lobe of the characteristic histological features of a secretory gland is thus explained. It is, in fact, a neurohaemal organ, where the neurohypophysial hormones are stored, prior to release into the blood stream.

Filamentous material can sometimes be seen in some of the ergastoplasmic cisternae of the cells. This is thought to be an inactive protein precursor of the hormones, one suggestion being that the active hormones are released from this protein within the granules, during their transport through the cytoplasm. There is an obvious analogy here with the production of insulin by the breakdown of the precursor pro-insulin.

But in any case the synthetic processes are complicated by the existence of a substance called neurophysin, in addition to the hormones. This cystine-rich protein forms non-covalent complexes with the polypeptide hormones, and is located with them within the elementary granules. Two major fractions, neurophysin I and II, have been isolated, and of these, I is associated with oxytocin and II with vasopressin. The explanation of the existence of neurophysins is not clear. One suggestion is that each hormone and its neurophysin are jointly the products of the precursor protein, the molecule of this being cleaved within the granule during final processing. Evidence supporting this is that hormones and neurophysins are stored within the granules in unit stoichiometric ratio. Moreover, there is a strain of rat which has hereditary diabetes insipidus, resulting from a genetic disability preventing the synthesis of vasopressin. One of the neurophysins is also lacking in this rat, which is what would be expected if synthesis of the two polypeptides, neurophysin and vasopressin, were directed by the same loci. As to the functions of neurophysins, which clearly recall the storage protein found in the chromaffin granules of the adrenal medulla (p. 190), it may be that they hold the hormones within the granules and protect them from enzymic degradation. However, the neurophysins are said to be released into the circulation, and this is more difficult to explain, for they have no known systemic function. Thus some unknown function may remain to be discovered.

An essential step in this analysis of the mode of origin of the neurohypophysial hormones is to show a clear correlation between the distribution of the neurosecretory material and of the hormonal activity. This can readily be done. Typical activity can be detected in the hypothalamus, as well as in the pituitary stalk, while if the stalk is transected it can be shown that the accumulation of neurosecretory material at the proximal end of the incision is paralleled by an increase in the yield of activity at the same point. Moreover, conditions such as deprivation of water, or heavy salt intake, which result in the discharge of vasopressin, can be shown to be accompanied by a discharge of neurosecretory material from the neural lobe. Thus, if a rat is caused to drink 2·5% salt solution for thirteen days, its pituitary will be completely devoid of the material at the end of that time. If the demand for vasopressin is then reduced, by allowing the animal to drink tap water, the neurosecretory material rapidly accumulates and reaches a more or less normal condition in a few days.

The evidence is given further precision by study of the elementary granules. Centrifugates that are rich in these are correspondingly rich in hormonal activity. Moreover, density-gradient separation of the granules into two size groups indicates that oxytocin is located in one size and vassopressin in the other. This is an important finding, because it can be projected back to the cells themselves. The results of selective damage to the paraventricular nucleus in rats suggests that this nucleus is the main source of oxytocin, for there is depletion of this hormone in the rat and the cat after bilateral lesion of the nuclei. Moreover, extraction of the hypothalamic nuclei in a number of mammalian species suggests that relatively more oxytocin is present in the paraventricular nucleus, and more vasopressin in the supraoptic nucleus. Such differential distribution would make it easier to understand how the two hormones could be released independently of each other, but the evidence for it needs strengthening.

It is possible that a similar situation obtains in fish, for two types of cell have been distinguished in the eel; one with less electron-dense granules, with a mean diameter of 1627 ± 31 Å, and the other with denser granules, 2150 ± 30 Å in diameter. It may be that this indicates a segregation of the two hormones (vasotocin and isotocin in teleosts) in different cell types, and it could also be that the two types observed correspond with two types of fibre seen in the neurohypophysis of these animals. These possibilities need much further probing, but the mere formulation of them shows how necessary it is to consider the hypothalamus and pituitary as a whole.

Further clarification of the organization and mode of functioning of this system in mammals is given by the use of radioactive amino acids, combined with autoradiography and chemical separation. (Fig. 5.11). Thus, intraventricular injection of labelled [3H]tyrosine or [35S]cysteine is followed by the early appearance of 35S in the hypothalamic nuclei. The hypothalamus is shown by chemical assay to be maximally labelled 1 hour after the injection, the level subsequently falling. By contrast, radioactivity is not detectable within the neural lobe until after 1 hour, and thereafter it continues to increase to a plateau after 24 hours. Isolation of the hormones from the gland shows that both oxytocin and vasopressin are being secreted in labelled form. Further analysis suggests that the hormones can be synthesized and transported into the neural lobe in 1–2 hours, at a minimum rate of transport of 1–2 mm/hour. The initial lag is ascribed to the need for synthesizing the precursor in the endoplasmic reticulum. It has been suggested that perhaps the first radioactive material to reach the neural lobe is the protein, maturation of the hormones from this precursor

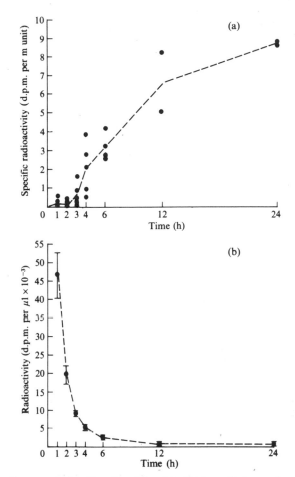

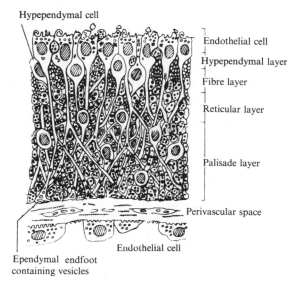

FIG. 5.11. (a) Specific radioactivity of the highly purified oxytocin-like peptide from goldfish at various times after intraventricular injection of [³H]tyrosine; (b) radioactivity remaining in samples of fluid covering the brain taken at various times after intraventricular injection of [³H]tyrosine. (From Jones, Peter, and Pickering (1973). *Gen. comp. Endocrin.* **20**.)

FIG. 5.12. Diagram of the fine structure of the rat median eminence. (From Kobayashi and Matsui (1969). In *Frontiers of endocrinology* (eds W. F. Ganong and L. Martin). Oxford University Press.)

vacuoles suggestive either of secretory or absorptive activity.

Beneath the ependymal and hypependymal layers is the inner zone, containing in its outer region a layer of fine nerve fibres, mostly belonging to the supra-optico-hypophysial tract, on its way to the neural lobe. Under this is a reticular layer, formed of a network of nerve fibres, some of which are Gomori-positive and others Gomori-negative. Glial cells are also present, in both the regions of this zone.

The outermost layer of the median eminence is the palisade layer, which consists of Gomori-positive and Gomori-negative nerve fibres, together with processes of the ependymal cells and glial cells. This layer is invaded by capillaries forming the primary plexus of the hypophysial portal system. The cell processes end against these vessels, so that the ependymal cells could have a functional relationship with them. Gomori-positive material is known to be secreted into the third ventricle, and it has been suggested, therefore, that such material might be taken up by the ependymal cells, passed along the cell processes to the capillaries, and through these into the adenohypophysis. This is one route by which chemical regulation might be exerted on the pituitary gland, but its reality has not been established. A much more clearly defined route is by the nerve

being completed during transport, as well as within the perikaryon.

5.5. Neurosecretion and the median eminence

The neural lobe is the posterior neurohaemal centre of the neurohypophysis. The median eminence (Fig. 5.12) constitutes an anterior and functionally distinct neurohaemal centre, which is composed in tetrapods of a characteristic series of layers. Lining the infundibular recess is an ependymal layer, formed of a single layer of endothelial cells, beneath which there may be a hypependymal layer formed of one or two layers of cells. The ependymal cells contain (in the rat, for example) PAS-positive material, while electron microscopy discloses microvilli and small fibres of the median eminence, which have terminals ending in close relation to the capillaries.

These nerve fibres constitute a varied population, with a corresponding variety of nerve endings, which can be related to the two types of neurosecretory fibre (type A and type B) that we have already mentioned. Many of the fibres are Gomori-positive ones, some entering the eminence from the hypothalamo-hypophysial tract. Others are Gomori-negative, easily overlooked in light-microscope sections, because their secretion is not stained by the standard neurosecretory techniques. Electron microscopy, however, shows membrane-bound granules in both types of fibres, with a diversity of size. Some are large granules, in which two types may be distinguished: a larger type, within the range 1800–500 Å in diameter, and a smaller type, with a diameter of about 1200 Å. Such large granules are characteristic of the Gomori-positive fibres, both in the median eminence and in the neural lobe. The fibres containing them are type A fibres, and are further distinguished into type A^1 (with larger granules) and type A^2 (with smaller ones). Their endings are described as peptidergic, because it is supposed that in general these endings contain a peptide secretion, as they clearly do in the neural lobe. However, it does not follow that these fibres are releasing neurohypophysial hormonal molecules in the median eminence. Some of these fibres may be passing on to the neural lobe, while others may be releasing material chemically different from neurohypophysial hormones. For example, the Gomori-positive material in the amphibian median eminence stains differently from that of the neural lobe, which suggests that in this instance, at least, the eminence is receiving a special category of material.

A second category of granules, also with an electron-dense core, has a diameter of about 1000 Å. These granules, which are particularly characteristic of the median eminence, are thought to be contained in the Gomori-negative fibres, and to carry monoamines such as noradrenaline, dopamine, and serotonin, which are detectable within the eminence. These are type B fibres, and their endings are described as aminergic. Evidence for this interpretation is given by the Falck technique of formalin-induced fluorescence, which reveals a rich monoamine content in the nerve fibres of the inner zone, while monoamine oxidase can also be demonstrated. Further evidence is that these fibres can be shown to take up noradrenaline and dopamine. The use of radioactively labelled noradrenaline, followed by

electron microscopy, has shown in *Rana esculenta*, for example, that labelled amine is located in fibres with dense-core granules of this size range.

A third category of inclusion comprises electron-lucent vesicles, of a size of about 500 Å. These are less easy to interpret, but it is supposed that they may contain acetylcholine, which is normally associated with such bodies. Alternatively, some of them may be developing or discharged stages of electron-dense granules. Obviously, it is difficult to de-limit different types of granule with assurance when dealing with such a complex situation, and for this reason the classification outlined above should be accepted with reserve. However, the functional diversity of the secretory products detectable in one way or another within the median eminence is not in doubt. Of course, the secretions need not all function at the same site. We shall see later that some of them must be the releasing factors which pass into the hypophysial portal system for transmission into the pars distalis, but it is possible that the catecholamines function locally, and are involved in stimulating the release of other secretions.

Some of the Gomori-positive fibres, but not necessarily all of them, probably arise in the supra-optic and paraventricular nuclei. The source of the aminergic ones is more obscure, but many are thought to arise within a crescent-shaped area of the hypothalamus which includes the arcuate nucleus of mammals, and its homologue in teleost fish, the nucleus lateralis tuberis. The cells of the arcuate nucleus show formalin-induced fluorescence, which regresses after the median eminence has been injured by local lesions, but other parts of the hypothalamus may also be involved.

The crescent-shaped area is also the region where the inhibiting and releasing hormones which regulate adenohypophysial function (pp. 127, 173, 206) are thought to arise. Evidence for this is that pituitary (adenohypophysial) transplants inserted into this area maintain their histological organization, whereas they de-differentiate if inserted elsewhere. For this reason, the area has been called the hypophysiotropic area (Fig. 5.13). It agrees, in a general way, with evidence as to the localization of these hormones that has been obtained in experiments involving lesions and electrical stimulation, but more precise definition is still needed. The fact is that our knowledge of the chemistry of hypothalamic neurosecretions is far in advance of our anatomical understanding of their sources. Obvious difficulties in this field of study are are the complex neural anatomy of the forebrain, the paucity of specific staining techniques, the diffi-

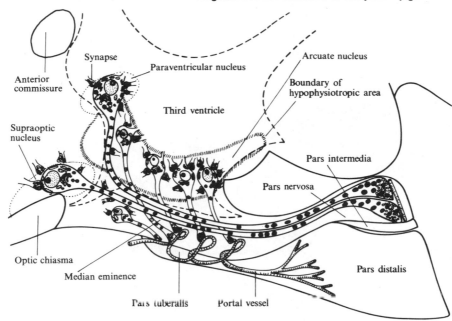

FIG. 5.13. Diagram of the neurosecretory systems of the mammalian pituitary gland. (By permission of D. Zambrano.)

culty of placing lesions with sufficient precision, and the likelihood that the effect of electrical stimulation will overstep synaptic boundaries. Immunohistochemical studies, based on the use of pure releasing factors coupled to larger molecules, may well yield decisive evidence.

5.6. The pituitary gland of the Cyclostomata

The adenohypophysis of lampreys (Figs 5.14 and 5.15) develops as a solid ingrowth which at first is connected with the olfactory sac by a solid nasohypophysial stalk. Later it separates from this, and at metamorphosis the stalk hollows out to form a sac which passes back from the olfactory organ to underlie the pituitary. This sac has often been regarded as a persistent hypophysial cavity, which, if it were correctly so interpreted, would be unique in its complete separation from the adenohypophysis. However, the facts of its development indicate that it may be a secondary feature of the organization of these animals.

The adenohypophysis becomes a flattened organ, divided by connective tissue septa into three regions, the rostral pars distalis, the proximal pars distalis, and the pars intermedia. (Alternatively, these regions have been called respectively the pro-, meso-, and meta-adenohypophysis, but these terms are now less favoured.) Cytological differentiation is meagre in the larva, but in the adult the rostral pars distalis

contains many cyanophil cells. These are probably gonadotropic, since they show increased activity with the approach of sexual maturity, and since hypophysectomy indicates that the pituitary exerts some control over gonadal development. The pars intermedia, which contains carminophil cells, is so called on the assumption that it secretes melanophore-stimulating hormone; the assumption is justified by the permanent pallor which results when this region of the gland is destroyed. Nothing very definite is known about other possible adenohypophysial functions. In general, the cytological differentiation is less advanced than in higher vertebrates, and the existence of other adenohypophysial hormones remains to be clearly established. Immunohistochemical tests for corticotropin are negative, and experiments have failed to give convincing evidence for the presence of thyrotropin.

A neurohypophysis can be identified in both larva and adult, and, to preserve uniformity of nomenclature, is best termed an infundibulum. It has a very simple form, with no differentiated infundibular process, and is simply a depression of the floor of the third ventricle, which is here composed of a layer of elongated ependymal cells. Amongst these run nerve fibres which contain Gomori-positive material, and which are hypothalamic neurosecretory fibres. Here, as in other non-mammalian vertebrates, the fibres are derived from the preoptic nuclei,

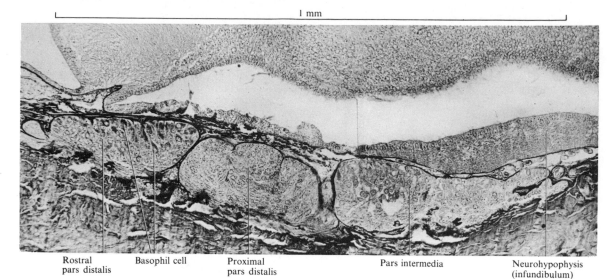

| 1 mm |

Rostral pars distalis   Basophil cell   Proximal pars distalis   Pars intermedia   Neurohypophysis (infundibulum)

Pineal body   Choroid plexus   Subcommissural organ   Third ventricle

Preoptic nucleus

Posterior hypothalamic neurosecretory nucleus
Infundibular recess
Neurohypophysis
Pars intermedia
Preoptic hypophysial neurosecretory tract
Proximal pars distalis
Neurosecretory ending
Rostral pars distalis

Blood vessel
Optic chiasma
Naso-pharyngeal stalk

FIG. 5.14. (a) Sagittal section of the pituitary region of a pre-metamorphic larval lamprey. (From van de Kamer and Schreurs (1959). *Z. Zellforsch.* **49**.) (b) Diagram of the same, showing neurosecretory relationships. (From Oztan and Gorbman (1960). *J. Morph.* **106**.)

which are the homologues of the separate supraoptic and paraventricular nuclei of mammals, but a small posterior nucleus is also present in the larva.

The adenohypophysis is closely applied to the neurohypophysis, which suggests that the close functional association between these two regions, so important in mammals, is already established at this early stage of vertebrate evolution. The two regions are separated by connective tissue, which is thinnest posteriorly, and in this run blood vessels which supply the ventral surface of the neurohypophysis, and also penetrate into the adenohypophysis. There is no median eminence. These vessels, however, could perhaps provide limited chemical communication between the two regions, and hence could provide a basis for neural regulation of the pars

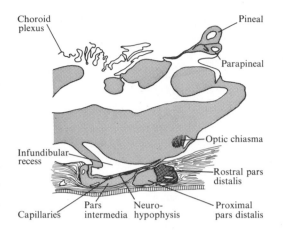

FIG. 5.15. Diagram of the pituitary region of an adult lamprey (*Lampetra fluviatilis*). (From Lanzing (1959). *Uitgeversmaatschappij Neerlandia, Utrecht.*)

distalis, always assuming that the cells of the latter lack secretomotor innervation, which has yet to be proved. That some control of the pars intermedia by the central nervous system must exist is clearly indicated by the melanophore responses in these animals (p. 214), but we do not know how this control is exerted.

The cytological differentiation of the adenohypophysis of *Myxine* (Fig. 5.16) is as limited as in lampreys, but the neurohypophysis is better developed, projecting backwards as a hollow lobe in a manner recalling the embryonic condition of the infundibular process of higher forms. It receives the product of neurosecretory fibres running from the preoptic nuclei, but some of their product is released in the floor of the hypothalamus immediately anterior to the infundibular process. The outer surface is conspicuously folded and vascularized at this point, and it

has been suggested that this may indicate a rudimentary median eminence, which has not otherwise been identified in cyclostomes. From this region small vessels penetrate the connective tissue that separates the adenohypophysis from the neurohypophysis, so that there is a meagre basis for a vascular link.

Evidently the organization of the cyclostome pituitary is in most respects less advanced than that of gnathostomes. This is in accord with our general conception of agnathans as being the more primitive in organization. But it is to be remembered that to dismiss them as primitive without further qualification is probably a serious over-simplification. They have a long evolutionary history behind them, fossil remains of lampreys, much like present-day ones, being known from deposits 280 million years old. Moreover, their mode of life is highly specialized, and myxinoids, in particular, must be insulated in their deep-sea habitat from most environmental signals. We can confidently conclude that there is a great deal still to be learned about the endocrine organization of these important and fascinating animals.

5.7. The pituitary gland of fish

The adenohypophysis of elasmobranchs (Fig. 5.17) develops as a hollow Rathke's pouch, its tip giving rise to the pars intermedia; this interdigitates so closely with the neurohypophysis that the resulting complex is termed the neuro–intermediate lobe. The pars distalis differentiates into a ventral lobe and a rostral lobe, the latter projecting forwards towards the optic chiasma. The functional organization of the

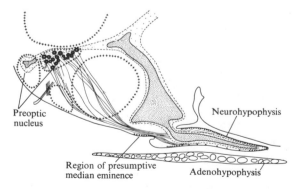

FIG. 5.16. Diagrammatic median reconstruction of the hypothalamus and pituitary gland of *Myxine glutinosa*. (From Olsson (1959). *Z. Zellforsch.* **51**.)

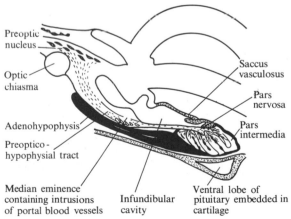

FIG. 5.17. Diagram of the hypothalamus and pituitary gland, in parasagittal section, of the dogfish, *Scyliorhinus caniculus*. (From Perks (1969). In *Fish physiology*, Vol. 2 (eds W. S. Hoar and D. J. Randall). Academic Press, New York.)

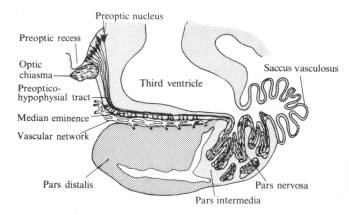

FIG. 5.18. The hypothalamus and pituitary gland of the sturgeon, *Acipenser*. (After Polenov, from Perks (1961). In *Fish physiology*, Vol. 2 (eds W. S. Hoar and D. J. Randall). Academic Press, New York.)

pars distalis is undoubtedly more advanced than is that of the cyclostome gland; experimental studies suggest a division of function between its two regions, with gonadotropin and thyrotropin production localized in the ventral lobe, and corticotropin production in the rostral lobe. These, however, are matters that need much further study.

Control of the adenohypophysis seems, in principle, to resemble the mammalian pattern. The pars intermedia is innervated by fibres entering from the neural lobe. These are type A and type B fibres, which have been shown to have secretomotor junctions with the cells that are presumed to secrete melanophore-stimulating hormone. Type A fibres are sometimes applied to the bases of these cells, and type B fibres to their apices, which suggests that in these instances production of the secretion is regulated basally by peptidergic control, while release of

the hormone is regulated apically by aminergic control. A small median eminence is present, associated with a portal system. This implies that pars distalis functions are regulated by neurohumoral factors, but nothing is yet known of the nature of these, and even their presence is inferential. An unexplained feature of the system is that some of the portal blood is conveyed to the neurointermediate lobe.

The adenohypophysis of teleosts usually develops as a solid ingrowth, as in the lamprey and in Amphibia, although the immature herring has an open Rathke's pouch which later becomes reduced to a strand of tissue. In the more primitive sturgeon a hypophysial cavity remains conspicuous even in the adult (Fig. 5.18), and tubular extensions of it penetrate into the glandular tissue. In the lower Actinopterygii, as also in teleosts, the adenohypophysis becomes differentiated into three regions. These are

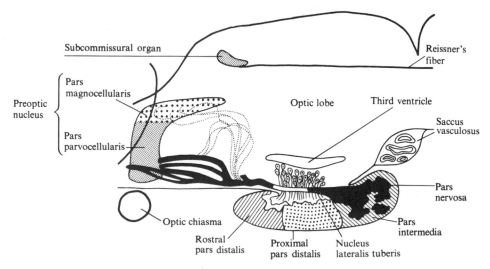

FIG. 5.19. Hypothalamus and pituitary gland of the eel. *Anguilla anguilla*. Neurosecretory tracts from the preoptic nucleus are shown in black and as dotted lines. (From Perks (1961). In *Fish physiology*, Vol. 2 (eds W. S. Hoar and D. J. Randall). Academic Press, New York.)

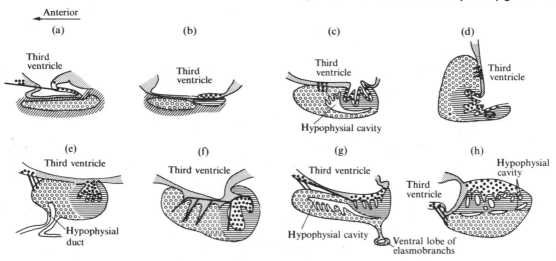

FIG. 5.20. Diagrammatic midsagittal sections to illustrate the main features of pituitary structure in the different fish groups. In all diagrams, anterior is to the left. (a) Myxinoid; (b) lamprey; (c) *Acipenser*; (d) *Amia*; (e) *Polypterus*; (f) teleost; (g) elasmobranch; (h) dipnoan (lung-fish). Small dots, nervous tissue; large solid dots, stainable neurosecretory material; large open dots, pars distalis; horizontal lines, pars intermedia; thick black lines, blood vessels which appear to convey neurosecretory material to the adenohypophysis or (myxinoid) to the neurohypophysis; oblique hatching, connective tissue. (From Ball and Baker (1969). In *Fish physiology*, Vol. 2 (eds W. S. Hoar and D. J. Randall). Academic Press, New York.)

called the rostral pars distalis (formerly called the pro-adenohypophysis), the proximal pars distalis (meso-adenohypophysis), and the pars intermedia (meta-adenohypophysis). No homology is implied with the correspondingly named parts of the lamprey's pituitary, the terminology being for descriptive convenience. The pars intermedia is an exception to this reservation, however, for it is the source of melanophore-stimulating hormone; as usual in vertebrates, it is in close contact with the neurohypophysis.

In teleosts (Fig. 5.19), as in fish generally, a saccus vasculosus is attached to the floor of the brain close to the pituitary; it arises from the infundibulum, but has no endocrine function. The infundibulum also gives rise to the neurohypophysis. A complex pattern of neurosecretory tracts extends through this from the preoptic nucleus (Fig. 5.19) but, in teleosts, and in contrast to other vertebrates, an infundibular process and stem are not separately identifiable, and a true neural lobe (in the sense of a region with independent vascularization) is not differentiated. A notable feature of teleosts, and a point of contrast with elasmobranchs, is-that there is no median eminence in the anterior region of the neurohypophysis.

This absence of a median eminence calls for explanation, but is not difficult to understand if consideration is given to more primitive actinopterygians, such as *Polypterus, Acipenser, Amia,* and

Lepisosteus (Fig. 5.20). In these fish there is a rostral and proximal pars distalis, and a pars intermedia, just as in teleosts, but in addition there is a median eminence (Fig. 5.21) which, while very small, conforms to the usual gnathostome pattern in giving rise to portal vessels which discharge into the pars distalis. Comparison of these pituitaries with the gland of teleosts suggests that in the latter group the median eminence region has invaginated into the pars distalis. As a result, all the blood for the adenohypophysis passes first through capillaries in the neurohypophysis, and then into vessels serving the pars distalis and pars intermedia. This arrangement, found in no other vertebrate group, might seem to suggest a reduction in precision of the regulating system, and this could well be so were it not for another peculiar feature. This is that in teleosts there is direct innervation of the cells of the pars distalis, an arrangement which is also without parallel in any other major group.

The fibres concerned in this innervation are neurosecretory ones, both type A and type B. The type B ones are thought to arise in the nucleus lateralis tuberis, which, as already noted, is the homologue of the arcuate nucleus of mammals. The relations between the nerve endings and the secretory cells are of several types (cf. p. 61). Some fibres have neurovascular junctions (ending, that is to say, on capillary vessels). Others (in *Hippocampus*, for example) make

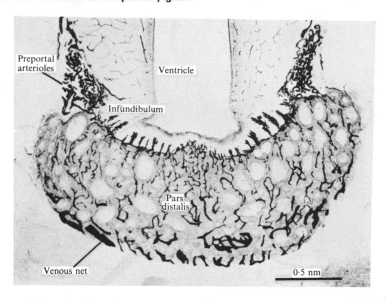

FIG. 5.21. Photomicrograph of a 50 μm thick section through the median eminence of *Amia*, superior to the level of the neuro-intermediate lobe (cf. Fig. 5.20(a), after india-ink vascular perfusion. The arrow indicates groups of capillary loops (capillary glomeruloids) which form the primary capillary bed of the median eminence. These penetrate the infundibulum perpendicularly, and continue as short portal vessels into the pars distalis, which is vascularized solely from the portal system. Scale 0·5 mm. (From Lagios (1970). *Gen. comp. Endocrin.* **15**.)

synaptoid connections with the secretory cells, while in the tench the endings are separated from the secretory cells by only a basement membrane. That some of these fibres must mediate the regulation of some, at least, of the pars distalis activities seems self-evident, and this has been shown to be so by lesion studies. Lesions of the preoptic nucleus do not affect thyrotropin or gonadotropin content, so that the neurohypophysial hormones cannot be involved in regulation of the output of these hormones. Lesions of the anterior region of the nucleus lateralis tuberis, however, produce hyperthyroidism, while in the posterior part they also have this effect and in addition reduce gonadal activity.

Regulation of the pars intermedia is similar to that found in elasmobranchs, as far as can be judged from ultrastructural studies. Type A and type B fibres enter it from the neurohypophysis, and innervate its secretory cells with one or other of the three types of ending found in the pars distalis. Type A fibres (presumably peptidergic) are distinguishable in the eel into type A^1 (granules 1200 Å in diameter) and type A^2 (1700 Å in diameter). The type B fibres, not visible by light microscopy because they are not stainable by the Gomori stains, are presumed to be aminergic.

The pars distalis of teleosts shows a pronounced regional localization of cell types (Fig. 5.22), and for

this reason is particularly suited for studies of the correlation of these types with specific hormones, along lines similar to those that we have already

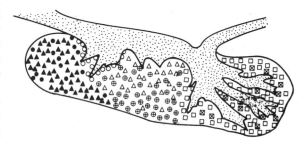

FIG. 5.22. Diagrammatic median section of the pituitary of a teleost (*Anguilla*), showing the distribution of the cell types in the adenohypophysis. ● Basophils of the rostral pars distalis; ⊕ Basophils of the proximal pars distalis; ○ lead haematoxylin positive cells of the rostral pars distalis; ▲ acidophils of the rostral pars distalis; △ acidophils of the proximal pars distalis; ⊠ basophils of the pars intermedia; □ PAS-negative cells of the pars intermedia. (From van Oordt (1968). In *Perspectives in endocrinology* (eds E. J. W. Barrington and C. B. Jørgensen). Academic Press, New York.)

discussed in relation to mammalian pituitary organization, including electron microscopy (Fig. 5.23). PAS-positive cells in the upper part of the proximal pars distalis of *Anguilla* and *Poecilia* (two genera well studied from this point of view) are identifiable

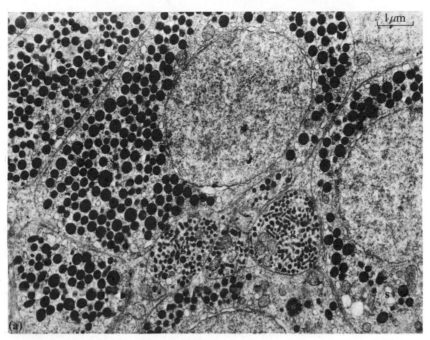

FIG. 5.23. Electron micrographs of the pars distalis of the pituitary of the eel, *Anguilla anguilla*, showing distinctive cell types (cf. Fig. 5.22). Rostral pars distalis in (a); proximal pars distalis in (b), (c), and (d).

(a) g_1, gonadotropin cell; two types are recognizable, the one shown here having electron-dense vesicles, *ca.* 1900 Å diameter; s, somatotropin cell, with spherical or slightly oval vesicles, *ca.* 4000 Å diameter.

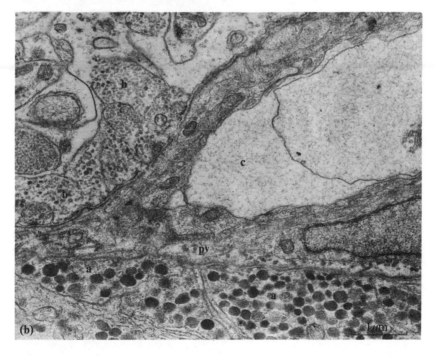

(b) a, corticotropin cell, evenly packed with electron-dense vesicles, *ca.* 2000–500 Å diameter; b, type B fibre (cf. p. 61); c, capillary; pv, perivascular space.

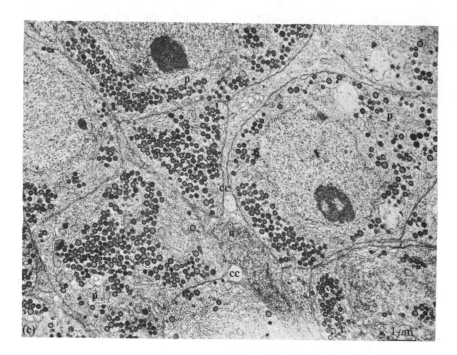

(c) cc, connecting canal; these canals lead from the centre of the glandular follicles to the intervascular channels; n, neck cell; function unknown, but perhaps regulating the size of the connecting canals; p, prolactin cell, conical, with narrow extremity bordering the central space of the follicle, and with vesicles, *ca.* 2800 Å diameter, which are sometimes paler at their centres.

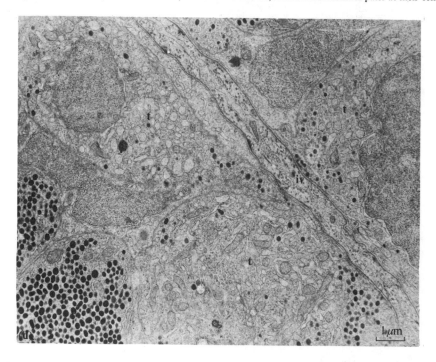

(d) t, thyrotropin cells at the periphery of the follicle, bordering an intervascular channel (iv). (From Knowles and Vollrath (1966). *Phil. Trans. R. Soc. B* **250**.)

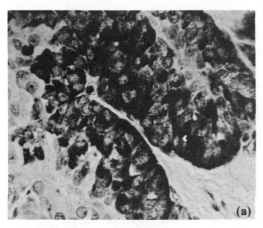 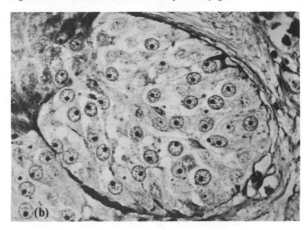

FIG. 5.24. (a) Corticotropin-secreting cells in the pituitary gland of a normal eel in fresh water, stained with lead haematoxylin. (cf. Fig. 5.22). (b) The same region, similarly stained, in an adrenalectomized eel, killed 8 days after adrenalectomy. The cells are degranulated, except for a thin rim of granules at the cell periphery, and the nuclei and nucleoli are hypertrophied. (Photographs by courtesy of M. Olivereau.)

as thyrotropic cells because they become degranulated when fish are immersed in goitrogen solution. Moreover, when the pituitary is ectopically grafted into the muscle of the body wall, these cells (in contrast to others to be mentioned later) persist, and, in correlation with this, the thyroid remains fully active.

PAS-positive gonadotropic cells are identifiable in the ventral regions of the proximal pars distalis, and are similarly located in *Salmo*, their function in the latter being indicated by their scarcity in yearling (sexually immature) fish, and their abundance in mature ones. In *Poecilia*, which is a live-bearing fish, changes in these cells can be correlated with stages of the reproductive cycle. For example, gonadotropins stimulate the second (vitellogenic) phase of oocyte growth. In *Poecilia* with ectopic pituitary grafts, the ovaries regress and the eggs show no vitellogenesis. In correlation with this, the gonadotropic cells in the grafts are chromophobe and evidently inactive. Further, hypophysectomy does not affect gestation or the birth of the young; in correlation with this, the gonadotropic cells of normal fish are small and inactive during these phases, indicating that they have no effect upon them. Whether two types of gonadotropic cell are present in fish, or in any non-mammalian vertebrate, is uncertain. Indeed, it is uncertain whether or not FSH and LH are two separate entities in non-mammalian vertebrates.

As regards acidophils, prolactin-secreting cells are readily identifiable in teleost fish, with secretion granules resembling those of many mammals in being strongly erythrosinophilic. In *Poecilia*, these cells occupy most of the rostral lobe of the pars distalis, as they also do in *Anguilla*. The identification of their function rests not only upon their staining, but on their immunofluorescent reaction to prolactin antibody raised in the rabbit, and on a correlation with the known effect of the hormone on ion balance. Both in *Fundulus* and in *Lebistes* these cells look relatively inactive in sea-water animals and active in fresh-water ones. Hypophysectomized *Poecilia* die in fresh water, but fish with ectopic grafts of the pars distalis can survive; this survival is correlated with the persistence in the grafts of active prolactin cells. Further, the salmon, *Salmo salar*, shows great activity and mitosis in these cells when the fish return to estuaries on their spawning migration.

A second type of acidophil, staining with orange G, is distributed over the same region as the thyrotropic cells. These acidophils are considered to produce somatotropin, although the evidence is less precise because these cells are less responsive to experimental stimulation. However, hypophysectomized fish with an ectopic graft show a reduced growth rate, and these cells in *Poecilia* are correspondingly reduced.

Finally, corticotropin-secreting cells have been convincingly identified in the teleost pituitary by the use of metopirone (Fig. 5.24). These cells, which stain readily with lead haematoxylin, are arranged, both in *Poecilia* and *Anguilla*, as a palisade along the inner edge of the rostral pars distalis, where this is in contact with the pars nervosa. Metopirone treatment results in hypertrophy of these cells, accompanied by a rounding and enlargement of the nucleus.

Supporting evidence comes from ectopic grafts of the pituitary in *Poecilia*. Active corticotropin cells are recognizable in these grafts, but they are fewer than in normal glands, and, in correlation with this, the adrenal cortex is less well developed than in control fish.

The uniformity of the results obtained from mammals and teleosts in this field of study is very impressive. It is true that they are obtained from only a few species, but these, in evolutionary terms, are so widely separated that the uniformity gives a good basis for the belief that vertebrate pituitaries have a common plan of cytological differentiation in the pars distalis.

Neither the elasmobranchs nor the actinopterygians are on the direct line of ascent to tetrapods. This gives particular importance to studies of the pituitary of the Crossopterygii, for this group contains two Subclasses, the Rhipidistia and the Dipnoi, of which the Rhipidistia were certainly ancestral to the terrestrial vertebrates. The Dipnoi (lung-fish) have followed an independent line of evolution, but are nevertheless sufficiently close to the tetrapods to parallel them in many features of organization. *Latimeria*, the only surviving rhipidistian, has a pituitary with some actinopterygian features, for it has a rostral and proximal pars distalis, and a neuro-intermediate complex; there is also a median eminence and a portal system. It is, of course, a highly specialized fish, and it is difficult to evaluate the significance of these features without knowledge of the pituitary organization of the extinct osteolepids, which, of all the crossopterygians, stood closest to the tetrapods.

The pituitary of the Dipnoi, however, is undoubtedly very amphibian in its form (Fig. 5.25(a)). The adenohypophysis arises as a solid ingrowth, which then develops a cavity by splitting, this cavity persisting in the fully formed gland. The pars intermedia lies above the cavity, and is penetrated by outgrowths from the neurohypophysis, the two forming a neurointermediate lobe. Two cell types are recognizable in the pars intermedia. The pars distalis, which lies below the cavity, contains cyanophil and acidophil cells, which can be differentiated into five types. Little is known of their function, but they resemble the cell types of the amphibian gland, and similarity of function can reasonably be assumed. A true saccus vasculosus is not present; the region from which this develops in other fish has presumably become merged into the main pituitary gland, as it has in tetrapods. Finally, a median eminence is present, constituted by a region in the postoptic

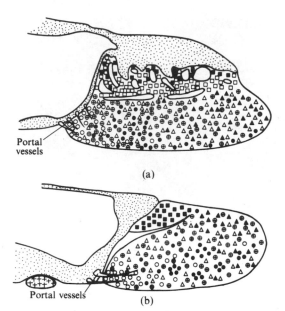

FIG. 5.25. Diagrams of median sections of the pituitary of (a), *Protopterus* and (b), an anuran, showing the distribution of the cell types in the adenohypophysis. ● basophils type 1 (thyrotropin-producing; cf. Fig. 5.27(a) and (b)); ⊕ Basophils type 2, ○ basophils type 3 (perhaps gonadotropin-producing); △ acidophils type 1 (perhaps somatotropin-producing); ▲ acidophils type 2 (perhaps corticotropin- or prolactin-producing, but cf. Fig. 5.27 (a) and (b), where the A1 cells are the equivalent of these); ■ Basophils of pars intermedia; □ PAS-negative cells of pars intermedia; + Chromophobes of pars tuberalis. (From van Oordt (1968). In *Perspectives in endocrinology*. Academic Press, London and New York.)

ventricular floor where the external surface is indented by capillaries. In general, the dipnoan gland is almost identical in organization with that of amphibians (Fig. 5.25(b)), a resemblance all the more striking in that the pituitaries of primitive actinopterygians conform so closely to the teleost type. This is in conformity with the evidence, drawn from so many sources, that actinopterygians and crossopterygians, which supposedly had a remote common origin, must have diverged at a very early stage of their history.

5.8. The pituitary gland of Tetrapoda

In Amphibia, as in lampreys and some actinopterygians, the adenohypophysis arises as a solid ingrowth; a convenient circumstance, which made possible the classic experiments involving the adenohypophysectomy of tadpoles at an early stage of their development. The more dorsal part of this rudiment becomes closely applied to the floor of the diencephalon and develops into the pars intermedia; the remainder forms the pars distalis, in such a way that this comes to form the more posterior part of the

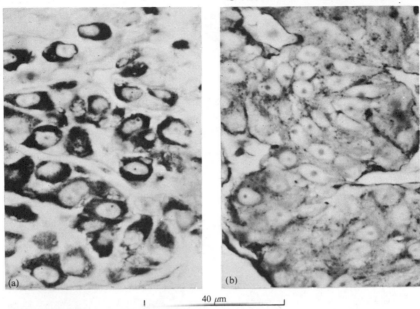

FIG. 5.26. Cell types in the amphibian pituitary. (a) granulated thyrotropin-producing cells in the pituitary of a *Xenopus laevis* larva; (b) degranulated and hypertrophied cells in a larva treated with propylthiouracil. Aldehyde–fuchsin. (From van Oordt (1968).)

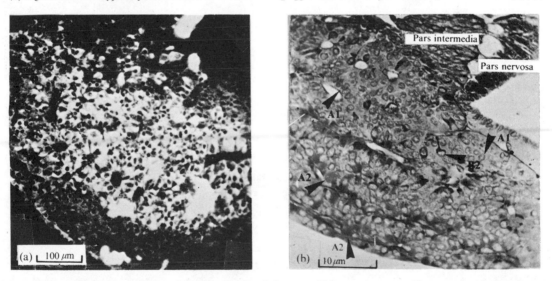

FIG. 5.27. (a) Paramedial sagittal section of the pars distalis of the newt, *Triturus cristatus carnifex*, treated with fluorescent anti-prolactin globulin. The light-grey fluorescent reaction, appearing white in the photograph, is localized in the dorsocentral region. The large white patches are artifacts. (b) A similar section, stained to show the cell types. A1, acidophil cells, pale grey (= acidophils type 2 of Fig. 5.26); A2, acidophil cells, dark grey (= acidophils type 1 of Fig. 5.26); B2, basophil cells, black. Higher magnification would show that the antigen–antibody complex is present only in the A1 cells, which are thus the prolactin-secreting ones. Susa fixation; staining method of Herlant. (From Vellano *et al.* (1973). *Gen. comp. Endocrin.* **20.**)

gland. The pars tuberalis is sometimes reduced or absent. The adenohypophysial cells reach a stage of cytological differentiation which is fully comparable with that of mammals and teleosts. Descriptive and experimental studies reveal three types of basophil and two types of acidophil (Fig. 5.26). The functions of these need further clarification, but the basophils are probably concerned with the secretion of thyrotropin (Fig. 5.26(a) and (b)) and gonadotropins, while the acidophils secrete prolactin (Fig. 5.27(a)

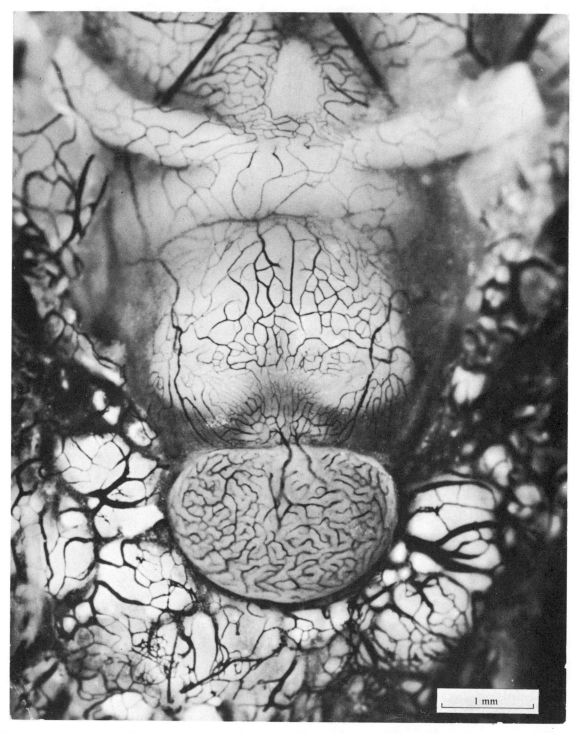

1 mm

FɪG. 5.28. Hypothalamus and pituitary gland of the toad, *Bufo bufo*, in ventral view, after injection of the blood vessels with an india-ink–gelatine suspension. The optic chiasma is above (anterior) and the pars distalis below (posterior), with the hypothalamus lying between them. The median eminence is at the posterior end of the hypothalamus, and two hypophysial portal vessels run downwards (posteriorly) from it to the pars distalis. (From Jørgensen *et al.* (1960). *Comp. Biochem. Physiol.* **1**.)

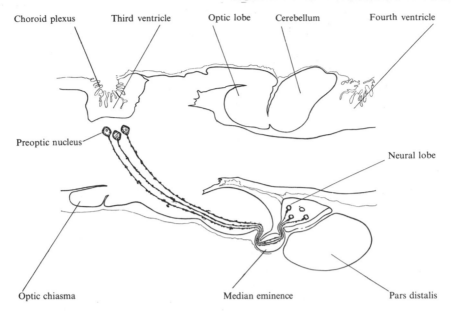

Choroid plexus   Third ventricle   Optic lobe   Cerebellum   Fourth ventricle

Preoptic nucleus

Neural lobe

Optic chiasma   Median eminence   Pars distalis

FIG. 5.29. Diagram of the hypothalamico-neurohypophysial system in the toad, *Bufo arenarum*. (From Gerschenfeld *et al.* (1960). *Endocrin.* **66**.)

and (b)), and perhaps somatotropin and cortico-tropin.

The neurohypophysis gives rise to a neural lobe, in the sense of a region that receives a blood supply separate from that to the adenohypophysis. There is also a well-defined median eminence, with a primary capillary plexus in its thick outer layer (Fig. 5.28). From this arise portal vessels which run into the pars distalis, giving rise there to a secondary plexus. The blood supply of the pars distalis is derived almost entirely from this system, although the vessels of the neural lobe do have some small degree of communication with it.

Neurosecretory fibres, arising from cells in the nucleus preopticus, run in a preoptico-hypophysial tract (Fig. 5.29) which is at first divided into two sections; these then unite into one median tract which passes backwards through the thin inner layer of the median eminence to enter the neural lobe, where the fibres end around its blood vessels. Some of these fibres, however, enter the outer layer of the median eminence, where their endings are oriented in a very clearly defined radial pattern around the capillaries of the primary plexus. Doubtless other fibres in the median eminence arise elsewhere in the hypo-thalamus. Indications of the functional significance of the median eminence emerge from the results of experiments on grafted pituitaries. Thus it has been shown that the pars distalis of the toad will remain

functional if it is grafted on to the eminence, but will regress into inactivity if grafted on to other parts of the brain. Clearly this supports the view that the median eminence is concerned here, as in mammals, with the transmission of chemical signals to the pars distalis. So also does the further observation that if the median eminence is removed, and the pars distalis grafted into its place, the pars distalis will become functional. This is presumably because it receives chemical signals from the cut ends of the fibres that were originally associated with the eminence.

The organization of the amphibian gland, together with the advantage of being able to study its develop-ment during the active larval stage, has made possible a particularly thorough analysis of the mode of regulation of the pars intermedia. Conventional nerve fibres and neurosecretory ones enter the pars inter-media from the neurohypophysis, and, not sur-prisingly, experimental data favour the existence of neural rather than humoral regulation. The depend-ence of the pars intermedia upon the neurohypo-physis is obvious throughout the vertebrates, from agnathans upwards, and we have already seen some of the evidence for this. In anurans, as in mammals, the intermedia does not develop unless there is con-tact with the infundibulum. In *Hyla regilla* no inter-media develops if the adenohypophysis is ectopically transplanted before it has established contact with the neurohypophysis; only the pars distalis forms.

The pars intermedia does, however, develop if transplanting is delayed until after contact has been established. This illustrates what is called, in embryological terminology, an inductive action of the neurohypophysis. Once the pars intermedia has differentiated, however, it can function independently of any connection with the central nervous system. Ectopic transplants, or severing of the pituitary stalk, in either the anuran tadpole or adult frog, results in darkening of the skin; this indicates a release of melanocyte-stimulating hormone, and shows that the pars intermedia is normally inhibited by the neurohypophysial influence. The same conclusion follows from experiments in which the anterior hypothalamus (including the nucleus preopticus) has been removed from tadpoles of *Xenopus*; this causes regression of the neural lobe, but hypertrophy of the pars intermedia, with consequential darkening of the body.

The inference from these and similar experiments is that control of the pars intermedia in amphibians is neural, as it evidently is also in fish, and probably in lampreys. We have seen that in mammals there is believed to be humoral control; nothing certain is known of this in amphibians, although the possibility that it does occur cannot be excluded by the results of these experiments. Much remains to be learned about the functioning and regulation of the pars intermedia throughout the vertebrates.

The pituitary of amniotes, which has already been considered in some detail in its mammalian form, shows, in these animals as a whole, a rather uniform organization. An exception is that birds (Fig. 5.30) lack a pars intermedia (as, of course, do certain mammals). The neural lobe is independently vascularized in amniotes, a portal system is present, and in birds all blood entering the pars distalis must pass through that system (Fig. 5.30). In some reptiles, however, the pars distalis may receive in addition a direct blood supply, as may also occur in mammals.

Varying degrees of histological differentiation are shown by the neurohypophysis. In its simplest form, as found in *Sphenodon* and in certain lacertilians and chelonians, its organization is virtually uniform throughout its length, with a continuous lumen and with little difference between the neural lobe and the median eminence. Its wall at this stage is composed of an internal lining of ependyma, a neurosecretory layer of fibres, and an outer glandular layer in which a colloid-like secretion is seen; pituicytes are absent and the blood vessels confined to the outer surface. In other reptiles, including various snakes, the neural lobe becomes compact and solid, the median eminence is thickened, and the capillary vessels sink into

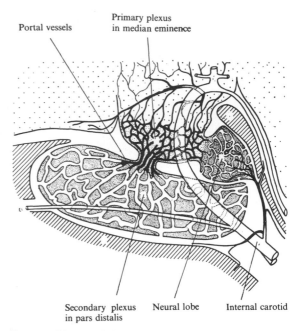

FIG. 5.30. Diagram of the blood supply of the pituitary gland of *Columba livia*. (From Wingstrand (1951). *The structure and development of the avian pituitary*. Lund, Gleerup.)

it, while pituicytes become conspicuous, perhaps derived from ependymal cells and perhaps sharing some secretory function with them.

Somewhat similar variations are found in birds, but in mammals the neurohypophysis is always of a more complex type of organization. The Monotremata, as might be expected, have the simplest and presumably most primitive structure, but even in them the neural lobe is well defined with thickened walls, and its lumen may be much reduced. Not the least important aspect of such variations of pattern is that they remind us that the relatively few mammalian types on which most research effort has been concentrated are the end result of lengthy evolutionary developments and that our generalizations regarding pituitary organization and function will be insecurely based until simpler and more primitive stages have been taken fully into account.

5.9. The pituitary gland and the Protochordata

We have seen that the cyclostomes have a pituitary gland which, while simpler in the details of its organization than is that of gnathostomes, already possesses the fundamentally important characteristic of an adenohypophysis and neurohypophysis in close association. This association, then, must be a primary feature of vertebrate organization, and must have appeared at a very early stage of the evolution of the group. So we must turn to the protochordates to seek for further information regarding the possible origin of the pituitary gland.

As far as amphioxus is concerned, there are two organs which merit some consideration, Hatschek's pit (Fig. 5.31) and the infundibular organ (Fig. 5.32).

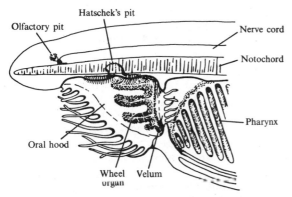

FIG. 5.31. Left side of the head of a young amphioxus, with the left body-wall, oral hood, and wall of pharynx cut away. (From Goodrich (1971). *Q. Jl microsp. Sci.* **62**.)

The former, an invagination situated just in front of the velum, forms part of the animal's filter-feeding mechanism, but there is sound embryological evidence to justify regarding it as a possible homologue of the adenohypophysis. The argument was first clearly formulated by Goodrich, who pointed out that Hatschek's pit takes its origin in part from the pre-oral pit, an ectodermal depression which develops in the early larva on the left side of the head and acquires an opening into the left member of the first pair of coelomic sacs. At metamorphosis this opening is lost, and the preoral pit spreads out to form the wheel organ. It contributes also to Hatschek's pit,

which is derived partly from the preoral pit and partly from the temporary connection of this with the coelomic sac. The asymmetry of the preoral pit is a secondary consequence of the asymmetry of the larva. If normal bilateral symmetry were restored, the pit would lie in essentially the position of Rathke's pouch in the vertebrate embryo, and would presumably have connections with both left and right members of the anterior pair of coelomic pouches. It is this latter feature which provides the most cogent argument for homologizing the pit with Rathke's pouch, for open connections exist between this and the first pair of coelomic cavities in the embryo of *Torpedo*. This can hardly be a chance coincidence; indeed, closed vestiges of such connections are a transient feature of the developing pituitary of the duck, which suggests that they must be a deep-seated feature of vertebrate organization.

As regards the infundibular organ, this is situated in the floor of the cerebral vesicle towards its posterior end (Fig. 5.32). It consists of slender cells which are believed to be primary sense cells, having one or two flagella at their free ends and being continued basally into nerve fibres. They contain granules, which stain with chrome-alum–haematoxylin, and which are thought to be secreted into the cavity of the vesicle, where they contribute to the formation of Reissner's fibre, a structure that is characteristic of the central canal of the vertebrate nervous system. In vertebrates it is derived from a dorsally situated subcommissural organ, but the situation in amphioxus may indicate the more primitive mode of origin, since in teleost embryos it has been shown to arise first from another group of cells, the flexural organ, situated ventrally in the mid-brain, and to establish later its permanent dorsal relationship. All of these cells, those of the subcommissural organ and of the flexural organ as well as those of the infundibular organ of amphioxus,

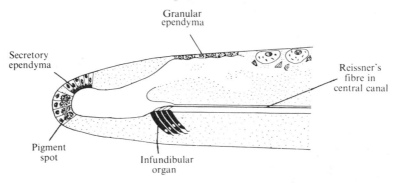

FIG. 5.32. Diagram of the anterior end of the nervous system of amphioxus. (From Olsson and Wingstrand (1954). *Univ. Bergen Årb.* 14.)

possess granules which stain with chrome-alum–haematoxylin, and it has therefore been suggested that they may be the surviving parts of an originally more widely distributed secretory region in the vertebrate brain. Furthermore, it has been suggested that the neurosecretory cells of the hypothalamus might also have been derived in this way, the implication here being that cells originally ependymal in position and secretory in function might have passed inwards, away from the ventricular lining, and have added nervous functions to their original secretory one.

This conception is speculative, and it must always be remembered that the staining of cell inclusions with chrome-alum–haematoxylin is no evidence at all for their homology or, indeed, for their secretory nature. Nevertheless, it is of interest to find such widespread evidence of secretory activity in the central nervous system, and to find it already established at the protochordate level.

It is, however, the situation in the Tunicata which has in the past attracted the greater amount of attention from investigators. The evolutionary interpretation of these animals is complicated by the fact that they undergo a profound metamorphosis from a free-swimming larva, and a much-favoured view as to the origin of vertebrates derives them from this larval stage by a process of neoteny. Leaving this difficult issue on one side, however, it is noteworthy that the nerve ganglion of the adult tunicate is commonly associated with a neural gland, which opens into the anterior end of the pharynx by means of a short duct (Fig. 5.33). A number of investigators, impressed by the superficial resemblance between this neural complex and the pituitary complex of vertebrates, have tested the former for the presence of pituitary hormones and have claimed evidence for the presence of oxytocic, vasopressor, antidiuretic, and melanocyte-stimulating principles. Unfortunately, these claims have not survived critical examination. Similar effects can be obtained from other tissues of tunicates and also from other animals, while the oxytocin-like principle differs in its chemical and pharmacological properties from true oxytocin. To take only one other illustration, the supposed antidiuretic activity of dried extract of the ascidian *Pyura* is only one two-hundred-thousandth of that of mammalian dried powder, so that it can hardly be regarded as a specific physiological property of the material. In short, the earlier reports seem not to have paid sufficient regard to the fact that all tissue extracts may be expected to display some degree of pharmacological activity, a source of error on which we have already had occasion to comment. While, therefore, the homology of the neural complex with the pituitary complex is not actually disproved by these results, it still awaits experimental confirmation. This, however, need not exclude it from our present consideration, for speculation regarding its possible relationship with the pituitary can be approached from another point of view.

The histological structure of Hatschek's pit is complex, and it has been suggested more than once that both it and the neural gland of tunicates might be sensitive to materials in the sea-water passing into the pharynx, and that by responding in some way to secretions of other individuals of the species they might regulate sexual maturation and spawning. We comment elsewhere (p. 1) on this type of communication system, and it is attractive to reflect that an organ so concerned might have become

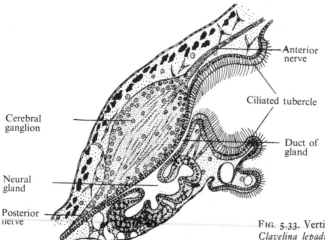

Cerebral ganglion

Neural gland

Posterior nerve

Anterior nerve

Ciliated tubercle

Duct of gland

FIG. 5.33. Vertical section of neural complex of the ascidian, *Clavelina lepadiformis*. (From Grasse (1948). *Traite de zoologie*, Vol. 11. Nasson et Cie, Paris.)

closed off from the outside world and have evolved into an internally secreting gland responding to chemical influences received now from the central nervous system. It would not be difficult to elaborate such a speculation in some detail, but it seems wiser for the present to treat it as no more than a general guide for future investigation. The presence of a preoral ciliary organ at the base of the proboscis of the hemichordate Enteropneusta, a group closely related to the protochordates, suggests that a tendency for the development of a sensory invagination in this region may well have been common to all the early chordate groups, and may then have been inherited by the vertebrates. Such a common inheritance might have expressed itself in markedly divergent ways in different groups, depending upon their adaptive needs. Because of this, and because our knowledge of the early chordates is at best fragmentary, it is perhaps unlikely that we shall ever achieve a satisfactory interpretation of the early history of the pituitary gland. Further research, however, should certainly be directed towards testing the hypotheses outlined above, and, if necessary, suggesting alternatives to take their place.

6

The neurohypophysial hormones

6.1. 'Pitocin' and 'pitressin'

The neurohypophysial hormones, as we have already seen, are neurosecretory products originating in the hypothalamus. Their cells of origin are concentrated, in mammals, into two pairs of nuclei, the supraoptic nuclei and the paraventricular nuclei; in lower verte-brates these are represented by a single pair, the preoptic nuclei (Figs 5.17, 5.18, and 5.19). From these points, the hormones are passed along the axons of the neurosecretory cells into the neural lobe, which is the neurohaemal organ where they are stored, and from where they are released into the blood stream. However, studies of these hormones were initiated at a time when the pituitary gland was regarded as composed of an 'anterior lobe' and a 'posterior lobe' (p. 62). It is because of this that the earlier literature commonly refers to them as 'posterior lobe' hormones, present in 'posterior lobe' extracts.

The neurohypophysial hormones have four main actions in mammals. These comprise a raising of blood pressure (vasopressor action), and ejection of milk from the mammary glands (milk-ejection or milk-letdown action), uterine contraction (oxytocic action) and a reduction in flow of urine (anti-diuretic action). In earlier investigations use was made of crude 'posterior lobe' extracts which had been separated into two fractions: 'oxytocin' (marketed as Pitocin), containing the bulk of the oxytocic and milk-ejection activities; and 'vasopressin' (marketed as Pitressin), containing the bulk of the vasopressor and anti-diuretic activities. Later, it became clear that these activities were actually localized in the neurohypophysis, and the hormones responsible for them have now been fully characterized. However, before we consider the evidence for this, we must examine the actions themselves more closely.

We shall be considering later the consequences of the discovery by Oliver and Schäfer in 1895 of the vasopressor action of adrenal extracts. Later, while pursuing similar investigations into the effects of other glands, they found that intravenous injections of extracts of the pituitary also produced a rapid rise of blood pressure, which could be maintained for many minutes. As with the adrenal effect, the rise resulted from the combination of vasoconstriction with augmentation of the heart beat, and appeared to be due to a peripheral action rather than to a central reflex, for it occurred even if the spinal cord was cut or the medulla destroyed. This was the vaso-pressor action to which we have referred, and which provides a bioassay procedure (Fig. 6.1).

As regards the action on the mammary glands, this contributes to the second of the two main phases of lactation; this is milk removal, the first phase being milk secretion. Milk removal involves two stages, the first (which is the phase with which we are now con-cerned) being the active ejection of milk from the alveoli and finer ducts of the mammary glands into the larger ducts; this is a result of contraction of the myoepithelial cells of the alveoli. The second is the withdrawal of the milk by the act of suckling or by the hand of the milker; this is a purely passive phase as far as the mother is concerned.

Earlier workers, again including Schäfer, had noted that the injection of 'posterior lobe' extracts could evoke active ejection. Pressure changes associ-ated with this are the basis of a bioassay, using the lactating rabbit (Fig. 6.2). It was further shown that normal ejection could be abolished in the nursing bitch by anaesthesia (Fig. 6.3), and that this in-hibition could be overcome by injection of the extracts. At the time of these observations there was still a tendency to regard all the actions of 'posterior lobe' extracts as being pharmacological rather than physiological. The truly physiological status of this particular response did not emerge until 1941, when it was shown that application of the normal milking stimulus to a cow would bring about ejection from a denervated half of an udder as well as from the other half, which retained its normal innervation. It was further shown that the ejection of milk could be evoked from an isolated udder which had itself been

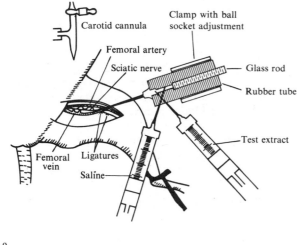

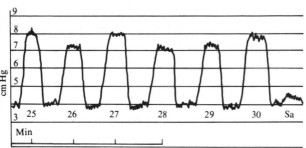

FIG. 6.1. *Above*, apparatus used for recording the vasopressor action of the neurohypophysial hormones. Preparations are injected into the femoral vein, and the blood pressure recorded through a cannula inserted into the carotid artery. *Below*, tracing showing the results obtained. Abscissae, time; ordinates, blood pressure. The injections were: 25, 0·008 international units of a 'posterior lobe' extract; 26, 0·006; 27, 0·008; 28, 0·006; 29, 0·006; 30, 0·008; Sa, 0·2 ml saline. (From Landgrebe *et al.* (1946). *Proc. R. Soc. Edin.* B **62**.)

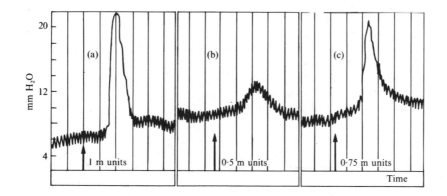

FIG. 6.2. The effect of intravenous injections of standard pituitary extract on the pressure in the mammary gland of a lactating rabbit; the animal weighed 1·8 kg, and was in the eighth day of lactation. The small regular waves represent respiratory movements. One division on the abscissa represents 2 s. (After Thorp (1962). *Methods in hormone research* (ed. R. I. Dorfman), Vol. 2. Academic Press, New York.)

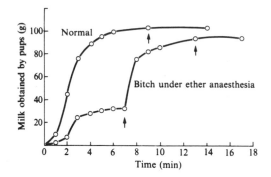

FIG. 6.3. Milk flow curves from a bitch under normal conditions and under ether anaesthesia. Arrows indicate injection of 'posterior lobe' extract. (From Cowie and Folley (1957). *The neurohypophysis* (ed. H. Heller). Butterworth, London.)

stimulated by milking. The hypothesis suggested by these results was that the milk-ejection response was dependent upon the stimulation of receptors by the act of suckling or milking; the resulting nerve impulses being transmitted to the brain, and bringing about the release of a hormone from the neurohypophysis. Such a pathway is often called a neuroendocrine reflex arc. In terms of control theory, this one is an example of positive feedback, since continuous stimulation of the teats prolongs the release of the milk. It contrasts with negative feedback, examples of which will be encountered later. In the present instance, the neuroendocrine reflex facilitates the conditioning of the mother to various external stimuli with which the milking process is associated.

Later evidence relevant to this hypothesis is that if a female rat is deprived of its neurohypophysis, her young are unable to obtain milk from her teats and will die of starvation. If, however, 'oxytocin' is injected into her they can secure the milk and can be reared at almost the normal rate. It has been shown, too, that milk ejection can be evoked in cows by the injection of 'oxytocin', and in ewes, goats, and rabbits by electrical stimulation of the neurosecretory fibres (Fig. 6.4), applied through electrodes implanted

in or close to the supraoptic nuclei or the median eminence (p. 64). That the hormone is present in the blood is indicated by milk ejection being evoked in a lactating animal when it is injected with blood taken from a goat that had been subjected to this electrical stimulation.

The oxytocic action was discovered by Dale, who has recorded how in 1906 he was comparing the effects of adrenaline and of 'posterior lobe' extracts upon the arterial blood pressure of the anaesthetized pregnant cat, and happened at the same time to be recording the activity of the uterine wall. As a result, he discovered that the pituitary extract produced a powerful contraction of the uterine muscle. The physiological significance of this oxytocic response (which provides another bioassay, Fig. 6.5) is still

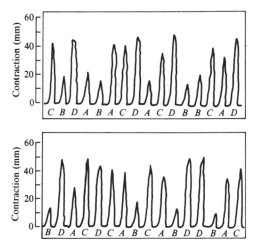

FIG. 6.5. An assay for oxytocin. The record shows 32 contractions of a rat's uterus. The contractions are responses to four different doses of pituitary; *A*, *B*, *C*, and *D*, each of which is given once in each group of 4 contractions. There are 8 groups in all. $A = 0.05$ units, $B = 0.04$ units, $C = 0.064$ units, and $D = 0.08$ units. *B* and *C* were treated as 'standard'. *A* and *D* were treated as 'unknown'. $A:D = B:C = 5:8$. Estimate of unknown:standard $= 1.25$. True value of unknown:standard $= 0.05/0.04 = 1.25$. A dose was put into the bath every 4 min and washed out after 45 s. Weight of rat 140 g. Temperature 34–6 °C. Load on uterus 1.3 g. Total experimental time 4 hours. (From Holton (1948). *Br. J. Pharmacol.* 3.)

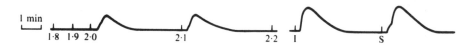

FIG. 6.4. Tracings of kymograph records of milk-ejection responses to electrical stimulation of the median eminence and infundibular stem in an anaesthetized rabbit. The stimuli were applied for $\frac{1}{4}$ min in the vertical plane of the median eminence; the figures give the depth (in cm) of the electrode tip below the surface of the skull (cf. Fig. 7.22). A moderate response is obtained at 2·0 cm and 2·1 cm depth, but none at 1·8 cm, 1·9 cm, and 2·2 cm. Stimulation of the infundibular stem (S) gives a greater response which is similar to that following the injection (I) of 50 m units of whole pituitary extract. (From Cross and Harris (1952). *J. Endocrin.* 8.)

doubtful (as is also true of the vasopressor response), although it is certain that oxytocin is released from the pituitary during labour, and it is therefore used in obstetrical practice. An indication that the response is truly physiological is that the sensitivity of the uterus to the hormone increases towards the end of labour in some mammals; this is a result of the uterus being affected by changes in the output of ovarian hormones.

Meanwhile, Schäfer and others had been studying another property of these pituitary extracts, for it had now been found that intravenous injection of them into anaesthetized animals resulted in increased diuresis. There is found in man a condition known as diabetes insipidus, in which excessive urine production is accompanied by a thirst so tormenting that afflicted individuals have been known to drink as much as thirty litres of water per day. Their urine lacks the sugary taste characteristic of the urine of diabetes mellitus (p. 24), and it is this fact which gives the name to this condition. Attention was called in 1912 to the frequent association of diabetes insipidus with injury to the pituitary gland, but it was at first assumed that such injury, by irritation of the glandular tissue, evoked an over-production of a diuretic principle. When, however, investigators came to examine the effect of injecting 'posterior lobe' extracts into patients suffering from the disorder, there emerged the unexpected discovery that these injections actually alleviated diabetes insipidus, whereas on the above hypothesis the diuresis should, if anything, have been increased.

It is now known that the hormone concerned is actually antidiuretic, that diabetes insipidus results from a lack of it, and that the spectacular alleviating effect of the injections is a practical application of replacement therapy. The diuretic action which had been observed in the earlier injection experiments was probably a secondary and artificial effect, associated with the influence of anaesthesia upon the functioning of the kidney. The hypothesis that had been based upon this action was reasonable in the light of the knowledge then available, but the episode demonstrates very clearly how important it is to consider very carefully all of the conditions that are operative during a physiological experiment.

Conclusive evidence of the release from the neurohypophysis of an antidiuretic hormone, and of the direct action of this upon the kidney tubules, came in part from the study of isolated preparations of the heart, lung, and kidney of the dog. If these are perfused with blood, there results a considerable diuresis, which can be inhibited by the addition to the perfusing fluid of 'posterior lobe' extract. It can be shown that this inhibition is not accompanied by any significant reduction of the rate of flow of blood through the kidney, so that the extract must be exerting a direct and specific action upon the kidney itself rather than upon its blood supply. Further, inhibition can also be produced by including the head of the dog in the perfusion circuit, the implication being that the inhibition is here a result of the addition to the blood of the secretion released from the pituitary. Our understanding of the mode of action of the hormone is less complete. The current view of the mode of functioning of the mammalian kidney is that active reabsorption of sodium occurs in the proximal convoluted tubule of the mammalian nephron (Fig. 6.6), and is accompanied by a passive

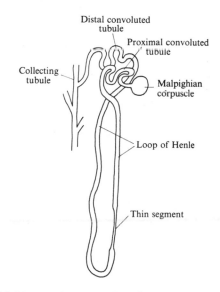

FIG. 6.6. Diagram of a nephron from the cortex of a mammalian kidney.

diffusion of water; these processes are thought to be unaffected by the antidiuretic hormone. In the distal convoluted tubule, and in the ascending limb of Henle's loop, there is a further active reabsorption of sodium, but the amount of water absorbed there, and perhaps also in the collecting tubule, is variable, and is thought to be regulated by the action of that hormone upon cell permeability, the resultant composition of the urine reflecting the state of water balance of the animal. These two types of water reabsorption are referred to respectively as obligatory and facultative; it has been suggested that the latter may also take place in the first (descending) limb of Henle's loop and in the collecting tubules, and that at these sites. too, it may be regulated by the antidiuretic hormone. The operation of the facultative reabsorption is well seen if a hypertonic solution is injected into the carotid artery of an experimental animal. This brings about an antidiuresis, which is supposedly evoked by the release of the hormone. This release, it is thought, may be a consequence of the stimulation of osmo-receptors in the forebrain, or may perhaps result from the direct response of the neurosecretory cells to the osmotic composition of their blood supply.

6.2. Oxytocin and the vasopressins

The isolation of two distinct fractions from neurohypophysial extracts left unanswered the question whether there were two distinct hormones, or whether the chemical procedures had broken up an originally single substance which carried all the activity. The problem was resolved from 1949 onwards by the success of du Vigneaud, another Nobel laureate, in isolating from the pituitary glands of cattle two pure hormones. With the pioneer studies of Sanger as an example, it proved possible to determine the molecular structure of these, as a result of which they were shown to be nonapeptide amides of closely similar pattern, each being formed of a cyclic pentapeptide with a tripeptide amide side chain. They are called oxytocin and vasopressin, which are the trivial names that were already well-established before the hormones had been chemically characterized. Corresponding trivial names have been given to the related hormones that were discovered afterwards and that we shall be considering later. An international recommendation has, however, been made for the appropriate chemical nomenclature of these molecules. The ruling is that, in a polypeptide with the trivial name X, the semitrivial name of a derivative of it should be q-new amino acid-X, where q is the number of the substituted amino acid in the polypeptide chain. In shortened form, this becomes new amino acid^q-X. This nomenclature is used in Fig. 6.7. In the text it is usually used once, and the trivial names used thereafter for convenience.

The primary structure of oxytocin and vasopressin is shown in Fig. 6.7, from which it will be seen that they have seven amino acids in common. Vasopressin differs from oxytocin in having phenylalanine replacing isoleucine at position 3 in the ring, and arginine replacing leucine at position 8 in the side chain. In this form it is commonly called arginine vasopressin but, more strictly, should be termed 8-arginine-vasopressin, or, in abbreviated form, Arg^8-vasopressin.

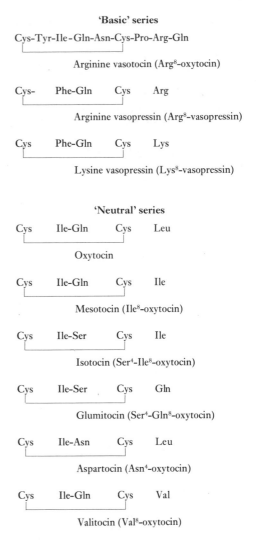

FIG. 6.7. Structural formulae of the neurohypophysial hormones.

The biological properties of these two hormones can be measured in a series of standard bioassays, using mammal oxytocic, milk-ejection, vasopressor, and antidiuretic effects. Additional properties can also be used, including fowl vasopressor, fowl and turtle oxytocic (i.e. oviduct contraction), and frog-bladder effects. The last-named property will be discussed in the next section. Data from these bioassays give a quantitative pharmacological spectrum which is characteristic for each molecule (Table 6.1). They show that rat oxytocic and rabbit milk-ejection effects are mainly the property of oxytocin, and that rat vasopressor and dog antidiuretic effects are mainly the property of vasopressin. In addition, oxytocin shows a small amount of vasopressor and anti-diuretic action, amounting to 1–2 per cent of the activity of pure vasopressin, while the latter shows a small amount of oxytocic and milk-ejection activity. Such a spectrum gives a good first approximation to the identification of the hormonal content of a pituitary extract, but is not adequate for complete identification; the biological differences are not always sharply defined, and can readily be obscured by contaminants. The information therefore needs to be supplemented by chemical characterization of the molecule, which involves determining electrophoretic and chromatographic migrations, and amino-acid composition.

TABLE 6.1

Pharmacological spectra of neurohypophysial hormones
(Data collected from various sources by Heller and
Pickering (1961). *J. Physiol.* **155**.)

Assay method	Arginine vasotocin	Arginine vasopressin	Lysine vasopressin	Oxytocin
Rat uterus	40	20–25	15–20	360, 415
Rat blood pressure	71	400–450	270–340	< 10, 3·8
Rat antidiuresis	71	400–450	110–140	diuretic
Rabbit milk ejection	119	70–80	50–60	371
Hen oviduct	1630	320	29	29
Frog water balance	2600	—	—	(360)
Frog bladder	7800	21	< 5	360

Arginine vasopressin has been identified in at least one species from each of six orders of eutherian mammals (Primates, Cetacea, Perissodactyla, Artiodactyla, Rodentia, and Lagomorpha), and may be regarded, on present information, as the normal vasopressin of mammals. An exception, however, is provided by the suborder Suiformes, some members of which secrete lysine vasopressin. This hormone, which has also been identified in a Peruvian strain of mouse (*Mus musculus*), differs from arginine vasopressin by having lysine substituted for arginine at position 8. It is therefore 8-lysine-vasopressin, or, in abbreviated form Lys[8]-vasopressin, but is commonly called lysine vasopressin. The domestic pig (*Sus scrofa domestica*) secretes only this hormone, and not arginine vasopressin; many thousands of pituitaries from this species have been extracted, but the latter hormone has never been found. The African warthog (*Phacochoerus aethiopicus*) also secretes lysine vasopressin, but differs from the pig in secreting arginine vasopressin as well; some individuals secrete either one or the other, while some secrete both. The same may be true of the New World collared peccary (*Tayassu ungulatus*), in which lysine vasopressin occurs.

The supposition is that lysine has been substituted for arginine in these species as a result of mutation in the relevant codon. The domestic pig must now be homozygous for the new allele, whereas both alleles persist in the warthog and, supposedly, in the peccary. These latter two species thus provide examples of polymorphism, which can be defined as the existence of two or more forms in a species, in such proportions that the rarest cannot be maintained by recurrent mutation alone. An alternative wording would be that there are at least two alleles with frequencies greater than 0·01 per cent. The evolutionary implication of these definitions is that the polymorphism must be maintained by selection pressure, the simplest case being that the heterozygote has some selective advantage over either homozygotes. In this instance, nothing is known for certain of any selective advantage associated with one or other of the two forms of vasopressin. Some adaptation has certainly occurred, however, for the antidiuretic activity of the lysine analogue in the pig and the Peruvian mouse is about as high as that of the arginine analogue, although it is less active in mammalian species which secrete only arginine vasopressin. More general aspects of such molecular variation will be discussed later (p. 101).

The hippopotamus is another living member of the order Suiformes, and it, too, has been said to secrete lysine vasopressin. This, however, has been denied, and it now seems probable that it conforms to the normal mammalian pattern. A conclusion suggested by these facts is that there is a close genetic relationship between the pig and the warthog and the peccary, and that they have either inherited the lysine vasopressin allele from a common ancestor, or have developed it independently as a result of that close relationship. The hippopotamus, which has not developed or inherited this allele, would then be less closely related to them than they are to each other. This view conforms with certain other characteristics, including its subdivided stomach and its lack of a caecum, all of which suggest that it is somewhat intermediate between the other Suiformes and the remaining members of the order Artiodactyla (camels and ruminants), none of which is known to secrete lysine vasopressin. This can be held to justify one view of suiform classification, which is to place the pigs and peccaries in an infraorder Palaeodonta and the hippopotamuses in another group, the infraorder Ancodonta. An alternative view which has also had support is to place the pigs, peccaries, and hippopotamus in three separate families, called respectively the Suidae, the Dicotylidae, and the Hippopotamidae. Current views on the distribution of lysine vasopressin clearly do not support this view quite so strongly, but it is obvious that evidence drawn from one hormonal molecule is extremely tenuous. A much broader range of information is needed to determine taxonomic relationships. And it is obvious that if this particular molecule occurs in the mice of a Peruvian village, it may occur in other mammals as well, if only as a genetic variant in natural populations.

6.3. Water balance in Amphibia

Neurohypophysial hormones are present throughout the vertebrates, but the ecological and physiological problems facing the lower forms are very different from those encountered by mammals, and the hormones themselves are different as well. This is exemplified very clearly in the regulation of water balance in Amphibia: animals which do not drink, and which have a highly permeable skin that is therefore a critical limiting factor in their water uptake.

Terrestrial frogs and toads have a remarkable capacity for increasing the uptake of water through their skin. The first indication that the neurohypophysis was involved in this emerged from the work of Brunn, who showed in 1921 that if 'posterior lobe' extract was injected into the lymph sac, and the animal kept in water, the result was an increase in weight up to as much as 20 per cent in five to ten hours. This 'Brunn effect' (or water-balance response) is a result of the accumulation of water (mostly retained in the lymph spaces). It depends in part upon the action of the extract in promoting the movement of water through the skin along the osmotic gradient, accompanied by the active uptake of sodium (natriferic effect). These skin responses, which can be demonstrated in the isolated tissue as well as in the intact animal, are not, however, the only factors involved in the effect.

It can be demonstrated, by cannulating the cloaca of a toad, that the uptake of water is accompanied by a reduction in the rate of flow of urine, so that the kidney must be cooperating with the skin in building up the excess of water. We have seen that in mammals an antidiuretic effect is brought about by the action of vasopressin on the distal segment of the nephron, and it is believed that in amphibians also the antidiuresis is mediated by a tubule response. In addition, there is probably constriction of the arterioles of the glomerulus, which reduces the amount of fluid available for filtration.

Yet another factor is the uptake of water through the wall of the bladder. This also is under the control of the neurohypophysis, as can be shown by tying off the cloaca of a frog and then leaving the animal in water for some hours. During this time it will gain in weight because water will enter the body through the skin and will be unable to escape. It accumulates in the bladder, and the amount of urine found there will be approximately equivalent to the water taken in. If, however, 'posterior lobe' extract is injected at the end of this period and the animal left for another two hours, it is found that the water content of the bladder has decreased. This is due to the passage of the water through the bladder wall in response to the neurohypophysial hormone, an effect which can be demonstrated in the isolated bladder of the bullfrog.

Neurohypophysial extracts can therefore influence the water balance of anurans by action at three points: the skin, the kidney, and the bladder. This represents a complex of adaptive mechanisms which are of the greatest importance to the group in the terrestrial phase of their lives. So long as the animals are in water, their main problem is to get rid of the excess that enters by osmotic flow, but on land they are faced with the problem of desiccation, and this becomes increasingly acute as they become increasingly terrestrial in habit. It is in this context that the adaptive value of the water-balance response becomes clear, for different genera vary in the intensity of their responses, and these variations, which depend in part upon variations in the sensitivity of the target organs (p. 2), can be related to their mode of life.

For example, the highly terrestrial toad shows a much greater degree of water uptake after 'posterior lobe' injections than does the less terrestrial frog, while the fully aquatic *Xenopus* is unable to increase its water uptake after dehydration, and shows virtually no antidiuretic response to neurohypophysial extracts. Even more striking data emerge from a comparison of the water-balance responses of two genera of Australian frogs. Amongst four species of *Neobatrachus*, it is those from drier areas that take up water more readily. No such correlation is found in four species of *Heleioporus*, probably because they dig burrows in which they are well protected from water loss.

Urodeles have been less thoroughly studied, but they certainly exhibit water-balance responses on the principles outlined above. For example, the responses of the fully aquatic *Necturus* and larval *Ambystoma* yield weight increases of only 2–6 per cent, whereas those of the terrestrial *Salamandra maculosa* and of other terrestrial newts range from 14–20 per cent. The pattern of effector action in urodeles is, however, different from that found in anurans, and varies in ways that are not directly related to habitat. In *Necturus*, *Triturus*, and *Ambystoma*, for example, the response is effected solely by the kidney, unaccompanied by any response from the skin or bladder. In *Salamandra*, by contrast, the bladder is the effector organ, with no response from either the skin or the kidney.

In the earlier investigations of water balance, it was uncertain whether or not the active agent was identical with one or other of the mammalian neurohypophysial hormones. In 1941, however, it was shown that the effect of extracts of frog pituitaries on water uptake was not proportional to their mammalian antidiuretic (Fig. 6.8(a)), oxytocic (Fig. 6.8(b)), and vasopressor activities; it appeared, therefore, that an entirely distinct 'water-balance principle' might be concerned. Later it was shown that either pure oxytocin or vasopressin can evoke water reabsorption from the bladder of the frog, and that oxytocin is the more potent of the two. Yet it was difficult to see how oxytocin could be identical with the 'water-balance principle', for large doses of it were required in comparison with the small amounts of frog pituitary extract which would produce similar responses. In other words, it became necessary to postulate the existence in the frog pituitary of a hormone with a pharmacological spectrum different from those of the mammalian hormones. It is here that the study of synthetic analogues proved of extraordinary interest.

One of these was arginine vasotocin (Arg[8]-oxytocin), so called because the vasopressin side chain is here combined with the oxytocin ring (Fig. 6.7). As might be expected, this substance shows the properties of the natural mammalian hormones, but in quite different ratios (Table 6.1). These properties agreed so closely with those required of the postulated 'water-balance principle' that it immediately seemed likely that the latter was, in fact, arginine vasotocin, and this was later confirmed when it was chemically identified in amphibian pituitary extracts. That this analogue is indeed a true vertebrate hormone, not only in amphibians, but probably in all non-mammalian vertebrates, has now been amply established. It thus provides the remarkable situation of a widely distributed vertebrate hormone being first discovered and characterized as a synthetic product in advance of its isolation from biological material. We will now consider the evidence for this broader conclusion in more detail, together with the

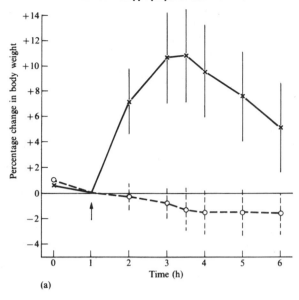

(a)

FIG. 6.8. (a) The difference between the mean percentage changes in weight of 20 frogs produced by the injection into each of the extract of a single frog pituitary gland ($\times$——$\times$) and of 10 m units pitressin (O– – –O). Injections at the time marked by arrow. Vertical lines indicate the standard errors. The pitressin (a) has no effect, although the maximum antidiuretic activity of a frog pituitary gland has been found to equal only 5 m units pitressin.

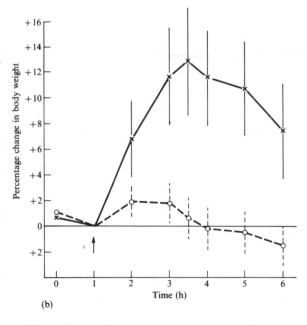

(b)

(b) A similar experiment, but with 40 m units pitocin substituted for 10 m units pitressin. The pitocin has little effect, although the oxytocic activity of a frog pituitary gland had been found to be considerably less than the equivalent of 40 m units pitocin. (From Heller (1941). *J. Physiol.* **100**.)

further and fundamentally important findings to which it has given rise.

6.4. Distribution of the neurohypophysial hormones in vertebrates

Early in the study of the properties and distribution of arginine vasotocin it was found that there was high water-balance activity in the pituitaries of *Petromyzon marinus*, *Pollachius virens* (pollack), *Bufo americanus*, *Rana catesbeiana*, and *Chelone mydas* (green turtle).

elasmobranchs, but it now seems probable that it is indeed secreted in both elasmobranchs and in holocephalans. It has not been identified in any adult mammal, but it has been found in the pituitaries of the foetuses of the pig, sheep, seal, and guinea-pig. Evidently, then, it is a very ancient hormone, and one of great molecular stability. It must have been replaced by arginine vasopressin at some stage in the evolution of mammals—perhaps at an early stage—for it is thought, on pharmaco-

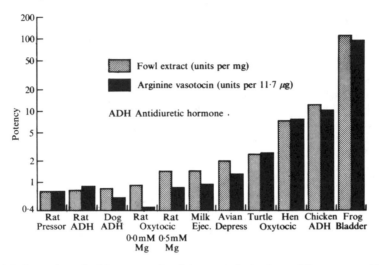

FIG. 6.9. Potencies of fowl neurohypophysial extract and arginine vasotocin in eleven different assays. The potencies are plotted logarithmically, with scales adjusted to approximate pressor activities. (From Munsick *et al.* (1960). *Endocrin.* **66**.)

This gave some presumptive indication that other species, as well as amphibians, might be secreting this hormone. Further, it was found that the pharmacological properties of neurohypophysial extracts of the fowl (*Gallus domesticus*) were not what would be expected from a combination of the two mammalian hormones, but that they could be accounted for on the assumption that the hormones actually secreted in this animal were oxytocin and arginine vasotocin. The results (Fig. 6.9) showed close correspondence between the spectra of the fowl extract and of arginine vasotocin, the differences being ascribable to the presence in the extracts of small amounts of oxytocin. This conclusion was confirmed by the isolation of arginine vasotocin from the fowl's pituitary, and its chemical characterization.

A range of similar pharmacological and chemical studies have now convincingly shown that arginine vasotocin is present in all non-mammalian species that have been studied, belonging to agnathans, fish, amphibians, reptiles, and birds (Fig. 6.13). At first it seemed doubtful whether it was present in

logical evidence, to be present in monotremes and marsupials. If we accept the view that the evolution of mammals was polyphyletic, with monotremes originating independently of the other two groups, this implies an early appearance of the new hormone in therapsid reptiles (perhaps 200–230 million years ago), or, of course, some degree of parallel evolution.

Arginine vasotocin, arginine vasopressin, and arginine lysopressin are termed the 'basic' neurohypophysial hormones, owing to their arginine or lysine content. Contrasting with them, and presenting more complex evolutionary problems, are a group of 'neutral' hormones, of which we have so far only considered oxytocin. Pharmacological and chromatographic evidence, not yet confirmed by chemical identification, indicates that only arginine vasotocin, and no other molecule, is present in the cyclostomes, but all gnathostomes so far studied possess at least one hormone of each group.

Three 'neutral' hormones (Fig. 6.7) have so far been chemically characterized in the elasmobranchs:

glumitocin (Ser[4], Gln[8]-oxytocin) in *Raja* spp., and valitocin (Val[8]-oxytocin) and aspartocin (Asn[4]-oxytocin) in the dogfish *Squalus acanthias*. The corresponding hormone in the holocephalan *Chimaera* is said to be oxytocin. The difference between these two groups, if confirmed, would be in line with the view that the classes Elasmobranchi and Holocephali have had a long independent history following a remote (and hypothetical) common origin.

Teleost fish secrete a 'neutral' hormone that is not found outside actinopterygians. This hormone was at first called ichthyotocin, but it was later characterized as Ser[4],Ile[8]-oxytocin, and is now called isotocin, in reference to its isoleucine content (Fig. 6.7). It has also been chemically identified in the palaeopterygian *Polypterus*, which indicates that it is a primitive feature of the class Actinopterygii.

The third major group of extant fish, the subclass Dipnoi (lung-fish), are closely related, within the class Crossopterygii, to the subclass Rhipidistia, from which the tetrapods evolved. Lung-fish, while not themselves ancestral to tetrapods, show many resemblances to amphibians, and may therefore be expected to show some parallelism with them in their neurohypophysial hormones, as we have seen that they do in their pituitary organization in general (p. 82). This expectation proves justified, for their 'neutral' hormone is mesotocin (Ile[8]-oxytocin), which has

been chemically characterized in *Protopterus*; also in the amphibians *Rana* and *Bufo*; the snakes *Vipera*, *Naja* (cobra), and *Elaphe*; the lizard *Iguana*; and, amongst birds, in the chicken, goose, and turkey. The situation is complicated, however, by some evidence (not clear-cut) indicating that both mesotocin and oxytocin may coexist in the lung fish *Lepidosiren*, in some anurans, and in *Naja*, while earlier chemical evidence (now apparently rejected) had indicated that oxytocin was also present in chickens. These complications are as yet unresolved. In part they arise because it is difficult to distinguish these two hormones on pharmacological criteria (Fig. 6.10), but it is impossible to exclude the possibility that many non-mammalian tetrapods may be polymorphic in this respect.

At present, however, it can be argued that during the emergence of mammals there was a double change in the neurohypophysial hormones. One change, for which the evidence is clear-cut, was the substitution of arginine vasopressin for arginine vasotocin. Arginine vasopressin has the higher antidiuretic and vasopressor activity of the two, and a much reduced oxytocin and milk-ejection activity (Fig. 6.10). Functionally, therefore, this change may be regarded as the substitution of a physiologically more specialized molecule for one that is more generalized in its properties. The other change, for which the evidence

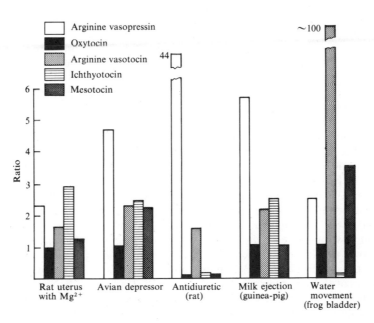

FIG. 6.10. Histograms of the pharmacological spectra of neurohypophysial hormones (cf. Table 6.1). The potency ratios are relative to the action of the hormones on the isolated rat uterus in the absence of Mg^{2+} ions. (From Heller and Pickering (1970). In *International encyclopaedia of pharmacology and therapeutics*, §41, Vol. 1, p. 59–79 (eds H. Heller and B. T. Pickering). Pergamon Press, Oxford.)

is less complete, was the substitution of oxytocin for mesotocin. This, however, would have involved very little change in biological properties (Fig. 6.10), and it is difficult to account for it. It should be remembered, however, that the evolutionary history of these 'neutral' hormones is much less easy to define at present than is that of the 'basic' line.

6.5. Some principles of molecular evolution

Information regarding the distribution of the neurohypophysial hormones in vertebrates is still very restricted. Nevertheless, it is well worth while examining its evolutionary implications. Several attempts have already been made to outline a phylogenetic history of the hormones and, not surprisingly, these have always had to be modified in the light of further discoveries. This is likely enough to be the fate of the interpretation to be suggested here, but the attempt can readily be justified. Not only does it have its own intrinsic interest; it also provides a good model for the interpretation of the evolution of polypeptide and protein hormones in general. We shall therefore approach the problem along a broad front. This will inevitably raise difficult issues of molecular biology and of evolutionary genetics, but these can only be touched upon in very general terms.

A fundamental assumption, deriving from our knowledge of the genetic code, is that amino-acid substitutions in polypeptide and protein molecules are the result of gene mutations, which, in many cases, can be ascribed to single base changes in the relevant cistrons, or to a series of such changes. There is, however, an immediate difficulty when we attempt to translate this assumption into phylogenetic terms, for we cannot be sure that evolution has necessarily followed what, in theory, may seem to be the simplest route. One complication arises from the so-called degeneracy of the genetic code, which permits an amino acid to be specified by more than one triplet codon. This allows the occurrence of 'silent' or 'same-sense' mutations; that is, base changes which do not alter the specification of the amino acid, and which therefore leave the polypeptide unaltered. Another obvious complication is the possibility of reverse mutations, which will leave no trace in the amino-acid sequences that are available for our study.

However, leaving these difficulties aside, it is obvious from inspection of the molecular variants of hormones that not all sites in a polypeptide chain are equally prone to substitution. Some are invariant; others are conservative, in the sense that they are only rarely substituted (Fig. 3.12, p. 36). One reason for this is that only certain substitutions are acceptable ones, in terms of natural selection. Other substitutions, although they may seem theoretically possible, will be forbidden, because their effects would be disadvantageous; they will therefore be rejected by natural selection. Some mutations may be acceptable because their effect is neutral or harmless, although estimates of the evolutionary significance of such mutations are matters of current controversy into which we shall not enter. Other substitutions may be acceptable because they confer functional advantages, and will therefore be favoured by natural selection. Here, however, it should be borne in mind that the properties of a molecule depend very much upon its tertiary structure; acceptability and advantage may thus depend not merely on the biochemical properties of particular amino acids, but also on their structural effects and their interactions with neighbouring loci.

Favoured mutations can provide the basis for evolutionary change, but usually only on a small scale, with the fundamental properties of the molecule remaining unaltered. We have seen examples in the variants of the mammalian insulin and somatotropin molecules. It must be admitted, however, that these particular variations are difficult to account for in terms of selective advantage, unless it is that they are needed to ensure self-recognition and the maintenance of functional efficiency in the evolving internal environment. Substitution sites in the mammalian insulin molecules are restricted, and the mutations have little phylogenetic relevance; the insulin of the dog and of the two species of whale are identical, while these two whale insulins differ from that of a third whale species. On the other hand, comparison of mammalian insulins with those of fish certainly reveals marked phylogenetic divergence, such as might well be expected (Table 3.2).

One highly significant fact is that the section of the mammalian pro-insulin molecule which connects the future A- and B-chains has many substitutions, in contrast to the few in the A- and B- regions. Bovine and porcine pro-insulins, for example, differ at 36 per cent of the sites in the connecting region, whereas their insulins differ at only 2 out of the 51 sites. Even the lengths of the connecting regions are different, for there are 30 amino acids in the bovine link and 33 in the porcine. We may ascribe these features to the linking region having few structural requirements, its sole function being to link the A- and B-regions; few substitutions, therefore, will be forbidden.

An extension of this type of molecular variation is the existence of two or more acceptable alleles at a single locus, with individuals in a population carrying either one or both of two distinct forms of the molecule. This is polymorphism, as we defined it on p. 95. It is a widespread phenomenon, by no means confined to hormones, but affecting also, for example, many enzymes, the polymorphic forms of which are termed isozymes. Whether it conforms in any particular case to classical Darwinian theory (p. 95), or whether it is a chance consequence of the establishment of mutation by genetic drift, is often not clear, and the distribution of arginine and lysine vasopressin in certain populations of Suiformes illustrates the difficulty. Genetic investigations on a wide front may be expected to clarify the problem, but in the meantime it is well to bear in mind that hormonal polymorphism may be associated with subtle adaptive properties that have not yet been defined by the procedures so far available for their study.

Finally, there is another type of molecular variation which has much greater potential for large-scale evolutionary change, and for the emergence of new endocrine activities. This is gene duplication, which makes it possible for one gene to be concerned with the specification of the already established molecule, while its replicate gene is free to accept mutations which can lead to the specification of a new molecule with new properties. Such mutations may be termed alterative mutations, as compared with conservative ones that have only minimal effects upon the properties of the molecule. Gene duplication can originate in two ways. First, it can result from unequal exchange between two chromatids of the same chromosome (so-called tandem duplication). This is thought to have only limited evolutionary potential, because both genes may be expected to remain under the control of the diffusing products of the same regulator gene, and this will tend to prevent the emergence of new properties at the new locus. Secondly, however, gene duplication can result from tetraploidy (i.e. duplication of a set of chromosomes), which has much greater evolutionary potential, because it involves the duplication of both the structural gene and its regulator gene.

On the above argument, a case could be made for regarding tetraploidy as an essential mechanism for the provision of an adequate source of evolutionary novelty, and this case finds support in estimates of genome size, which indicate considerable increase during the evolution of the phylum Chordata. In the ascidian *Ciona*, it is only 6 per cent of the mammalian size, and in amphioxus it is 17 per cent. In the lamprey (*Lampetra planeri*), it is 40 per cent, while in teleost fish it ranges from 14 per cent in the puffer

(*Spheroides maculatus*) to 90 per cent in the coho salmon (*Oncorhynchus kisutch*). In this phylum the process probably reached its limits during the evolution of fish. It could occur in them because their sex-determining mechanism is not strongly differentiated. In reptiles, birds, and mammals, on the other hand, where the sex chromosomes are sharply differentiated, tetraploidy becomes more difficult, because it is likely to lead to imbalance of the sex-determining mechanism. It is essential for males to produce sperm of the genetic constitution 2AXX or 2AYY, and there is no way of ensuring that this will happen.

Clear-cut evidence of gene duplication, as distinct from multiple allelism, is seen when the results of population sampling indicate that *every* individual possesses *both* molecular variants. One illustration is the existence of two insulin molecules in the rat. In this instance the duplication has not led to any known adaptive divergence of the two molecules, but it is the possibility that such divergence may follow gene duplication that gives the process its great evolutionary potential. As we shall see later, it must surely be the explanation of the establishment of two series of neurohypophysial polypeptides in the gnathostome vertebrates.

Molecules that have evolved in this way are said to be homologous, using the terminology that is familiar at the level of whole-animal studies. We mean by this that similarities in amino-acid sequences (isology) are a consequence of derivation from a common ancestral pattern, with subsequent divergence. To establish homology convincingly, it is desirable to be able to show that the similarities are greater than could be ascribed to chance, and that only a minimal number of the invariant sites are required for the functioning of the molecule. If all the identical sites are required for functioning, then the similarities may be due to analogy, which is defined as similarity in structure resulting from similarity in function. It is fair to add that, in an endocrinological context, the case for homology is strengthened if the two hormones are secreted in the same tissue, or in closely related tissues. This is obviously the case with the neurohypophysial hormones.

It will be helpful to mention here certain other hormones which illustrate the application of this principle of evolution by diversification from a common molecular origin after gene duplication. These are the hormones of the gastro-intestinal tract (p. 20), corticotropin and the melanophore-stimulating hormones (pp. 205, 213), and somatotropin, prolactin, and human placental lactogen (p. 123). We shall see that in all these instances it may be assumed that selection has favoured the divergence of the products of duplication so as to give two or more distinct hormones, with different functions.

6.6 Molecular evolution and the neurohypophysial hormones

We may now illustrate these general principles by applying them in more detail to the neurohypophysial hormones. Taking first the simpler situation presented by the 'basic' molecules (Fig. 6.11), we can

Arginine vasotocin	Arginine vasopressin	Lysine vasopressin
3-isoleucine AUC $\longrightarrow$ AUU $\longrightarrow$	3-phenylalanine UUC UUU	
	8-arginine AGA $\longrightarrow$ AGG $\longrightarrow$	8-lysine AAA AAG

FIG. 6.11. Possible paths of molecular evolution in the 'basic' series of neurohypophysial hormones.

postulate that the evolutionary series began with arginine vasotocin, that this mutated to arginine vasopressin during the emergence of mammals, and that this mutated again to lysine vasopressin in certain groups. Reference to the genetic code shows that each of these steps can, in theory, be effected by a single base change. Either of two codons specifying isoleucine can change in this way to give the codon for arginine. The subsequent substitution of lysine for arginine could be effected equally simply, starting, however, with one of two different codons for this amino acid. This substitution of one set of arginine codons for another could be attributed to 'silent mutation', as explained above.

The origin of the second line of evolution, comprising the 'neutral' molecules, must be ascribed to gene duplication, since agnathans have only the one 'basic' molecule. Presumably this duplication occurred when gnathostomes separated from their agnathan ancestors. (We are assuming, for the sake of simplicity, that there has not been a loss of a 'neutral' hormone during the history of the living cyclostomes, although the possibility of this cannot be excluded.) The interpretation of the subsequent history of the 'neutral' hormones depends upon whether mesotocin or oxytocin is regarded as the first of the two molecules to have appeared. The wide distribution of mesotocin in lower forms suggests that it is the more primitive, and that oxytocin evolved from it. Against this view, however, is the existence of oxytocin in holocephalans, which could be held to suggest that it is this molecule which is the more primitive one.

If we adopt the first view, it is possible to derive mesotocin from arginine vasotocin by a single base change, a further base change then giving rise to oxytocin (Fig. 6.12). If we adopt the second view (that oxytocin is the more primitive), it is necessary to invoke the intervention of silent mutations, for oxytocin cannot be derived from arginine vasotocin by only one base change. Thereafter, however, a single change will transform oxytocin into mesotocin. But if this second alternative was indeed the true course of events, how do we then derive the oxytocin of mammals? One suggestion is that this molecule, established early in the vertebrate line, might have persisted without change in the line leading to mammals. We have seen that the possibility of oxytocin being present in lung-fish and reptiles cannot be wholly excluded, and we obviously do not know whether or not it was present in the rhipidistian ancestors of tetrapods. Alternatively, it is possible that mesotocin, having evolved from oxytocin, might

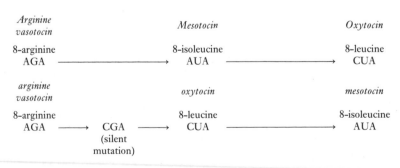

FIG. 6.12. Possible paths of molecular evolution in the 'neutral' series of neurohypophysial hormones.

then have mutated back to oxytocin through a single base change. We have no way of deciding between these possibilities on present evidence.

These arguments are highly theoretical. Moreover, they do not account for the evolution of the other hormones of the 'basic' series, which raises difficult issues that are outside our present scope. In any case, it is obvious that fact gleaned from a few dozen of the 50 000 or so living species of vertebrates cannot possibly provide a complete phylogenetic history at the molecular level; too much theorizing at this level of knowledge is apt to be unproductive. Even if the evidence were more complete, it would still be difficult to judge what allowance should be made for reverse mutation, parallel mutation, and silent mutation. Moreover, it is far from clear that we are justified in assuming that the history of the neurohypophysial hormones must comprise a continuous line of hormonally active peptides. We cannot exclude the possibility that gene duplication may have resulted in the production of inactive peptides that underwent successive mutations until they gave rise to newly active molecules, which then came again under the influence of natural selection.

It is worth noting also that some 200 analogues of oxytocin and vasopressin have been synthesized, and their biological properties studied. It is an impressive figure, yet the calculated number of nonapeptide analogues that might theoretically be produced is of the order of 512 billion. It may be unwise then, to say the least, to assume that the few neurohypophysial hormones which have so far been chemically characterized in vertebrates are the only ones actually present in them. Others may also exist, without being distinguishable by their biological properties in the only tests that our ingenuity has so far devised. The difficulty in distinguishing oxytocin from mesotocin is a case in point.

The uncertainties, it must in fairness be added, are not confined to molecular analysis, for the much richer resources of comparative anatomy and palaeontology are insufficient to establish with certainty the relationships of the main groups of fish. It is possible that elasmobranchs and holocephalans were derived from a common chondrichthyan ancestry, and the Dipnoi (lung-fish) and actinopterygians from a common osteicthyan ancestry. It may even be that cartilaginous and bony fish ultimately diverged from a common fish-like ancestor, but none of these supposed ancestral stocks can be identified, and they certainly have no living representatives. Clearly there is no assistance here for divining the relationships between, for example, the oxytocin of holocephalans

and the glumitocin, valitocin, and aspartocin of elasmobranchs, or the relative antiquity of oxytocin and mesotocin. Simpson has argued that molecular phylogeny needs to be confirmed by being tested against a framework provided by comparative anatomical data, but in this instance even the framework itself is only of limited value.

What we can tentatively conclude on present evidence is that cyclostomes have only one neurohypophysial hormone, and that each major group of gnathostomes has at least two, which are either peculiar to it, or shared with groups that are believed to have evolved from it (Fig. 6.13). Further, we can trace two main lines of molecular evolution of these hormones, although the course of events in the 'neutral' line is still very uncertain. We would suppose, according to the conventional view of evolutionary change, that the molecular variations established in these two lines have been determined by natural selection acting on random mutation. Yet the implication that new neurohypophysial molecules have evolved in adaptation to new needs, and to improve prospects of survival, is by no means self-evidently correct. An extreme example is given by the amphibians. Their need to conserve water is mediated by arginine vasotocin, but this did not evolve in relation to this need. It is supposedly the most ancient hormone in the whole neurohypophysial series, and the amphibians simply turned an old hormone to new use. This was rendered possible by adaptation of target tissues (in this instance the skin, kidney, and bladder), according to the principle that we discuss elsewhere (p. 180).

Seen from this point of view, these hormones show remarkable stability, in contrast to the readiness with which the molecular chemist can produce such a wide range of analogues. It is possible, however, to suggest a reason for this stability, arising from the principle that endocrine regulation depends upon mutual adaptation of hormone and target. A hormone fulfils functions that are part of a complex system of regulatory responses, in which are involved interactions with other hormones, as well as co-ordinated responses of a diversity of targets. A change in the hormonal molecule, with consequent changes in its properties, would be likely to throw the whole system out of alignment. Mutations that would produce such changes would be unacceptable (p. 100), and would be rejected by natural selection. In general, then, one may suppose that evolutionary change in the endocrine system is most likely to proceed by keeping the molecule unaltered, and by modifying instead the properties of those targets that

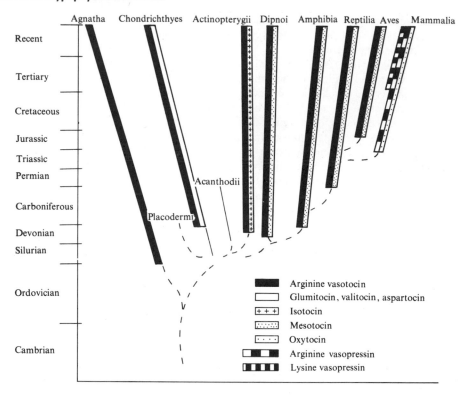

FIG. 6.13. A phylogenetic tree of the main vertebrate groups, to which has been added the distribution of the hypothalamic neuro-hypophysial hormones. The distribution indicated is an extrapolation from the information available for a small number of species. *Long dashes in bars*, arginine vasopressin; *black*, arginine vasotocin; *white*, glumitocin; *crosses*, ichthyotocin; *short dashes in bars*, lysine vasopressin; *close dots*, mesotocin; *spaced dots*, oxytocin.

are needed to contribute to the new adaptive requirements.

But if this is so, why have these neurohypophysial hormones varied at all? The question is difficult to answer. We have seen that these hormones must have played an important part in the adaptation of vertebrates to terrestrial life, but how far were these functions established before this adventure was undertaken? Conditions in fish are clearly critical for this analysis. Unfortunately, however, it has not yet been possible to demonstrate clearly a physiological role for the neurohypophysial hormones in these animals. This is partly because the mammalian hormones were commonly used in earlier work, so that any responses elicited may have been only pharmacological. More recently it has been possible to use arginine vasotocin, so that the situation is improved.

One fact clearly established is that there is no water-balance response in cyclostomes or fish; this seems to be an exclusively amphibian adaptation, evolved in response to their peculiar needs. Some effects upon ion and water fluxes have been observed,

however, in these lower forms. Arginine vasotocin increases sodium loss in lampreys, mainly by an action on the kidney which results in an increase of sodium in the urine. Other hormones, however, such as oxytocin, also have this effect. In teleosts, the effects of injections of arginine vasotocin vary with the dose; higher ones promote diuresis, whereas lower ones are antidiuretic. Here, too, there is also an action on sodium flux; extrarenal flux is increased in fresh-water fish and outflux increased in sea-water ones. The physiological significance of these scattered results is at present wholly obscure. Information is too limited, and derived from too few species, to permit generalization, and in any case there are other hormones that are certainly involved in osmoregulatory responses in these aquatic animals. Doubtless, therefore, there is much hormonal interaction in this field, and these aspects will be examined further in other contexts (pp. 122, 202).

As far as the neurohypophysial hormones are concerned, we can only bear in mind at this stage that the several molecules may be adaptively advantageous in lower vertebrates in ways that we have not yet been able to detect because we do not know what to look for. It is also conceivable that polypeptide variation is a facet of the general evolution of protein specificity. If this is so, the variations may not be exclusively related to the establishment of new functions, but may reflect also the need to ensure the retention of the old ones. There is nothing simple about these biological problems, and there is nothing simple about molecular history.

Finally, we remarked earlier that discussion of the evolution of the neurohypophysial hormones provides a good model for considering the evolution of polypeptide hormones in general. Their value in this connection can be illustrated by returning to some of the hormones discussed in Chapters 2, 3, and 4. These hormones (gastrin, secretin, cholecystokinin, pancreozymin, and others) have many features in common. They are all polypeptides, they originate in the alimentary epithelium or its derivatives, certain of them share common structural features in the primary structure of their molecules, and they show some overlap in properties.

Substances with certain of these properties are already present in agnathans and, as we have seen, may be present in invertebrates as well. They have still to be chemically characterized, but it seems reasonable to conclude that the vertebrate alimentary tract possessed from a very early stage a capacity to secrete biologically active polypeptides. Consideration of the structural resemblances of the mammalian molecules suggests the further conclusion that these polypeptides became diversified in structure and function early in vertebrate history, in correlation with the progressive morphological and physiological specialization of the digestive system. There are no obvious structural resemblances between the molecules of secretin, CCK/PZ, and insulin; these, then,

may well have evolved along independent lines, as products of the secretory capacity of the alimentary tract. On the other hand, the remarkable resemblances between the molecules of secretin and glucagon (together with gastric inhibitory polypeptide and motilin) suggest, by analogy with the neurohypophysial hormones, that they may have evolved by diversification from a single ancestral type of molecule, after gene duplication. The same conclusion is suggested by the resemblances between gastrin and CCK/PZ, which might similarly have evolved from a common origin by gene duplication and diversification.

These arguments are speculative, yet they can fairly be said to be rooted in reality. Further, they suggest that the molecular diversification of polypeptide hormonal molecules may well have been a process of fundamental biological importance in ensuring evolutionary progress. For example, the capacity of the alimentary tract to secrete these polypeptides, and the potentiality for diversification which went with it, would have provided a pool of hormonal variability, capable of establishing new adaptive relationships with evolving target organs. Such a pool must have been of great survival value. How could the pancreas, for example, have evolved without the simultaneous elaboration of some mechanisms for co-ordinating its activity with the flow of material through the alimentary canal? The nervous system could doubtless have played a part, although its role in the lower vertebrates has not yet been adequately elucidated. But the potentiality for hormonal diversification, and thus for the continued improvement of chemical regulation of digestion and metabolism of the food, must have greatly facilitated the evolution of the vertebrates, and not least because of the demands imposed by their active and predatory mode of life.

7

Hormones and reproduction I

7.1. Steroid hormones

Steroids are widely distributed organic compounds that have a molecular structure based upon a four-ring system called the perhydro[1,2]cyclopenteno-phenanthrene nucleus. The sterols are one example. These are steroid alcohols, the most familiar being cholesterol; others are 7-dehydrocholesterol (present in the skin, and converted into a form of vitamin D by ultraviolet light) and ergosterol (present in yeast and moulds, and a precursor of vitamin D). Other examples of steroids are bile acids, plant glycosides called sapogenins and cardenolides (the last-named being of value in cardiac therapy and in the making of arrow poisons), and toad venom. In addition, steroids are used as hormones in vertebrates and in insects.

It is not clear whether other invertebrate groups secrete steroid hormones, although there is suggestive evidence, particularly from crustaceans and molluscs, that they may do. Many invertebrate tissues possess enzymes that can carry out one or other of the steps of vertebrate steroid biosynthesis, but it does not follow from this that they possess all the enzymes required for a typical vertebrate biosynthetic sequence. Moreover, the evidence often comes from *in vitro* studies with added precursors,

and it does not necessarily follow that such precursors are the natural substrates of the enzymes. Further, the identification of the products has not always satisfied the increasingly rigorous demands of this difficult branch of organic chemistry. What may be reasonably concluded is that some capacity either to produce steroids, or to metabolize them, is universal in living systems, and that the associated biosynthetic pathways were established at a very early stage of evolution. The functional significance of this is unknown. It may be that steroid products often function locally in the tissues or cells that manufacture them, and that this was the origin of their use as hormones. What is clear is that vertebrates, very early in their history, turned this capacity to the purposes of endocrine regulation, with the production of a series of hormones with wide-ranging functions.

An understanding of the chemistry of these biologically important compounds dates from 1932, when Rosenheim and King established the correct structural formula of cholesterol. King has told how, at the time when the formula deduced by Wieland and Windaus was proving unsatisfactory, he said to Rosenheim on the spur of the moment: 'why don't you take ring II in the Windaus–Wieland structure

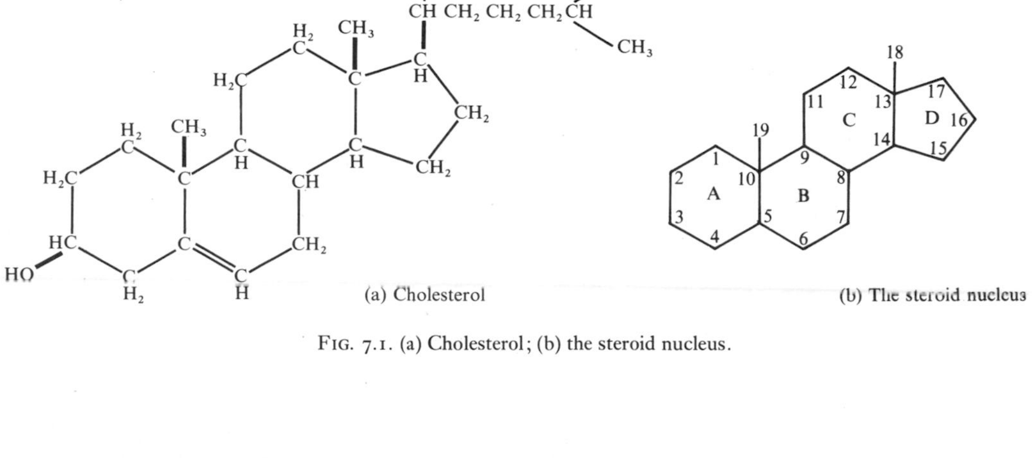

(a) Cholesterol

(b) The steroid nucleus

FIG. 7.1. (a) Cholesterol; (b) the steroid nucleus.

and put it on the other side of ring I so as to produce a potential chrysene structure?', and how Rosenheim took the problem home and returned the next morning to exclaim excitedly—'It fits, it fits!'.

The formula of cholesterol is shown in Fig. 7.1. For descriptive purposes the carbon atoms receive a conventional numbering which is shown in the figure; a side chain is attached at C-17, and methyl groups are attached in the angles at C-10 and C-13, although these are not necessarily always present in steroids. Side-chain carbon atoms are numbered from 20 onwards.

Steroids are regarded as being derived from one or other of five parent substances, cholane, cholestane, oestrane, androstane, and pregnane. These are modified by the incorporation of double bonds and substituent groups which are referred to by the prefixes or suffixes given in Table 7.1, the position of these being indicated by stating the carbon atom with which they are associated. Thus 1,3,5(10)-triene indicates the presence of double bonds between C-1 and C-2, C-3 and C-4, and C-5, and C-10, both numbers being given when the two atoms concerned are not consecutively numbered. Only one kind of substituent group in each compound is indicated by a suffix; the remainder are designated by prefixes, the decision as to which of the groups shall be selected for the suffix being determined by agreed convention.

TABLE 7.1

Some prefixes and suffixes used in steroid nomenclature

Group	Prefix	Suffix
Olefinic double bond, C:C	Δ†	ene
Hydroxyl, OH	hydroxy	ol
Carbonyl (keto), C:O	oxo	one

di, tri, tetra, penta = 2, 3, 4, 5
† This prefix is no longer correct in formal nomenclature

The stereochemistry of the molecule is an important aspect of its interpretation, for since there are eight asymmetric carbon atoms (at positions 3, 5, 9, 10, 14, and 17) it can theoretically exist in 256 (i.e. 2^8) stereoisomeric forms. In our analysis we shall be concerned with only a few of these, but it is well to remember that this complication greatly adds to the difficulty of synthesizing the steroid hormones. For graphical representation the nucleus is regarded as being planar and as lying in the plane of the paper; those groups which then lie below this plane are called α, and their bonds are drawn as broken lines, those, including the angle methyl groups, lying above this plane are called β, and their bonds are drawn as heavy continuous lines, while a wavy line shows that the configuration is unknown. The configuration of the substituent groups is indicated by the appropriate Greek letter placed before the term indicating their nature, while C-5 is always represented either as 5α or 5β, unless there is a double bond at this point, because the stereoisomerism at C-5 is particularly variable. Thus the systematic name for cholesterol is cholest-5-en-3β-ol, and for pregnanediol (Fig. 7.11) is 5β-pregnane-3α,20α-diol. In practice it is usually more convenient to refer to the steroid hormones by their trivial names, for the commonest of these are internationally accepted; to avoid confusion, however, it is well to quote the systematic name once in each article in which reference is made to a particular hormone.

The steroid hormones of vertebrates are secreted by the testis, ovary, and adrenocortical tissue, all of which are linked embryologically by their development from the coelomic epithelium. In addition, they are also secreted by the mammalian placenta, which makes an important contribution to the hormonal regulation of pregnancy. The various hormones are the products of metabolic pathways that have many features in common; so, as might be expected, the cells that secrete them have common features that facilitate their identification.

These cells (Fig. 7.2) have a well-developed endo-

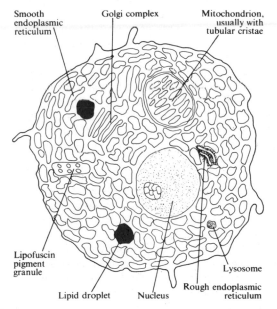

FIG. 7.2. Diagram of ultrastructure of steroid-secreting cell. (From *Research in Reproduction* 3, no. 5. International Planned Parenthood Association.)

plasmic reticulum, which is agranular, in contrast to the granular type found in protein-secreting cells, while their mitochondria are characterized by possessing tubular cristae. There is often much lipid material in the cytoplasm, demonstrable by the fat-soluble Sudan dyes, such as Sudan black; usually the lipid contains cholesterol, which is a precursor of the hormones. Variations in this lipid content may give a good indication of the functional state of the cells, and of cycles in hormone production. A particularly useful characteristic is the presence of the Δ^5-3β-hydroxysteroid dehydrogenase (3β-HSDH) system, which mediates the formation of Δ^4-ketosteroids, such as progesterone, from Δ^5-3β-hydroxysteroids, such as pregnenolone. In practice, this system is required for the biosynthesis of virtually all of the steroid hormones. Its presence (which can be visualized histochemically), in conjunction with cholesterol-positive lipid, thus gives a very firm basis for the identification of steroidogenic endocrine tissues.

The identification and quantitative assay of the steroid hormones themselves, however, is beset with technical difficulties. Two main types of procedure are available: *in vivo* and *in vitro*. *In vivo* procedures are especially valuable when it is possible to sample the effluent blood from an endocrine organ, but this may be quite impossible in lower animals, owing to their size, and to anatomical problems. In any case, there is always the difficulty that the titre of circulating steroids is very low.

In vitro procedures, involving the incubation of tissue in media containing appropriate precursors, is often more practicable, but here, too, there are many problems to be overcome. As with all incubations, the results may be confused by the accumulation of metabolites, although it may be possible to overcome this by using some type of continuous flow procedure. But there is a more fundamental difficulty. The fact that a tissue can metabolize a precursor into an identifiable product does no more than demonstrate that a particular enzyme system is present. It does not mean that this reaction necessarily takes place *in vivo*; to show that it does so, it is essential to demonstrate that the added precursor is one that is normally present in the tissue.

A basic difficulty in steroid investigations is that the hormones are only present in very small quantities, not only in the body fluids but also in the glands. The large amount of lipid in steroid-secreting tissues is misleading in this respect, for only very small amounts of the hormone may actually be stored, a situation especially characteristic of adrenocortical

tissue. Methods are thus required that permit the study of microgram or nanogram quantities. This has required the development of ultramicrochemical methods relying on various types of chromatography, on spectrometry, and on the use of isotopically-labelled reference compounds, in conjunction with highly sensitive and sophisticated counting equipment. Derivative formation is also valuable, particularly as used in the double-isotope derivative assay, which permits the measurement of steroids in amounts of 10^{-7}–10^{-10} g. Another sensitive procedure makes use of a system in which the steroid being investigated competes with a labelled authentic compound for the binding sites on a globulin (transcortin) that is found in blood plasma and that selectively binds steroid molecules. Displacement of the labelled steroid can be measured, and this gives a measure of the amount of the other steroid that is present.

Much of the earlier work on steroids, including those of the lower vertebrates and of the invertebrates, was carried out before these sensitive procedures had been developed, or were even practicable. The results of such valuable pioneer work are often highly suggestive, but the amount of completely convincing data, judged by the most rigorous standards, is still very small, and this, as we shall see, often makes generalization very difficult.

7.2. Reproduction and periodicity

Sexual reproduction involves in most animals a marked periodicity, the analysis of which has been the foundation of much of our present understanding of hormonal interactions in the vertebrates, and of the unique status of the pituitary gland.

The existence of sexual cycles arises in part from the fact that the production of germ cells, and the behavioural adaptations that are essential to ensure successful insemination, are physiologically exhausting and often necessitate a relatively quiescent period for recovery. This by itself, however, would not result in all sexually mature members of a population passing through the same phase of the cycle at about the same time, as they very often do. The need for this arises from the fact that conditions favourable for reproduction and, in particular, for the rearing of the young, are commonly restricted to a limited period of the year, determined by the nature of the climatic variations which the species encounters. We may therefore expect to find that these cycles are of a highly adaptive character.

Sexual periodicity, then, has a dual basis, and this is reflected in the physiological mechanisms by which

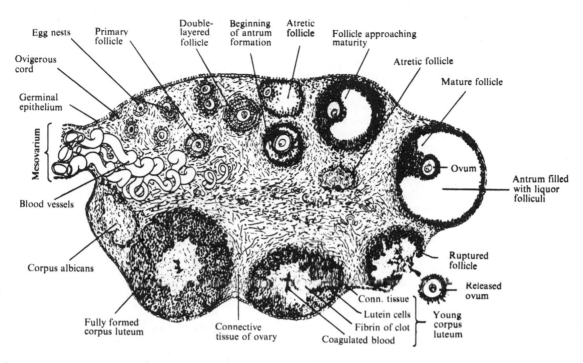

FIG. 7.3. Schematic diagram of a mammalian ovary, showing the sequence of events in the origin, growth, and rupture of the Graafian follicle, and the formation and retrogression of the corpus luteum. Follow clockwise around the ovary, starting at the mesovarium. (From Patten (1958). *Fundamentals of embryology.* McGraw-Hill, New York.)

it is controlled, for these depend in part upon endogenous factors (arising within the body) and in part upon exogenous ones (arising in the outside world). Important amongst the former are the gonadal hormones secreted by the ovary and testis, while the latter include a variety of stimuli such as those provided by temperature, daylight, rainfall, and the presence of other individuals, the relative importance of these depending upon the mode of life of the species concerned. Further, the pituitary gland is of central importance in effecting the co-ordination of these endogenous and exogenous factors, as a consequence of its being related to the outside world through the nervous system and receptors, and to the rest of the endocrine system by a complex pattern of hormonal interactions. In attempting an analysis of this situation we shall begin by considering the mammals, for it is research on that group which has so far provided the most complete data. We shall then turn to review some aspects of sexual periodicity in other vertebrates, to see how far the principles established for mammals can be regarded as of general applicability throughout the group.

7.3. The mammalian ovary

The ovary of mammals (Fig. 7.3) is formed of an outer cortex and an inner medulla, the latter small in extent and possessing large blood vessels. The cortex contains follicles in all stages of development, the smallest consisting of a single layer of flattened epithelial cells surrounding a primary oocyte; between the follicles extends a dense stroma containing spindle-shaped interstitial cells. Externally the cortex forms a dense tunica albuginea, composed of muscle cells and connective tissue, and external to this again is the germinal epithelium, continuous with the peritoneal epithelium and formed of more or less cubical cells, from which arise oogonia and follicle cells.

Far more follicles are formed than ever complete their development, and many undergo a regression called follicular atresia. Those that do complete it undergo immediately prior to ovulation an enormous enlargement, brought about by proliferation of the follicular epithelium and by the accumulation of fluid. Initially, the follicle cells become cubical or columnar, and multiply to form several layers, while a zona pellucida appears around the oocyte, perhaps by transformation of the cell membrane, and the surrounding stroma becomes organized into a theca. Later, the follicle becomes vesicular as a result of the increasing accumulation of fluid amongst its cells, and it thus becomes transformed into the mature Graafian follicle.

In its fully developed form, this consists of a peripheral layer, several cells thick, called the membrana granulosa; the latter encloses a cavity, the antrum, filled with the fluid, or liquor folliculi, into which projects a thickening of the granulosa. This thickening, the cumulus oöphorus, contains the much-enlarged oocyte, the cells immediately surrounding this being the corona radiata. Externally to the membrana granulosa, the theca has differentiated into the theca externa and the theca interna; the former is fibrous and seems to be primarily a supporting tissue, but the large cells of the theca interna contain cholesterol-rich lipid and give a strong 3β-HSDH reaction. For this reason, and because the lipid becomes depleted at the height of oestrus (p. 129), it seems likely that this tissue is the source of the ovarian oestrogen that we shall discuss later. The interstitial tissue, comprising epithelioid cells lying between the follicles, probably secretes ovarian androgens (p. 112).

When the oocyte has been discharged from the ovary, usually after the first maturation division, its follicle becomes transformed into an endocrine gland, the corpus luteum. This involves an enlargement of certain of the granulosa cells, which assume a polygonal shape, while lipoid droplets and lipochrome pigments accumulate in them; in this way they are transformed into the characteristic luteal cells, some of which also arise from the theca interna. A supporting framework is then formed around the cells by connective tissue and blood vessels, which extend inwards from the theca interna, and perhaps

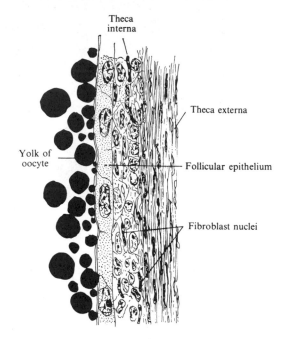

Fig. 7.4. The ovarian follicle of the platypus (*Ornithorhynchus*). (a) Follicular wall of oocyte, about 3 mm in diameter.

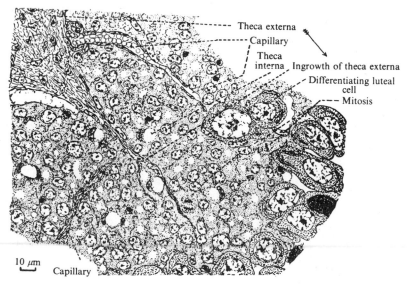

(b) Portion of wall of corpus luteum. (From Hill and Gatenby (1926). *Proc. zool. Soc. Lond.* **2**.)

also from the theca externa. This completes the development of an important endocrine gland, the essential features of which are already established in the Monotremata (Fig. 7.4). When its period of duty is ended (its function will be considered later), it degenerates into a whitish body, the corpus albicans, which sinks deeper into the ovarian stroma and eventually disappears.

7.4. Oestrogens

Brown-Séquard is said to have been the first to suggest, in 1889, that the ovary might be an internally secreting organ. It was at about this time that the therapeutic value of thyroid extracts was becoming established, and, following his suggestion, extensive use was optimistically made of extract of ovaries, but the attempts were premature and the results highly variable. Later and more successful developments derive from the studies of F. H. A. Marshall and Jolly on the reproductive system of the dog, as a result of which they expressed in 1906 the view that 'the ovary is an organ providing an internal secretion which is elaborated by the follicular epithelial cells or by the interstitial cells of the stroma. After ovulation, which takes place during oestrus, the corpus luteum is formed, and this organ provides a further secretion whose function is essential for the changes taking place during the attachment and development of the embryo in the first stages of pregnancy.'

This concept of the ovary as an endocrine organ won increasing acceptance during the early years of the century, but the turning-point in the investigation of its secretory activity came with the development by Allen and Doisy in 1923 of a simple and reliable bioassay method. This method, which owed much to the fact that these two investigators brought biological and biochemical experience into association, is another good example (p. 57) of the way in which biological research often waits upon the development of the proper tools. Coupled with the large expansion of research after the First World War, it initiated an intense concentration upon sexual endocrinology.

The method of Allen and Doisy depends upon the fact that the sexual activity of most female mammals is based upon the recurrence of an oestrous cycle (*oistros*, gadfly). In rats and mice the successive stages of this are characterized by clearly defined changes in the vaginal epithelium, so that by taking samples of this from the living animal, and by studying vaginal smear preparations made from them (Fig. 8.1, p. 129), it is possible to follow the whole course of the cycle. Moreover, this cycle is absent from sexually immature animals or from those which have undergone ovariectomy (removal of the ovaries). Thus, by injecting test substances into them and examining their vaginal smears, it is possible to determine which of the substances can evoke the cycle, those which have this property being termed oestrogens (estrogens in the U.S.A.).

Oestrogenic activity was readily demonstrable in ovarian extracts prepared with lipid solvents, but for a time investigators were still handicapped by the extreme difficulty of purifying the very small quantities of material which were available. Another important advance, however, was made in 1927 when Aschheim and Zondek showed that there was a large concentration of activity in the urine in pregnant women, for extracts obtained from this abundant source, and later from the urine of stallions and of pregnant mares, lent themselves much more satisfactorily to chemical processing.

The first oestrogen to be identified was oestrone (Fig. 7.5), the isolation of which in pure crystalline form was announced in 1929, while a second, the less active oestriol, was isolated in 1930. Both were obtained from human pregnancy urine, and are excretory products. In 1935, 12 mg of a much more potent oestrogen was isolated from four tons of pig ovaries, and it is this substance, 17β-oestradiol, which is the principal ovarian hormone of mammals. (There is asymmetry at C-17; 17α-oestradiol is also known, but is a much weaker oestrogen.) 17β-oestradiol is one of the essential factors in the regulation of the oestrous cycle (p. 129); in many mammals it increases the spontaneous activity of the uterine muscle, and it also promotes the development of the ductules of the mammary glands (p. 120) and the development and maintenance of the genital tract. The onset of puberty is marked by an increased output of this hormone. The result is an increase in growth rate of the uterus and vagina, the external genitalia, the mammae, the pelvis, and the pubic and axillary hair.

In discussions of such characters a distinction is sometimes made in both sexes between the primary sexual characters (the gonads), the accessory sexual characters (those, such as the male and female duct systems, which are of obvious and direct value in reproduction), and the secondary sexual characters (those—such as colour, plumage, antlers, hair distribution in the human, and, indeed, a whole host of features extending from the red belly of the stickleback to the leg elevation of the urinating male dog—which were thought at one time to have no obvious reproductive value). In fact, however, these second-

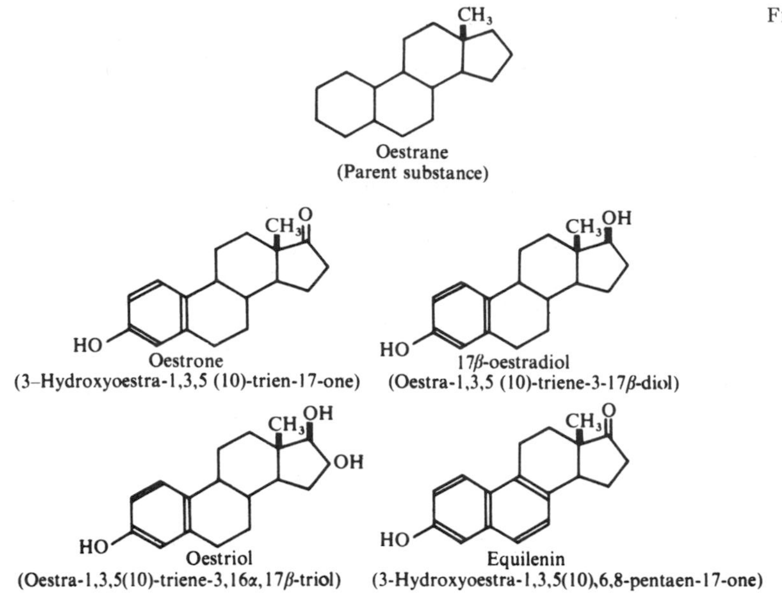

Oestrane
(Parent substance)

FIG. 7.5. Oestrogens.

Oestrone
(3–Hydroxyoestra-1,3,5 (10)-trien-17-one)

17β-oestradiol
(Oestra-1,3,5 (10)-triene-3-17β-diol)

Oestriol
(Oestra-1,3,5(10)-triene-3,16α,17β-triol)

Equilenin
(3-Hydroxyoestra-1,3,5(10),6,8-pentaen-17-one)

ary sexual characters often play a vital part in bringing the sexes together, in co-ordinating their sexual activity, and in ensuring successful fertilization. Thus the distinction between accessory and secondary characters is a false one, and it is not surprising to find that they are commonly under similar hormonal control through the gonads, although there are exceptions to this.

The structural formulae of the three oestrogens mentioned above are shown in Fig. 7.5. They contain eighteen carbon atoms and are therefore referred to as C_{18} steroids. Ring A (see Fig. 7.1, p. 106) is aromatic, the angle methyl group being absent from C-10, while the substitutent hydroxyl group at C-3 is phenolic. Oestrogens are formed by biosynthetic pathways (Fig. 7.6) which are common to all vertebrates, although there are quantitative and qualitative differences between species, and other variants are

also possible in particular groups. Cholesterol and the C_{21} compound pregnenolone are the principal precursors, as they are all of hormonal steroids, cholesterol being first formed from acetate and then transformed into pregnenolone. From pregnenolone are formed progesterone and then the C_{19} androgenic steroids, androstenedione and testosterone (Fig. 7.7). These are then aromatized to form the phenolic C_{18} oestrogens, probably with 19-hydroxytestosterone and 19-nortestosterone as intermediates (Fig. 7.8). 17β-oestradiol is metabolized into oestrone and oestriol, in part in the ovary but also in the liver, which is the main site of the intermediary metabolism of these compounds.

The ovary and the urine of females are not the only sources of oestrogens; they are also secreted in certain species by the testis and the adrenocortical tissue. Oestrone has been isolated from the urine of men, while in stallions it is the testis which is the tissue that is richest in oestrogens. The function of these substances in males is obscure, if, indeed, they have any functions at all, but we shall see that the oestrogens and androgens of the two sexes are chemically very closely related; indeed, some androgen is probably secreted by the interstitial tissue of the ovary. It is likely, and especially so in the adrenocortical tissue, that the biosynthetic activities of steroidogenic cells can be deflected into pathways leading to the production of substances different from those with which they are primarily concerned.

Oestrogens occur in plants as well as in animals,

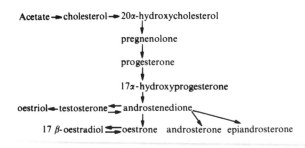

Acetate→cholesterol→20α-hydroxycholesterol

pregnenolone

progesterone

17α-hydroxyprogesterone

oestriol←testosterone⇄androstenedione

17 β-oestradiol⇄oestrone   androsterone epiandrosterone

FIG. 7.6. Biosynthesis of steroids, in simplified outline. Intermediate stages have been omitted.

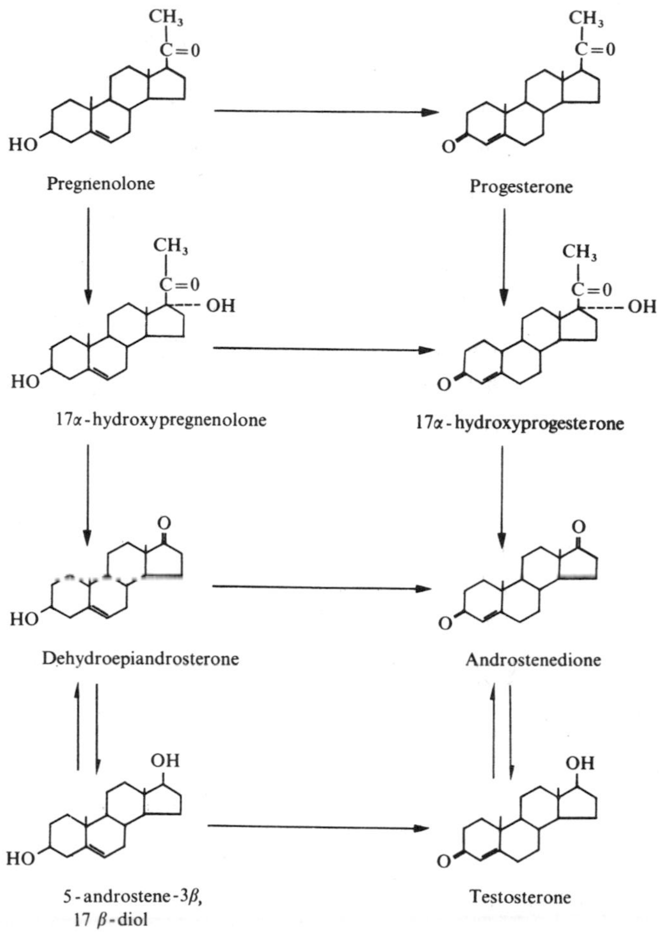

CH₃ structures...

FIG. 7.7. Biosynthesis of C_{19} steroids from C_{21} precursors in mammals. A similar sequence of reactions has been described for fishes, amphibians, reptiles, and birds. (From Sandor (1972). In *Steroids in non-mammalian vertebrates* (ed. D. R. Idler). Academic Press, New York.)

Pregnenolone — Progesterone

17α-hydroxypregnenolone — 17α-hydroxyprogesterone

Dehydroepiandrosterone — Androstenedione

5-androstene-3β, 17β-diol — Testosterone

ocstriol having been obtained from willow catkins and oestrone from palm kernels, but oestrogenic activity is not necessarily associated with the steroid nucleus, a point that is well illustrated by *Pueraria mirifica*. The tuberous roots of this Thailand plant have a remarkable reputation as rejuvenators and are capable, according to local tradition, of prolonging human life to as much as 280 years. Such value as they may have is probably dependent upon their considerable oestrogenic potency. The active substance, known as miroestrol (Fig. 7.9), has been obtained in a pure form and chemical studies have shown that it is not a steroid. The reason for its activity is not clear, but it has been suggested that it may be a chance consequence of some feature of its molecular pattern, the distance from 3-OH to 18-OH being very similar to that from 3-OH to 17-OH in the oestradiol molecule. However, this cannot always be the explanation of such a situation, as is shown by the

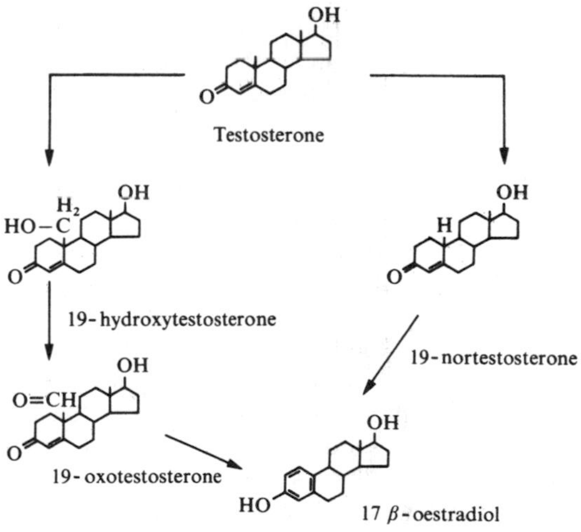

Testosterone

19-hydroxytestosterone

19-oxotestosterone

19-nortestosterone

17β-oestradiol

FIG. 7.8. Aromatization of C_{19} steroids to C_{18} steroids. (From Ozon (1972). In *Steroids in non-mammalian vertebrates* (ed. D. R. Idler). Academic Press, New York.)

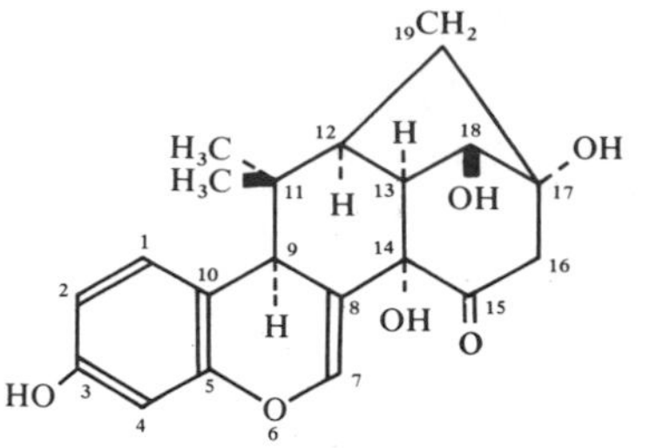

FIG. 7.9. Miroestrol. (From Cain (1960). *Nature* 188.)

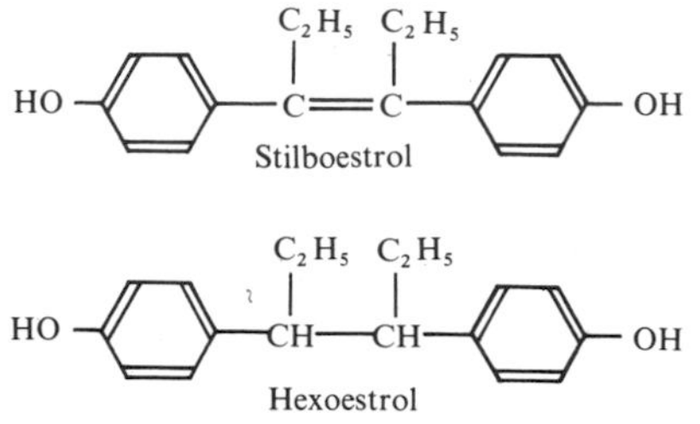

FIG. 7.10. Stilboestrol and hexoestrol.

synthetic compounds of the stilboestrol series (Fig. 7.10).

These are artificial oestrogens in the sense that they have the biological activity of oestrogens but do not occur under natural conditions. Unlike the naturally occurring hormones, they are highly active when taken by mouth, because they resist metabolism and inactivation in the liver. Therefore they have been used extensively for clinical treatment, particularly in the control of cancer of the prostate. They have also been used by the livestock industry, owing to the fact that their administration to poultry, by the insertion of a pellet under the skin, evokes changes in lipid metabolism; associated with these is an increased deposition of fat in the breast muscle and a bleaching of the flesh which combine to make old capons much more acceptable to the housewife. A different effect results from the addition of the substance to cattle feed, for this leads to increased stimulation of protein anabolism, with accelerated gain in weight and increased efficiency of feed conversion.

The molecular structure of the stilboestrols is substantially different from that of the steroids, and the explanation of their oestrogenic properties remains uncertain. There is no doubt, however, of the reality of these; they were sufficiently illustrated by the enlargement of the breasts and the sexual impotence which developed in male workers who were inadequately protected from the inhalation of

contaminated dust when the commercial manufacture of stilboestrol was first introduced. These effects, like the influence on the prostate, probably result in part from an interaction of this substance with the pituitary gland. Their occurrence, together with a possible risk of carcinogenic action, led to strict supervision of the use of artificial oestrogens in livestock production.

We have seen that, after ovulation, the Graafian follicle of the mammalian ovary becomes transformed into a corpus luteum. This is an endocrine gland, secreting the hormone progesterone (Fig. 7.11),

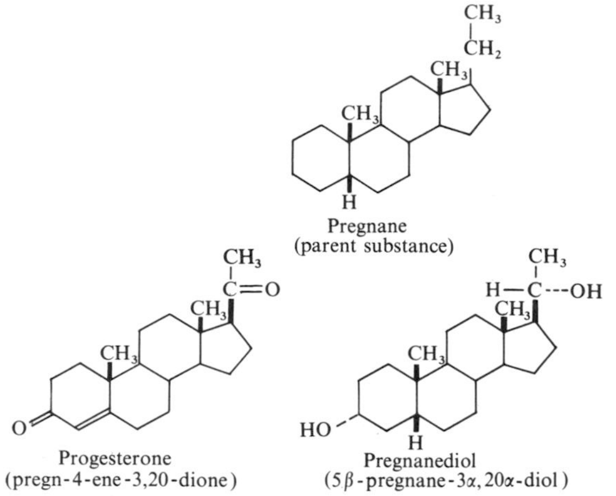

FIG. 7.11.

which is a C_{21} steroid and a diketone, with carbonyl groups at C-3 and C-20. The inactive steroid pregnanediol, present in urine, is a metabolic derivative of progesterone, and is formed by reduction in the liver. Progesterone promotes proliferation of the endometrium of the uterus in preparation for the implantation of the embryo, inhibits ovulation during pregnancy, and stimulates the growth of the mammary glandular tissue in preparation for lactation (p. 120). It is also responsible for the maintenance of pregnancy, so that in the mouse, for example, total ovariectomy at any stage of gestation is followed by abortion. In many species, however, the placenta is an important source of the hormone during the later stages of pregnancy (p. 146), so that fully functional corpora lutea may not then be present. Total removal of the ovaries in such species will only cause abortion if it is carried out during the earlier stages, before the endocrine functions of the placenta have become fully established.

Progesterone, being a precursor of androgens and

of corticosteroid hormones (Fig. 7.6), is produced throughout the vertebrates in both sexes. Evidently, therefore, mammals have introduced an already existing steroid metabolite into the regulation of their complicated reproductive cycle. Whether it has any hormonal function in non-mammalian forms is still uncertain (p. 143).

7.5. The mammalian testis and androgens

The outer wall of the mammalian testis is formed of a tough connective sheath, the tunica albuginea; this is covered on the outside by a mesothelium of the scrotal sac, and is continuous internally with a vascular layer, the tunica vasculosa. The main substance of the organ is formed of the much convoluted seminiferous tubules, which open through the rete testis into the epididymis, and through this into the vas deferens. The tubules are lined by the germinal epithelium, which is composed of two cell types, the spermatogonia and the Sertoli (sustentacular) cells. The latter (Fig. 7.12), which are interspersed with the spermatogonia, have been regarded as primarily nutritive, but there is increasing evidence that they are capable of androgen secretion. They have the ultrastructural features of steroidogenic cells, contain cholesterol-rich lipid and the 3β-HSDH system, and may well be responsible for the ability of isolated seminiferous tubules, incubated *in vitro*, to manufacture androstenedione and testosterone from progesterone. It is possible that their action *in vivo* is exerted locally upon germ cell production in the germinal epithelium.

Testicular steroidogenesis, however, with hormonal secretion into the blood stream, is mainly carried on by the interstitial (Leydig) cells, which are modified fibroblasts, readily seen as large polyhedral cells in the interstices of the tubules. They, too, have the ultrastructural and histochemical features of steroid-secreting tissue. Moreover, there is a close correlation between the state of development of this tissue and the sexual condition of the individual; one example of this is seen in Fig. 7.13. In man,

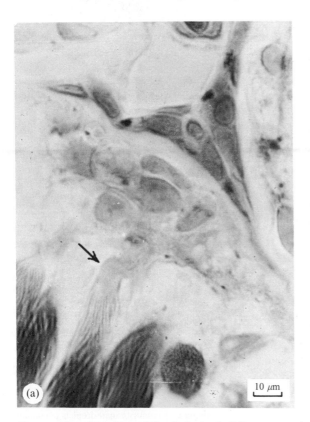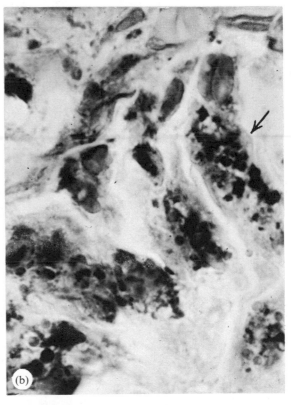

FIG. 7.12. Sertoli (sustentacular) cells (arrows) of *Rana temporaria*. In winter (a) they are generally without sudanophilic inclusions, but during the breeding season (b) they elongate and the cytoplasm becomes filled with sudanophilic droplets. Formol–saline, frozen, sudan black. (From Lofts and Bern, (1972). In *Steroids in nonmammalian vertebrates* (ed. D. R. Idler). Academic Press, New York and London.)

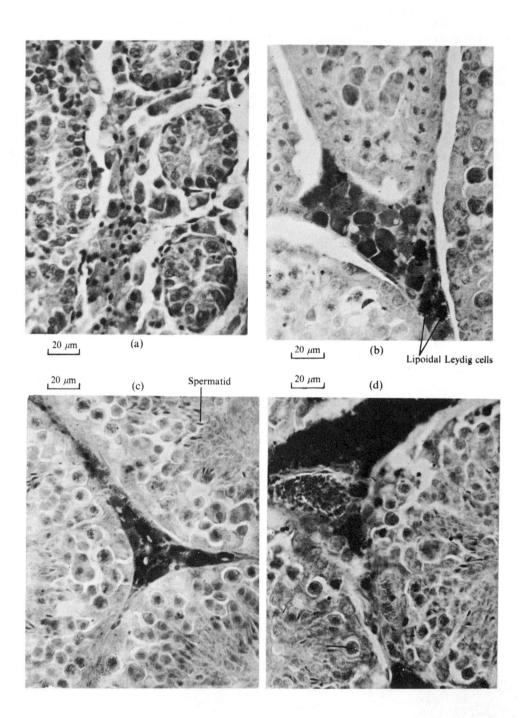

FIG. 7.13. Seasonal changes in the testis of the mole (*Talpa europaea*); this species is monoestrous, with a limited breeding season (in England) at the end of March. (a) Section of testis in early January; seminiferous tubules regressed, Leydig cells non-secretory. (b) Testis in February; spermatogenesis has begun and Leydig cells are beginning to accumulate lipid droplets (coloured here with Sudan black). (c) Testis in March; expansion of the tubules has constricted the interstitial tissue. (d) Testis in April; spermatogenesis is at its height and the Leydig cells are densely lipoidal. (From Lofts (1960). *Q. Jl microsp. Sci.* **101**.)

the interstitial tissue is well developed at birth, supposedly because of the action of maternal gonadotropins (p. 119); it soon reverts to fibroblast-like cells, and then develops once again at the onset of puberty.

The remarkable effects produced in mammals by the removal or degeneration of the testes have long been familiar in a variety of uses, as, for example, in the modification of the qualities of domestic livestock, or in the production of the male sopranos who, despite the penalty of excommunication associated with castration, were so characteristic a feature of the operatic stage and church choirs of eighteenth-century Italy. The credit for first recognizing that the testes were exerting an effect on the rest of the body through the blood stream is due to Berthold. John Hunter, in the eighteenth century, had shown that transplantation of these organs was a practicable operation. Berthold, reporting in 1849 the results of transplanting testes into four young castrated cocks, stated that two of the birds, with abdominal transplants, developed as normal cocks, whereas the other two, with no transplants, remained as capons. He did not interpret this as a result of the release from the transplanted testes of a specific secretion, nor could he have been expected to at that time. He did, however, conclude that the testes were exerting some influence upon the blood, and, through this, upon the rest of the body. He thus laid the foundations of the more specifically endocrine interpretation that gradually evolved later in the century, with the recognition of the regulatory functions of hormonal secretions.

Substances that show the masculinizing properties demonstrated by such transplantation experiments are known as androgens (*andros*, male), for their chief action is the promotion and maintenance of the male sexual characters (e.g. penis, prostate, seminal vesicles in mammals; comb and wattles in the fowl); these, like the corresponding characters of the female, usually atrophy in the absence of the gonads. In addition, the androgens stimulate the general growth of the body, and encourage nitrogen retention. The growth, under their influence, of the reduced comb

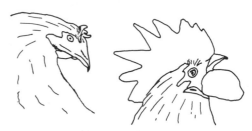

FIG. 7.14. *Left*, the head of a capon. *Right*, the head of the same animal after 22 daily injections of androsterone. (After Parkes (1935). *Biochem. J.* **29**.)

of the capon (Fig. 7.14) is the basis of a bioassay procedure. Testosterone, the most potent androgen, has been isolated from the mammalian testis, and may be the only male hormone actually produced in it in some species, although androstenedione has also been found in this organ. Two other androgens, androsterone and dehydroepiandrosterone, are present in urine as excretory products.

The molecular structure of these androgens is shown in Fig. 7.15. They are steroids, derived from the parent substance androstane, and, as we have already seen, are the precursors of the naturally occurring oestrogens, which they closely resemble in structure. They have angle methyl groups at C-10 and C-13, and an oxygen substituent instead of a side chain at C-17; they are therefore C_{19} steroids. Those with a carbonyl (ketone) group at C-17 (e.g. androstenedione) are referred to as 17-oxosteroids (formerly 17-ketosteroids). Like the oestrogens, they are largely inactive when given by mouth, because of inactivation by the liver, where they are conjugated with glucuronic or sulphonic acid. Methyl testosterone, however, which resists the liver's action, can be absorbed from the buccal mucosa. The biosynthetic pathways, related to those outlined earlier for the oestrogens, are shown in Fig. 7.7.

Many other androgenic steroids are known in addition to these three, derived either from natural sources or by synthesis. Included amongst them are a number (probably at least five) which have been isolated from the adrenocortical tissue (p. 206), and

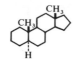

Androstane
(parent substance)

Testosterone
(17β-hydroxyandrost-4-en-3-one)

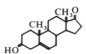

Androsterone
(3α-hydroxy-5α-androstan-17-one)

Dehydroepiandrosterone
(3β-hydroxyandrost-5-en-17-one)

FIG. 7.15. Androgens.

we shall see that over-production of these has an important bearing upon the development of sexual abnormalities. The clear-cut results of castration, however, show that these adrenocortical steroids cannot normally act in substitution for the male hormone secreted by the testis.

7.6 The pituitary gonadotropins

The effect of a hormone is rarely an island, entire of itself, and in the regulation of sexual periodicity the pituitary gland has a part to play no less important than that of the gonads. The first step in the analysis of this was taken with the discovery, dating from 1910, that while the 'posterior lobe' of the mammalian pituitary could be removed without adverse effects upon breeding, the removal of the 'anterior lobe' was followed by regression of the gonads and reproductive organs. (It is proper to refer to these two operations respectively as neurohypophysectomy and adenohypophysectomy, but it should be remembered that the pars intermedia will usually be included with the 'posterior lobe'. Hypophysectomy should strictly refer to the removal of the entire pituitary gland, although it is also used more loosely, with the extent of the operation left to be inferred from the context.)

The effect of hypophysectomy in mature male rats, for example, is a marked atrophy of the testes; spermatogonia persist and may show mitoses for some months but no mature germ cells are formed, while the interstitial tissue becomes inactive so that the accessory organs regress. In mammals such as the ferret, in which reproduction is restricted to a limited season, the effect depends upon the time of the year at which it is carried out; in winter the testes merely retain their inactive condition, but in the breeding season they regress in the same way as in the rat.

Comparable changes are found in females (Fig. 7.16); the ovary of the rat atrophies and the larger follicles degenerate at about the stage of antrum formation, although some growth of oocytes and primordial follicles can continue, a fact which indicates that these earlier stages are not under pituitary control. We have seen that classical endocrinological procedure, following the demonstration of the consequences of removal of a gland, is to carry out replacement therapy. From 1926 onwards, it was repeatedly shown that implants of 'anterior lobes' could alleviate the above effects in hypophysectomized rats and mice, or could induce precocious puberty in immature animals. Complete success is not always attained, but the testes of the hypophysectomized rat can be restored in this way to more or less normal activity, while ovulation can be induced in immature females and some degree of luteinization in hypophysectomized adults.

These results are a consequence of the production

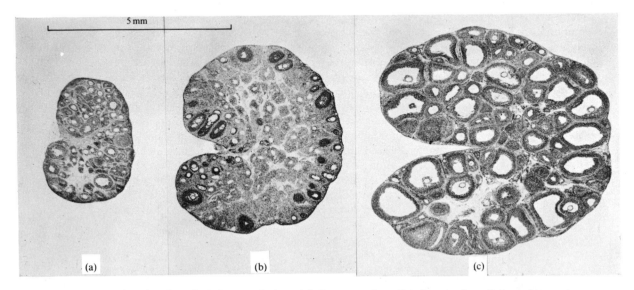

FIG. 7.16. Sections of ovaries of rats hypophysectomized at 26–8 days, 10–12 days after the operation; all three photographs are at the same magnification. (a) Untreated control. (b) LH treatment for 3 days; note that interstitial repair is the only result. (c) FSH treatment for 3 days; note the development of many follicles to medium and large size in the presence of deficient interstitial tissue. Haematoxylin and eosin. (From Simpson (1959). *Reproduction in domestic animals* (eds H. H. Cole and P. T. Cupps), Vol. 1. Academic Press, New York.)

by the pars distalis of gonadotropic hormones, or gonadotropins (*trope*, turn). The name refers to the orientation of the pituitary secretion towards the gonads; an alternative is gonadotrophic hormones, or gonadotrophins (*trophe*, nourishment). Two gonadotropins are secreted in mammals. One of these, follicle-stimulating hormone (FSH), is so-called because it promotes development of the ovarian follicles. This effect can be well demonstrated experimentally by the production of multiple follicles in immature hypophysectomized rats, but in these animals the follicles will not become luteinized. Nor will they secrete oestrogen (as evidenced by their vaginal smears), unless a very high dose of the hormone is used. In males, the hormone promotes the development of mature sperm, but produces no effect on the interstitial tissue, so that the accessory organs are unaffected.

The second gonadotropin is luteinizing hormone (LH), also known as interstitial-cell-stimulating hormone (ICSH), although the former name has priority. This hormone has no gonadotropic effect in immature females, but it completes the reproductive cycle in mature females by evoking ovulation and luteinization in those follicles that have reached the appropriate stage. In both sexes it promotes development of the interstitial tissue of the gonads. This results in growth of the accessory organs of the male, but those of the female are unaffected because, as we have noted, oestrogen is secreted by the follicles and not by the interstitial cells. The actions of the two gonadotropins are thus closely interlinked to ensure normal sexual development.

FSH and LH are glycoproteins, with a molecular weight of about 30 000, and with 15–18 per cent carbohydrate. The LH of the sheep has been particu-

larly well characterized. Its molecule is composed of two subunits, separable by counter-current distribution, each subunit being a polypeptide chain, called respectively LH-α and LH-β. The peptide sequences of the two subunits have been fully determined, and shown to be markedly different. The α-subunit (Fig. 7.17) is composed of 96 residues, with two carbohydrate moieties attached to asparagine residues at positions 56 and 82. The β-subunit (Fig. 7.18) is longer; it has 120 residues, with one carbohydrate moiety attached to an asparagine residue at position 13. When the two subunits are separated, they are inactive, at least with *in vivo* bioassays, but activity is restored when they are reunited.

Ovine FSH has been less well characterized, but it, too, has a subunit structure, with two markedly dissimilar subunits. Its carbohydrate moiety contains sialic acid, removal of which abolishes activity. It is likely that the subunit of FSH resembles the α-subunit of LH, but that their β-subunits are different, and that it is these latter that are mainly responsible for the specificity of the properties of the two hormones.

These facts are sufficiently remarkable, but what is even more so is that these two gonadotropin molecules closely resemble the third glycoprotein molecule secreted by the pars distalis. This is the molecule of the hormone thyrotropin (TSH, p. 170), which is also composed of two subunits. One of these (TSH-α) is almost identical in peptide sequence with LH-α (Fig. 7.17), while the other subunit (TSH-β) is characteristic of thyrotropin and unlike the subunits of the other two hormones, although regions of homology are present (Fig. 7.18). There is here an obvious implication of some pattern of molecular

H₂N-Phe-Pro-Asp-Gly-Glu-Phe-Thr-Met-Gln-Gly-Cys-Pro-Glu-Cys-Lys-Leu-
10

Lys-Glu-Asn-Lys-Tyr-Phe-Ser-Lys-Pro-Asp-Ala-Pro-Ile-Tyr-Gln-Cys-
20   30

Met-Gly-Cys-Cys-Phe-Ser-Arg-Ala-Tyr-Pro-Thr-Pro-Ala-Arg-Ser-Lys-
40

CHO
|
Lys-Thr-Met-Leu-Val-Pro-Lys-Asn-Ile-Thr-Ser-Glu-Ala-Thr-Cys-Cys-
50   60

Val-Ala-Lys-Ala-Phe-Thr-Lys-Ala-Thr-Val-Met-Gly-Asn-Val-Arg-Val-
70   80

CHO   TSH-α: Cys-Ser-
|
Glx-Asn-His-Thi-Glu-Cys-His-Ser-Cys-Thr-Cys-Tyr-Tyr-His-Lys-Ser-COOH
90

Fig. 7.17. Amino-acid sequence of ovine LH-α and bovine TSH-α (After Papkoff (1972). *Gen. comp. Endocrin.*, Suppl. 3 (eds W. S. Hoar and H. A. Bern).)

$$H_2N\text{-Ser-Arg-Gly-Pro-Leu-Arg-Pro-}\boxed{\text{Leu-Cys}}\text{-Glu-Pro-Ile-Asn-Ala-Thr-Leu-Ala-Ala-}$$
$$H_2N\text{-Phe-}\boxed{\text{Cys-Ile}}\text{-Pro-Thr-Glu-Tyr-Met-Met-His-Val-Glu-}$$

18
12

Glu-$\boxed{\text{Lys-Glu-Ala-Cys}}$-Pro-$\boxed{\text{Val-Cys-}}$ Ile-Thr-Phe-$\boxed{\text{Thr-Thr}}$-Ser- Ile-$\boxed{\text{Gly-Ala-Tyr-Cys}}$-
Arg-$\boxed{\text{Lys-Glu-Cys-Ala}}$-Tyr-$\boxed{\text{Cys-Leu-Thr-}}$ Ile-Asn-$\boxed{\text{Thr-Thr}}$-Val-Cys-$\boxed{\text{Ala-Gly-Tyr-Cys}}$-

37
31

Cys-Pro-Ser-Met-Lys-Arg-Val-Leu-Pro-Val-Pro-$\boxed{\text{Pro}}$-Leu- Ile-Pro-Met-Pro-$\boxed{\text{Gln}}$-
Met-Thr-Arg-Asx-Val-Asx-Gly-Lys-Leu-Phe-Leu-$\boxed{\text{Pro}}$-Lys-Tyr-Ala-Leu-Ser-$\boxed{\text{Gln}}$-

55
49

Arg-$\boxed{\text{Val-Cys-Thr-Tyr-His-Gln-Leu}}$- Arg-Phe-Ala- Ser-Val-Arg-$\boxed{\text{Leu-Pro-Gly-Pro-Cys}}$-
Asp-$\boxed{\text{Val-Cys-Thr-Tyr-Arg-Asp-Phe}}$-Met-Tyr-Lys-Thr-Ala-Gln-$\boxed{\text{Ile-Pro-Gly-Cys-Pro}}$-

74
68

Pro-Val-Asp-Pro-Gly-Met-Val-$\boxed{\text{Ser-Phe-Pro-Val-Ala-Leu-Ser-Cys-His}}$-Gly-Pro-
Arg-His-Val-Thr-Pro-Tyr-Phe-$\boxed{\text{Ser-Tyr-Pro-Val-Ala-} \text{Ile-Ser-Cys-Lys}}$-Cys-Gly-

92
86

Cys-$\boxed{\text{Cys}}$-Arg-Leu-Ser-Ser-$\boxed{\text{Thr-Asp-Cys}}$-Gly-Pro-Gly-Arg-Thr-Glu-Pro-Leu-Ala-
Lys-$\boxed{\text{Cys}}$-Asx-Thr-Asx-Tyr-$\boxed{\text{Ser-Asx-Cys}}$- Ile-His-Glu-Ala- Ile-Lys-Thr-Asn-Tyr-

110
104

$\boxed{\text{Cys}}$-Asp-His-$\boxed{\text{Pro}}$-Pro-Leu-Pro-Asp- Ile-Leu-COOH
$\boxed{\text{Cys}}$-Thr-Lys-$\boxed{\text{Pro}}$-Gln-Lys-Ser-Tyr-Met-COOH

120
113

FIG. 7.18. Comparison of the sequence of LH-β and TSH-β. The TSH-β structure is aligned below the LH-β structure. Areas of homology are indicated by the boxed sequences. (After Papkoff (1972). *Gen. comp. Endocrin.*, Suppl. 3 (eds W. S. Hoar and H. A. Bern).) (Bovine TSH-β structure by Pierce *et al.* (1970).)

evolutionary relationship (p. 101). Perhaps all three of these glycoprotein hormones originated in a common ancestral molecule, represented now by the α-subunit, with which individually characterized subunits (the β-subunits) have become associated. The suggestion is speculative, and needs testing against a knowledge of the characteristics of the glycoprotein hormones of the lower vertebrates; this knowledge is still to be obtained.

7.7. Prolactin

A third gonadotropin hormone, additional to FSH and LH, is functional in the rat. This is prolactin, another pars distalis hormone, which is a polypeptide and not a glycoprotein. This hormone promotes and maintains the secretion of progesterone in the rat after the formation of the corpus luteum; because of this, the functioning of the corpus luteum in this animal is prolonged if prolactin is injected at the end of oestrus (p. 130). Prolactin is thus alternatively known as luteotropic hormone (LTH), but the term is only truly applicable to the rat, for it is doubtful whether prolactin has luteotropic functions in other

species. It does, however, play an important part in mammals generally, by contributing to the regulation of lactation.

Lactation, as exemplified in the rat, depends upon the actions of a number of hormones. Oestrogen, secreted under the stimulus of FSH and LH, co-operates with growth hormone and the cortico-steroids (themselves secreted under the stimulus of corticotropin, p. 205) to induce the growth of the mammary ductules. Prolactin then stimulates the corpora lutea to secrete progesterone, and the full development of the alveoli results from the combined action of prolactin, somatotropin, oestrogen, proges-terone, and the corticosteroids, with the cooperation of placental hormones (p. 145). The actual secretion of the milk is evoked predominantly by prolactin and the corticosteroids, the influence of oestrogen and progesterone diminishing at this stage. Finally, the ejection of the milk occurs as a result of the action of oxytocin. Thus some ten or more hormones may be said to cooperate in the production of milk in this animal. No doubt this is in part a consequence of the complex hormonal interactions that are involved

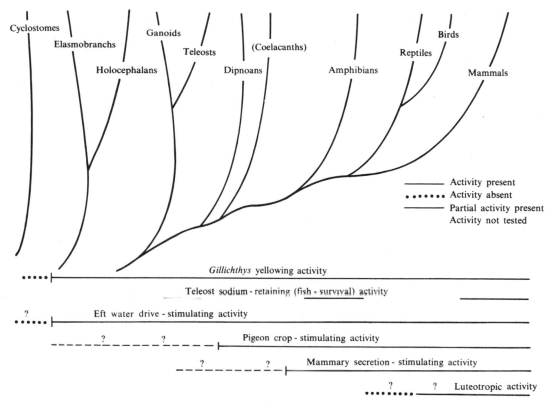

FIG. 7.19. Distribution of several of the activities of prolactin among the vertebrates. A scheme for the evolution of the hormone is proposed. (Modified from Bern and Nicoll (1968). *Rec. Prog. Hormone Res.* **24**. © 1967 by the American Association for the Advancement of Science.)

in the regulation of metabolism, for the synthetic activity of the mammary glands is bound to be influenced by this, but probably another factor is that these glands evolved late in the history of the vertebrates. It is thus understandable that their hormonal control would become enmeshed in the complexity that is so characteristic of the endocrine organization of the higher vertebrates.

In any case, it is certain that prolactin was not first evolved as a mammary hormone, for it exists throughout the gnathostomes, and is exceptional amongst the vertebrate hormones for the diversity of its functions. As many as eighty-two of these have been recorded, although probably not all of them are physiologically significant (Fig. 7.19).

Some of these functions are related to reproduction, and thus have something in common with the role of prolactin in lactation. Amongst these are the promotion of the secretion of 'crop milk' in pigeons, formed by proliferation of the lining of the crop in both sexes, and fed to the young by regurgitation. The resultant increase in weight of the crop, and

associated histological changes, are the bases for bioassay. The hormone also promotes broodiness and development of the naked and richly vascularized brood-spots formed in many birds at incubation. (The reduction of broodiness by selective breeding, involving both reduction of prolactin production and decreased sensitivity of the crop to its action, is an illustration of the practical application of the principles of endocrine evolution.)

Other reproductive functions are found in lower vertebrates. For example, in certain teleost fish (cichlids and catfishes), prolactin promotes the production, by cutaneous and buccal cells, of mucus which is used for feeding to the young. An example of another integumentary effect is the promotion of pigment synthesis in teleosts, and the potentiation of the action of melanocyte-stimulating hormone upon the proliferation of melanocytes in the teleost *Fundulus*.

Another action is exerted upon the immature terrestrial stages of certain newts *Triturus* (*Diemyctylus*) *viridescens* and *Triturus alpestris*. Administration of the hormone to hypophysectomized animals will induce within a few days a migration to water (the 'water-drive effect'); presumably, therefore, it promotes the normal reproductive migration of the young animals from land into water. The basis for this effect is not clear, but perhaps blood–electrolyte changes are one factor.

An influence upon electrolytes is certainly a factor in another action of prolactin, which is an effect upon osmoregulation in certain fish. For example, the cyprinodont *Poecilia* (*Mollienesia*) *latipinna* (the 'mollie' of the aquarist) is a fish which normally can live either in fresh water or in salt water. It cannot survive, however, in fresh water after hypophysectomy, although it can continue to live in normal or dilute sea water after this operation. The death in fresh water is associated with a marked decline in the level of blood sodium. Injections of ovine prolactin enable the operated fish to survive, and so also will an ectopic transplant of the pituitary gland (p. 81), for in these transplants the prolactin-secreting cells remain functional. Survival is associated with a restoration of normal blood-sodium levels (Table 7.2).

TABLE 7.2

Plasma sodium and potassium concentrations in adult female Poecilia latipinna. Means ± standard errors.

Treatment	No. of fish	Sodium (mequiv l⁻¹)	Potassium (mequiv l⁻¹)
1. Intact, 6 weeks in D.S.W.	10	$163 \cdot 3 \pm 0 \cdot 45$	—
2. Intact, reared in F.W.	9	$151 \cdot 3 \pm 1 \cdot 57$	—
3. Hypox 2 weeks, in D.S.W.	7	$160 \cdot 3 \pm 0 \cdot 82$	—
Group A. Fish killed 18–24 hours after transfer from D.S.W. to F.W.			
4. Intact	9	$129 \cdot 2 \pm 2 \cdot 73$	—
5. Hypox	5	$88 \cdot 1 \pm 2 \cdot 96$	—
Group B. Fish operated 3 days after transfer from D.S.W. to F.W., killed after 4 days			
6. Intact controls at 3 days	8	$148 \cdot 7 \pm 1 \cdot 25$	$9 \cdot 4 \pm 0 \cdot 27$
7. Sham hypox, injected CMC	7	$144 \cdot 7 \pm 0 \cdot 72$	$9 \cdot 5 \pm 0 \cdot 30$
8. Hypox, injected CMC	10	$111 \cdot 2 \pm 1 \cdot 34$	$9 \cdot 8 \pm 0 \cdot 92$
9. Hypox, injected prolactin	10	$141 \cdot 5 \pm 1 \cdot 81$	$9 \cdot 8 \pm 0 \cdot 66$

D.S.W., dilute sea water (12 parts per 1000); F.W., tap water; Hypox., hypophysectomized; CMC, 1% sodium carboxymethyl-cellulose in 0·6% NaCl solution (vehicle).

'*t*' test for sodium values: 1 and 2, $P < 0 \cdot 001$; 1 and 3, $P < 0 \cdot 01 > 0 \cdot 001$; 1 and 4, $P < 0 \cdot 001$; 2 and 4, $P < 0 \cdot 001$; 4 and 5, $P < 0 \cdot 001$; 2 and 6, $P = 0 \cdot 3$; 6 and 7, $P < 0 \cdot 005 > 0 \cdot 02$; 7 and 8, $P < 0 \cdot 001$; 7 and 9, $P < 0 \cdot 001$; 8 and 9, $P < 0 \cdot 001$.

The differences between the potassium values in Group B were not significant. (From Ball and Ensor (1965). *J. Endocrin.* **32**.)

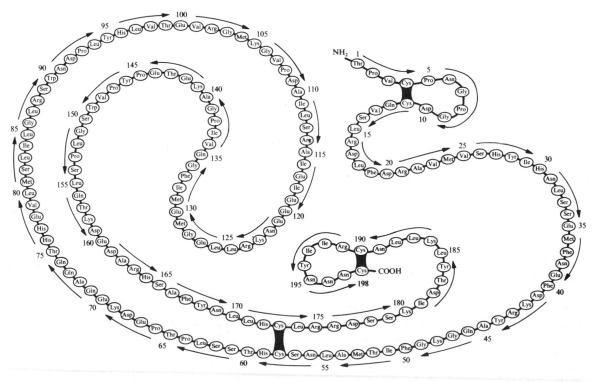

Fig. 7.20. The amino-acid sequence of ovine prolactin. (From Li (1972). *Growth and growth hormone* (eds A. Pecile and E. E. Müller). Excerpta Medica, Amsterdam.)

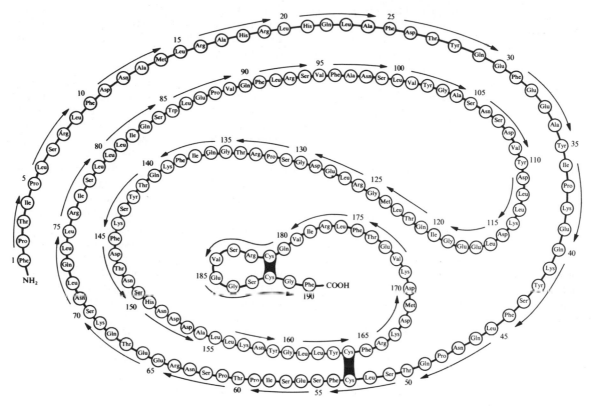

FIG. 7.21. The amino-acid sequence of human placental lactogen. (From Li (1972). *Growth and growth hormone* (eds A. Pecile and E. E. Müller). Excerpta Medica, Amsterdam.)

Finally, prolactin has important growth-promoting effects in all the major vertebrate groups; so much so, that at one time it was argued that it was itself the mammalian growth hormone. The action is well seen in amphibian tadpoles. In these it promotes increase in body weight and tail length, and tends to antagonize the action of thyroid hormones (p. 179) by preventing the onset of metamorphic climax and tail reduction. But perhaps the most striking aspect of this growth promotion is seen in man. Human somatotropin has an intrinsic lactogenic property, but it is uncertain whether or not there is a distinct pituitary prolactin. There is, however, in man a placental hormone (human placental lactogen) which is secreted in large quantities during pregnancy, and which influences maternal metabolism as well as the differentiation and development of the mammary glands. This hormone also has a growth-promoting action, but much less than that of the pituitary growth hormone.

In the light of discussions in earlier chapters, these cross relationships in hormonal properties suggest that there may be corresponding similarities in molecular structure, and this has proved to be so. Their existence has been established firmly by the determination of the peptide sequences of ovine prolactin (Fig. 7.20) and human placental lactogen (Fig. 7.21), which can thus be compared with the sequence of human growth hormone (p. 48). The two human hormones are strikingly similar. Each has 190 amino-acid residues, two disulphide bonds in the same positions, and 160 of the 190 residues identically situated. The total homology (p. 101), including identical residues and conservative replacements (judged by the chemical properties of the amino acids) is 96 per cent.

This is yet another example of close molecular resemblance which finds its only reasonable explanation in the concept of gene duplication, followed by divergence in molecular structure and function (p. 101). Prolactin and somatotropin must surely have had a common molecular ancestry. Much more evidence is needed in this field, and particularly from the lower vertebrates, but already one peculiar feature of prolactin is apparent, and one that differentiates it from the other polypeptide vertebrate hormones. Those that we have considered so far are hormones that have maintained stability of function; this is so of insulin, for example, despite the amino-acid substitutions which it has acquired. Prolactin, by contrast, has never become associated firmly with any one function. Rather, it seems to have been held in reserve, becoming involved in new functions at successive stages of evolution, in correlation with the appearance of new adaptional needs. We can suppose, by analogy with what we know of other hormones, that this has been accompanied by changes in the hormone itself, as well as in its targets, although we cannot be sure of this without knowledge of the peptide sequences of the prolactins of lower forms. It is very suggestive, however, that ovine prolactin can correct sodium balance in fish, whereas preparations of the fish hormone do not evoke a characteristic response from the crop of pigeons. Some histological change is detectable, but not the full secretory response evoked by the mammalian hormone, so that the fish hormone differs from the ovine in its biological properties.

On the other hand, the prolactin-secreting cells of the teleost pituitary can bind rabbit antiserum to ovine prolactin (p. 81). Probably, therefore, the fish hormone has immunological determinants that are similar to those of the mammalian hormone, but different biological determinants. To this must be added the fact that prolactins of lower forms do have some of the functions of the hormone of higher ones. For example, fish prolactin preparations evoke the water-drive effect in urodeles. It follows that in the higher groups use has been made of properties of the molecule that were already present in earlier stages of evolution, even though they may not have been used in those earlier stages. No other hormone better illustrates how the evolution of endocrine regulation has involved complex interactions of structure and function, in hormones as well as in their targets.

7.8. Neural regulation of gonadotropin secretion

The importance of the pituitary gland in the regulation of sexual periodicity in vertebrates is a consequence of its being functionally related both to the gonads and to the nervous system, and through the nervous system to the internal and external environment. An illustration of this is given by the rabbit.

Ovulation in this animal normally occurs at about ten hours after the stimulus provided by coitus. This response, which is mediated by the release of LH from the pars distalis, is an example of reproductive activity being influenced through the nervous system after the application of a specific stimulus, the time

interval being required for the mobilization of a concentration of the hormone adequate for evoking rupture of the follicles. What, then, are the pathways involved?

One step towards the answering of this question was taken in 1936, when Marshal and Verney showed that ovulation and pseudo-pregnancy (p. 130) could be produced in the rabbit if the animal was first etherized, and then electrical stimulation applied either to the brain or to the spinal cord. They dismissed the possibility that the nervous system was transmitting a signal direct to the ovaries, because it was already known that post-coital ovulation could occur even when the ovaries had been ectopically transplanted to abnormal positions, where they were deprived of any possible innervation. They therefore concluded that they had 'proved that nervous stimuli can act upon the anterior pituitary and change the functional activity of that organ and the character of its secretions in such a way as to alter and control certain of the phases of the oestrous cycle'.

Further suggestive evidence came from demonstrations of the dependence of the sexual rhythms of birds and mammals upon environmental stimuli, notably photoperiod; an aspect to which we shall return later. It was this evidence that led Marshall to argue that the anterior pituitary was 'playing the part of a liaison organ between the nervous system which is affected by stimuli from without and the endocrine system'. The dependence of adrenocortical activity upon emotional stress appeared to provide another illustration of this principle, while it already seemed probable, although at that time less certain, that the thyroid gland must also be under nervous regulation.

The argument was later greatly strengthened by the results of applying electrical stimulation to the hypothalamus of rabbits by remote control (see also p. 173). A small secondary coil is inserted so as to lie between the scalp and the skull; this coil carries an indifferent electrode that also lies beneath the skull, while a fine stimulating one passes downwards to the hypothalamus (Fig. 7.22). The stimulation is applied through a small primary coil, with the animal fastened in position; or, if it is preferred to avoid the stress of restraint, a large coil of three feet diameter can be used and the animal left free to move in its cage. Using this technique, it was possible to evoke ovulation in a rabbit by three minutes of stimulation, the most sensitive area of the hypothalamus being immediately above the anterior region of the median eminence. It was further shown that localized lesions of the hypothalamus, in corres-

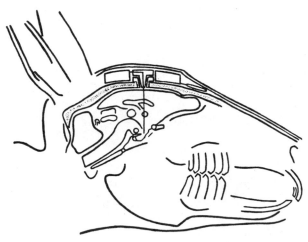

FIG. 7.22. Diagram of a sagittal section of a rabbit's head prepared for remote-control electrical stimulation. The stimulating electrode, insulated to the tip, is shown descending from the secondary coil unit through the corpus callosum and anterior commissure into the region of the tuber cinereum. (From Harris (1947). *Phil. Trans. R. Soc.* B 232.)

ponding areas of various mammals, would result in atrophy of the gonads, presumably because of a diminished output of gonadotropins. There was thus convincing evidence that the release of these hormones was determined by the activity of localized areas of the hypothalamus.

One way in which this dependence of the pituitary upon the hypothalamus might, in theory, be mediated is by direct innervation of the pars distalis of the adenohypophysis, but the evidence for this was never convincing, and with the use of electron microscopy it became clear that there was no innervation of the secretory cells of the pars distalis of mammals. (The situation in the pars intermedia of the adenohypophysis, as we have seen, is a separate issue.)

An alternative possibility was suggested by the peculiar vascularization of the pars distalis. As we have already seen (p. 65), the internal carotid arteries supply blood to a capillary plexus in the median eminence. From this plexus, portal vessels convey blood to the pars distalis, where they break up into a secondary plexus. The whole system forms the hypophysial portal system.

It was at first difficult to evaluate the significance of this system because of doubt as to which way the blood flowed in it. However, in due course it was established by direct observation, first in the living toad, and later in the rat, that the flow was from the brain into the pars distalis. This gave good foundation to the possibility that neural control might be mediated by chemical agents arising in the brain as a response to environmental signals, and passing into the pars distalis by the portal system.

This possibility was first ventilated in 1937 by Hinsey. He pointed out that it could be tested by sectioning the pituitary stalk, which would interrupt the supposed transmission, but, as he rightly commented, the results of sectioning were at that time baffling to interpret. Little, therefore, resulted from the suggestion, until Harris and Jacobsohn showed in 1952 that hypophysectomized rats could mate and give birth to young if they had received a pituitary transplant, provided that this was placed adjacent to the median eminence. If, however, it was placed under the temporal lobe, the animals became anoestrous, with reduced reproductive organs. Further clarification came when Harris showed that the difficulty of interpreting transections resulted from the regeneration of the sectioned vessels, which re-established communication between the hypothalamus and the adenohypophysis. Careful examination of thick sections of the stalk are needed to determine whether or not such regeneration has occurred. Given this post-surgical control, it was possible to show convincingly that the sexual cycle of the female ferret depended upon vascular communication between the hypothalamus and the adenohypophysis. Females could be brought into oestrus in winter by subjecting them to increased photoperiod, but this response was not obtained from animals in which the vessels had been interrupted and prevented from regenerating by the insertion of a plate. Oestrus did ensue, however, if the vessels regenerated around the edge of the plate.

No less cogent was the study by Everett of ectopic transplants of the pituitary (Fig. 7.23). These are transplants in which the organ concerned is moved to another region in the same individual. The pituitary de-differentiates if it is grafted under the kidney capsule, and eventually contains only cells that are slightly eosinophilic. These are the prolactin cells, which are inhibited by the influence of the central nervous system, and which pass into increased activity when they are removed from it (p. 69). The other secretory functions of the mammalian pars distalis depend upon the stimulatory influence of the brain. These functions are restored if the pars distalis is transplanted back to the region of the median eminence, so that its portal blood supply can be re-established.

Along these lines there has gradually been built up the conclusion, now firmly established, that pars **distalis functioning is regulated by chemical factors,**

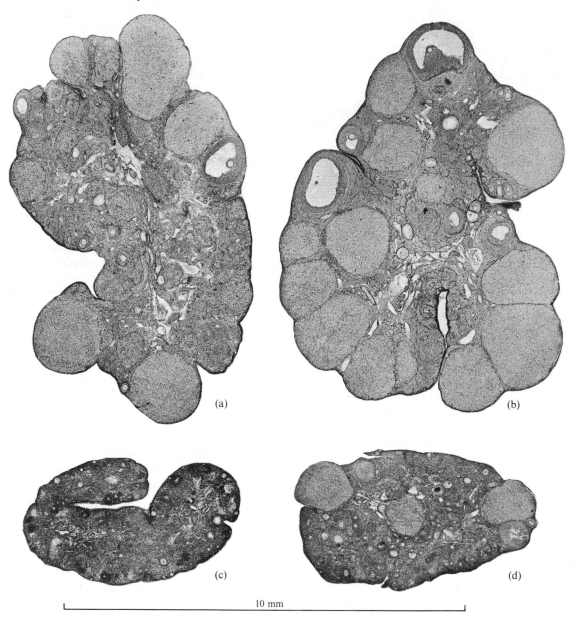

FIG. 7.23. The influence of pituitary transplantation upon ovarian activity in the rat; all four photographs are at the same magnification. (a) Ovary of a normal rat at pro-oestrus. (b) Ovary after re-transplantation of pituitary from renal capsule to a site under the median eminence; regular oestrous cycles have been resumed. (c) Atrophic ovary after retransplantation of pituitary from renal capsule to a site under the temporal lobe of the brain; note absence of corpora lutea. (d) Atrophic ovary after transplantation of pituitary to the renal capsule; the small corpora lutea are the result of transplanting during pro-oestrus. (From Nikitovitch-Winer and Everett (1958). *Endocrin.* **63**.)

originating in the hypothalamus, but distinct from the neurohypophysial hormones and constituting a separate group of neurosecretory hormones. The median eminence is their neurohaemal centre, providing for their passage from the hypothalamus into the pituitary gland through the hypophysial portal system. The development of this interpretation has been aided by the demonstration of the neurosecretory activity of the supraoptic and paraventricular nuclei. This, in conjunction with evidence of the passage of the neurohypophysial hormones down the pituitary stalk in neurosecretory axons, has suggested a model for a system which might be transporting other factors to the median eminence. Indeed, at one time it was thought that these neurohypophysial hormones actually might be the then hypothetical regulating factors, but spectacular chemical advances in this field have shown that this is not so.

Proof of the existence of these factors should rest ideally upon their identification and characterization in the portal blood, using biological, chemical, and physical criteria. It should also be demonstrated that blood containing one or other of these factors can influence the rate of release of a pars distalis hormone, and, of course, it is desirable to define the cells in which the secretions originate. These demanding criteria are not yet always fully satisfied, but the chemical evidence, in particular, has been carried a very long way, despite the call of the chemist for batches of 50 000 to 500 000 pieces of median eminence and adjacent regions. As a result, there is now satisfactory (and in some instances very good) evidence from mammals for at least nine of these hypothalamic factors (or hormones, as they may justly be called) regulating the release of the several adenohypophysial hormones, and perhaps in some cases regulating their synthesis as well. That the same is true, in principle, of other vertebrates is likely enough, but here the evidence is circumstantial and awaits more direct confirmation.

Somatotropin, prolactin, and MSH are perhaps regulated by dual systems, each comprising an inhibitory (or release-inhibiting) hormone (IH) and a releasing hormone (RH), but the existence of this dual control is still to be confirmed. The remaining hormones have each a releasing hormone only; these hormones are under inhibitory regulation through their feedback relationship with their target glands. Chemical studies in this field have been greatly advanced by the development of methods of bioassay and radio-immunoassay; in particular, the latter technique has made it possible to show that some of these hormones are released into the blood stream under physiological conditions, and that their release can be correlated with changes in activity of the target glands.

The evidence for the existence of thyrotropin-releasing hormone (TRH) and corticotropin-releasing hormone (CRH) will be referred to later (pp. 173, 206). As for the others, not all have been equally well characterized. A decapeptide which releases growth hormone (GH) has been synthesized, but certain experimental data show that this is probably

not the actual releasing hormone, if, indeed, this exists. A synthetic tetradecapeptide is, however, thought to be the inhibiting hormone (growth hormone inhibiting hormone GH-IH); this has great potentiality for the clinical treatment of acromegaly and giantism.

A tripeptide amide (Pro-Leu-Gly-NH$_2$), which is the COOH-terminal side chain of oxytocin, is one of two compounds which have been isolated from the hypothalamus, and which have been thought to be the inhibiting hormone for MSH (MIH), but the chemistry of this hormone and of the stimulating one (MRH) remains to be clarified. A prolactin-releasing hormone has been demonstrated experimentally in the hypothalamus of the rat, its concentration being decreased by suckling, and increased by tranquillizers (which may account for the secretion of milk sometimes observed in women after tranquillizer treatment). However, the chemical nature of this hormone, and of the supposed prolactin-inhibiting hormone, remains to be established.

(pyro)Glu-His-Trp-Ser-Tyr-Gly-Leu-Arg-Pro-Gly-NH$_2$

FIG. 7.24. FSH- and LH-releasing hormone. (Simplified from Schally *et al.* (1973). *Science* **179**.)

As regards sexual reproduction, however, the evidence for the intervention of at least one releasing hormone is particularly convincing. FSH-RH and LH-RH activities have been demonstrated in hypothalamic extracts of various mammals. Both show a decline in the rat at puberty, while there is a fall in level of LH-RH in the rat just before oestrus, this fall being correlated with the surge in the release of LH that is required to effect ovulation. Amongst other evidence may be mentioned an increase in the blood-level of LH-RH in the rat after electrical stimulation of the hypothalamus, and the detection of LH-RH activity in the blood of women at the middle of the menstrual cycle (p. 130).

LH-RH has been isolated and characterized as a polypeptide with ten amino acids (Fig. 7.24), this having been confirmed by synthesis. Its consequent availability in pure form has made it possible to test its properties both *in vivo* and *in vitro*. An unexpected result of this has been to show that the one factor is responsible for promoting the release of FSH as well as of LH. It is impossible to separate chemically the two activities, and that both are intrinsic to the molecule has been demonstrated by treating rat pituitaries *in vitro* with the synthetic compound. It is not easy to see how the preferential release of one or other of the two hormones can be mediated by one factor during the normal reproductive cycle, yet ovulation is certainly associated with a surge of LH. Conceivably there may be some interplay between this releasing hormone and the sex steroids, or between both of these and the pituitary gland.

The isolation and synthesis of this hormone (LH-RH/FSH-RH), and its testing by experiment, is the crucial evidence for chemical regulation of gonadotropin release. Its practical importance is that it may provide a means for treating infertility in man without the hazard of multiple births that is involved in gonadotropin treatment, while it could also be used for promoting fertility in domestic animals. Possibly, too, antagonists may be found which would bind competitively to the receptors of the releasing hormone, thus providing a new method of contraception.

7.9. Negative feedback control in mammalian reproduction

We have seen ample evidence of the influence of the pars distalis upon the gonads, by the discharge of gonadotropins and their transmission to the ovaries and the testes. Equally important, however, is the reciprocal influence of the gonads upon gonadotropin output. This can be demonstrated in many ways. For example, administration of oestrogen to immature female rats results in a development of corpora lutea which are clearly functional, for proliferation of the uterine endometrium also occurs (p. 114). This can only mean that the oestrogen is stimulating the secretion of LH. The effect falls off with prolonged administration, from which it follows that continued oestrogen administration eventually reduces LH output. Androgens and progestins also influence gonadotropin output. For example, a normal female rat, united in parabiotic union with a castrated male, develops an hypertrophied ovary, indicating that the output of gonadotropins from the male has increased in the absence of the restraining influence of its androgenic hormone. The injection of oestrogen, or, in larger doses, of androgen or progesterone, into the castrate abolishes this effect by inhibiting the secretion of its gonadotropins. This reciprocal action is reflected in the condition of the gonadotropin-secreting cells of the pars distalis, and we have earlier seen the importance of this

in interpreting the cytological organization of the gland.

The relationship thus revealed is an example of a negative feedback mechanism, which is a mode of regulation widespread in endocrine systems, and in physiological organization in general. In the present instance, an increase in output of gonadal hormones evokes a reduction in output of gonadotropins through a feedback loop provided by the blood stream. Thus the gonadal hormones restrain their own output, and it is in this sense that the feedback is a negative one (cf. p. 92). Expressed in the terminology of control systems, the hypothalamus is a sensor, detecting errors of misalignment. Information is fed from this to a servomotor, which is the pars distalis, and which regulates, by remote action, the final control element, which is the appropriate target gland.

What, however, is the pathway by which the signal actually reaches the pars distalis? Probably the gonadal steroids can have a direct action upon the pituitary cells, but there is also a less direct pathway, through the hypothalamus, and this is the more important one. The evidence for feedback action of the gonadal steroids on the hypothalamus is ample and diverse. For example, radio-isotopically labelled steroids are taken up by the hypothalamus, while lesions of the hypothalamus may suppress the feedback action which would normally follow prolonged steroid treatment. Other experimental procedures include the insertion of gonadal tissue, or of gonadal steroids, directly into the hypothalamus; a response, comparable to that produced by normal feedback, can then be detected in the pars distalis.

Thus the negative feedback loop involves not only the systemic circulation, but also the hypothalamic pathways that we have already analysed: the passage of LH-releasing factor from the hypothalamus, through the hypophysial portal system, into the pars distalis. It is because of this that reproductive cycles can be determined entirely by the interplay of gonadotropins and gonadal steroids, as we shall see them to be in the oestrous cycle of the unmated mouse or rat, and yet can also be determined or modulated by the interplay of the hormones with the external environment, through the central nervous system (cf. Fig. 9.34, p. 174). With these principles as a basis, we are now in a position to attempt some causal analysis of the sexual periodicity of mammals.

8

Hormones and reproduction II

8.1. Sexual periodicity in mammals

Sexual periodicity in the great majority of mammals is dominated by the oestrous cycle of the female. This cycle, which involves a series of changes in the reproductive system, culminates in oestrus or heat, the only period in which the female will permit insemination by the male. It will be convenient to consider first the situation in rats and mice, since these have been intensively analysed and have formed the material for so much experimentation. Here the mature unmated female exhibits a four- to six-day oestrous cycle which continues throughout the year, interrupted only by pregnancy; she is therefore said to be polyestrous all the year round. The cycle can be divided into four phases.

1. *Pro-oestrus* (lasting for 18 hours) is essentially a period of preparation, during which the ripening follicles grow and the output of oestrogen increases. Under the influence of this hormone the

wall of the uterus becomes hydrated and its cavity distended by fluid, while the vaginal epithelial cells multiply to form a thick layer from which the outermost cells are delaminated; thus the vaginal smear (p.111) characteristic of this stage is composed of nucleated cells without any leucocytes (Fig. 8.1). (A preliminary stage of some four hours during which these cells are not found in the smear is sometimes distinguished as pre-oestrus.) In the later stage of their growth, but not, apparently, in the earlier ones, the follicles are being stimulated by FSH, probably potentiated by LH in small quantities.

2. *Oestrus* (lasting for about 28 hours) is the period of sexual receptivity or heat, which results from the fact that the secretion of oestrogen reaches a climax during this phase. As the output of this hormone increases, it is thought to inhibit FSH output and to increase the output of LH; the latter then evokes ovulation, and the secretion of oestrogen diminishes.

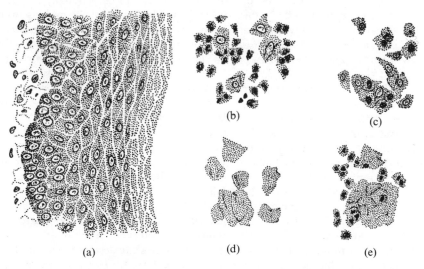

(a)

(b)

(c)

(d)

(e)

Fig. 8.1. The vaginal cycle in the white rat. (a) Vaginal wall at oestrus; the cells of the inner surface (right) are cornified and without nuclei. (b) Vaginal smear at dioestrus, containing epithelial cells (pale nuclei) and leucocytes (dark nuclei). (c) Just before oestrus the epithelial cells swell. (d) Smear at oestrus, showing cornified cells as in (a). (e) After oestrus the leucocytes return and the cornified cells disintegrate. (From Young (1957) (2nd edn, 1975). *The life of mammals*: Clarendon Press, Oxford.)

As a result of these interactions, the ova enter the oviducts at a time best calculated to ensure a good prospect of fertilization. During oestrus the uterine lumen remains distended, but there is some degeneration of its epithelium, while increasing cornification of the vaginal epithelium results in the vaginal smear consisting of cells which are cornified and non-nucleated (Fig. 8.1). In addition, those follicles which will be ovulated at the next oestrus begin their growth, while there are abundant mitoses in the germinal epithelium, but this does not necessarily represent the production of a new supply of oocytes. On the interpretation of oestrogens as mitotic stimulants, it has been suggested that this effect may be evoked by the high concentration of hormone present in the ovary and released from the follicular fluid at ovulation.

3. *Metoestrus* (lasting for about 8 hours) is marked by a heavy invasion of the vaginal epithelium by leucocytes; these therefore predominate in the vaginal smears, although they are accompanied by some cornified and some nucleated cells. The uterus meanwhile becomes reduced in size towards the resting stage characteristic of dioestrus, and there is by now a marked reduction of oestrogen secretion.

4. *Dioestrus* (lasting for about 53 hours) is a stage marked by the appearance of both nucleated epithelial cells and leucocytes in the vaginal smear (Fig. 8.1), and by the formation of corpora lutea. These, however, are virtually functionless in the rat and mouse and begin to degenerate at three days after ovulation, which accounts for the short duration of the oestrous cycle in these animals. In effect, the cycle in the unmated female of these species is a purely follicular one, determined by the time required to ripen a new set of follicles; the influence of a luteal phase is seen if the animal is mated, the extent of the influence then depending on whether or not pregnancy ensues. Without mating, dioestrus is followed by the pro-oestrus of a new cycle, with FSH secretion increasing again as a result of the reduction of oestrogen output; this simple type of cycle thus depends upon the reciprocal interaction of pituitary and ovarian secretions.

Pseudopregnancy (lasting for fourteen days in the rat) is the phase which results in the rat or mouse if copulation occurs without being followed by pregnancy; it is essentially a prolongation of dioestrus, with corpora lutea coming into function under the influence of prolactin (luteotropic hormone). It can be evoked by various artificial procedures which stimulate the effect of coitus, such as mechanical or electrical stimulation of the cervix uteri; a single electric shock during late pro-oestrus or oestrus is sufficient. The progesterone that is secreted during this phase stimulates proliferation in the glandular lining (endometrium) of the uterus; if this is now irritated, by the insertion of a thread, for example, it will respond by local growth which results in the production of nodules called deciduomata, a reaction which normally assists the implantation of the fertilized ovum. As we have seen, progesterone also prevents ovulation and hence the inception of a new oestrous cycle or the occurrence of superfoetation (the establishment of more than one generation of embryos in the uterus).

Pregnancy lasts for twenty-one to twenty-two days in the rat and, as already mentioned, the presence of the corpus luteum is needed to ensure its maintenance in this and certain other mammals (p. 114).

There are many variants of the oestrous cycle, and we can mention only a few here. The guinea-pig, like the rat and mouse, is polyoestrous all the year round, but its normal cycle corresponds to the pseudopregnant one of the latter. It includes, in other words, a functional luteal phase during which deciduomata can be induced in the uterus, and it is not modified by sterile mating, so that while in this animal the period of oestrus usually last for less than twelve hours, the whole cycle extends over some sixteen and a half days.

The cow and the sheep have several oestrous cycles during a restricted period of the year, this being followed by an inactive period called anoestrus; they are therefore said to be seasonally polyoestrous. For cows the modal length of the cycle is twenty-one to twenty-two days, and for sheep sixteen and a half to seventeen and a half days, oestrus lasting for less than one day in cows and for perhaps thirty to thirty-six hours in sheep. In contrast to these, the wild fox has only one oestrous cycle during the year, in the spring; it is thus monoestrous, with pro-oestrus and oestrus lasting about two weeks.

In man, apes, and monkeys, the characteristic menstrual cycle is determined by a sequence of events which is not fundamentally dissimilar from those governing the oestrous cycle (Fig. 8.2), but which falls into three phases.

1. *The follicular or proliferative phase* is accompanied by follicular growth and oestrogen secretion under the influence of FSH, the uterine endometrium meanwhile becoming greatly thickened and its glands enlarged. Ovulation normally occurs towards the end of this phase, at about the middle of the cycle, when there is a sharp increase in hormonal output (Fig. 8.3).

2. *The progestational or luteal phase* sets in at about one or two days after ovulation. Secretory droplets containing glycogen are discharged from the uterine epithelium, the enlarged glands become filled with

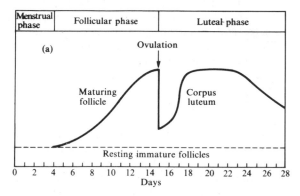

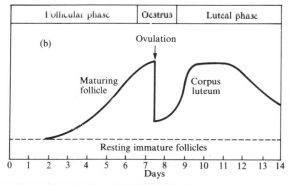

FIG. 8.2. Comparison of an oestrous cycle (*below*) with a human menstrual cycle (*above*), as reflected in the changes in size of the ovulating follicles. (From Bullough (1951). *Vertebrate sexual cycles.* Methuen, London.)

secretion, while the endometrium becomes increasingly thickened and oedematous. The uterus is now being maintained by progesterone, in readiness for the implantation of an embryo.

3. *Menstruation* terminates the progestational phase. It involves the discharge through the vagina of extravasated blood, fluid, and mucosa resulting from the collapse of the uterine endometrium, possibly because of a decline in the output of progesterone. Rapid regeneration follows, and leads to the inception of the next cycle.

In all of the above examples ovulation occurs spontaneously, in the absence of an external stimulus, as part of an endogenous rhythm, but in certain species, including the rabbit (p. 124), ferret, and cat, it will not take place without an exogenous stimulus supplied by coitus (or an artificial substitute for this); this is needed, as we have already seen, to evoke the release of LH. In the absence of this stimulus, the cycle is arrested at a period of prolonged oestrus which in the cat is followed by a quiescent phase, and this in its turn by another period of heat. In the rabbit, the female may remain in heat for up to five weeks in the absence of the male.

It will be apparent from this survey that the oestrous cycle of the female mammal depends upon an alternating ascendency of oestrogen and progesterone in those species in which the corpora lutea are active, and that one of the functions of the latter hormone is to induce what is in effect a temporary sterility. This is the basis of the contraceptive pill, which contains a mixture of synthetic oestrogen and progestogen. It provides a highly efficient method of contraception, with a failure rate of only 0·1 per

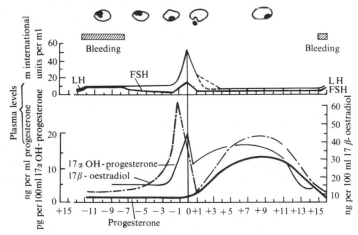

FIG. 8.3. Diagrammatic representation of the hormonal changes taking place during the human menstrual cycle, to show the relationships between ovulation and steroid hormone and gonadotropin secretion. (From Donovan and Lockhart (1972). *Modern trends in endocrinology*, Vol. 4 (eds F. G. Prunty and H. Gardiner-Hill). Butterworth, London.)

100 woman-years. Progestogen alone is unsatisfactory, as it results in irregular bleeding and gives an unacceptably high failure rate. The two compounds together complement each other, and act jointly to inhibit gonadotropin release. Ovulation is thus prevented, while there are other beneficial results as well; the cervical mucus is thicker and reduces sperm penetration, while the endometrium is rendered unsuitable for implantation.

This remarkable adaptive modification of a reproductive cycle is, of course, dependent upon the unique cultural evolutionary mechanism of the human species, but the adaptive character of sexual cycles in general is clearly seen in the modifications that the reproduction of other mammals may undergo in special circumstances. For example, the breeding season for Scotch black-faced sheep living in the Highlands may be restricted to only six weeks of the year, whereas Merino sheep in Australia, living in a much more favourable environment, are said to be able to breed throughout most of the twelve months. Presumably these differences reflect selective breeding working upon genetic variations, and again controlled by man, but one may suppose that, in the absence of his influence, such variations would be either encouraged or suppressed by the operation of natural selection. Thus the young of the red deer are commonly born in June, and it has been observed that those which for some reason or other are born later, in September or October, will often be unable to survive their first winter.

The influence of artificial conditions is well illustrated by the hypersexuality which, as Hediger has pointed out, is so often found in animals living in captivity. This is shown by excessive sexual activity in the pursuit of the female by the male, or by an extension of the oestrous period. It is probably due to a variety of circumstances, including the regular provision of food, the confined quarters, and the lack of diversionary interest. Whatever the precise cause, however, the results are certainly striking. Wild sows, which are normally in heat from November to January, and which give birth to young in April or May, have been known in captivity to have their litters in January or February, at a time when, in the wild state, the young inevitably would die of cold. The results in captivity may not be so disastrous, which explains why hypersexuality is a well-known feature of domestication. Three examples will illustrate this. The dog is monoestrous, but differs from the wild fox (p. 130) in having two cycles, one in early spring and one in autumn, these being separated by a period of anoestrous which last for an average of seven

months. The domestic rabbit can breed throughout most of the year under favourable conditions, while the wild one is restricted mainly to a period extending from January to June. The domestic cat may have several breeding periods during the year while the wild cat reproduces mainly during the spring, with perhaps another oestrous period later in the year.

These facts, implying as they do a subtle combination of rigidity and flexibility in reproductive cycles, emphasize the crucial importance of the pars distalis in acting as the intermediary between the exogenous and endogenous factors upon which these cycles are based. A few examples must serve to illustrate its operation. Sheep transferred across the equator from the northern to the southern hemisphere show a reversal of their reproductive cycle, so that they continue to breed at the appropriate season. This is because the declining autumnal photoperiod (i.e. the length of the daylight period during a single solar day) initiates the onset of the cycle; the same effect can be obtained under experimental conditions, by exposing sheep to increased illumination during the winter and decreased illumination during the summer.

Other mammals are stimulated to reproduction by the increasing photoperiod of early spring. An example is the ferret which can be brought into reproductive activity during winter, when it is normally sexually inactive, by exposure to increasing periods of artificial illumination during autumn. During the prolonged anoestrus the output of oestrogen is low, a situation which in the rat would result, as we have seen, in an increased output of FSH and the inception of a new oestrous cycle. Here, however, the gonadotropin output also remains low, and it is supposed that this is determined by some form of neural inhibition in the hypothalamus. On this interpretation, the effect of the increasing photoperiod is to remove this inhibition, with a consequent rise in the output of gonadotropin. Some support for this view is found in the observation that electrolytic lesions in the anterior hypothalamus of the anoestrous ferret will actually promote the precocious development of oestrus, presumably because they have removed the inhibitory influence.

It is possible that one of the factors involved in the regulation of mammalian reproductive photoperiodicity is the secretory activity of the pineal organ. We shall see (p. 211) that this influences the chromatophores of amphibian larvae through its production of melatonin. In mammals, the pineal has an antigonadotropic action, which is also mediated by melatonin, although other products of the organ have also been implicated in this. The action is enhanced in darkness, supposedly because the production of melatonin is then promoted by activation of an enzyme, hydroxyindole-O-methyl transferase, which is needed for its synthesis. That this effect is in some way associated with sexual condition is suggested by the results of a number of experiments. For example, the ovaries of rats maintained in darkness are 35 per cent smaller in intact animals than they are in pinealectomized ones. Clinically, too, it is suggestive that pineal tumours in young boys are associated with sexual maturity. Conceivably, then, the pineal might adjust the level of reproductive activity to seasonal changes, by transducing photostimulation into chemical secretion, which might then influence the nervous system. In principle, this conforms with evidence that the primitive photoreceptor cells of this organ have become transformed into secretory cells during the later history of the vertebrates. It is still far from certain that this organ is truly an endocrine gland, but at least our knowledge of it has progressed since the seventeenth century, when Descartes attributed to it a particularly close connection with the activities of the soul.

It should not be concluded from the examples so far given, that light is the only stimulus influencing reproductive periodicity in mammals. It is certainly an important one, at least in mid-latitude species, because of its predictive value, but various other factors, such as temperature, and the presence, behaviour, and numbers of other individuals, certainly play important parts.

An example from mammals is given by the population cycling in the snowshoe hare (*Lepus americanus*), which shows a 10-year cycle in Alberta. FSH and LH levels reach a peak in females in June and July, while FSH reaches peaks in April and June in the male. In 1970 and 1971 population density was high, and an adaptive response to this ensued, the breeding season being reduced to three litters instead of the usual four. This was accompanied by a sharp decrease in pituitary FSH levels in the females during August 1970. The precise cause of this adaptive response (more pleasing than infanticide) is not clear, but suggestive evidence comes from mice. In these animals, population density produces stress, which causes an increased output of corticotropin (p. 204). This is thought in some way to affect the output, or perhaps the action, of the gonadotropins, through the action of either corticotropin itself, or of the adrenocortical hormones that it regulates.

The way in which other factors may modulate the effect of photoperiod is shown by bilaterally castrating the snowshoe hare. This operation has no effect upon the pars distalis if it is carried out before the onset of the breeding season, presumably because at that time the hypothalamic–pituitary axis is insensitive to the gonadal steroid levels. It is thought that photoperiod switches on the hypothalamic–neurosecretory activity prior to the breeding season, and that this then stimulates the gonads through increased output of gonadotropins. Only then does the hypothalamus become sensitive to steroids, this permitting the final modulation of the onset of breeding.

These arguments reinforce our earlier conclusions that reproductive cycles depend for their efficiency upon control through the nervous system. Other examples can be given. The response of the ferret to increased illumination is abolished if the optic nerves are cut, showing that the propagation of nerve impulses through those nerves to the brain is an essential element of the reaction. Again, the oestrous cycle of the sheep can be shortened by subjecting the uterus to mechanical distension, but this effect is abolished if the distension is applied to a portion of the uterus which has been denervated; here also, then, nerve impulses must be passing centrally from the stimulated receptors. Our argument is that the final link in the chain of communication which leads to the release of gonadotropins from the pars distalis is the connection between this gland and the hypothalamus, to which these nerve impulses must be transmitted. The importance of this link is shown by the fact that coitus will not evoke ovulation in the rabbit if the connection between the pituitary gland and the brain has been completely severed, while ovulation can always be induced at any time simply by the injection of gonadotropins.

Another illustration of the influencing of reproductive cycles through the nervous system is provided by the action of pheromones. These are external secretions which convey information from one individual to another of the same species, and evoke (usually through olfactory receptors) specific reactions in the recipient. They thus differ from hormones, which are transmitted internally, and which evoke responses in the individual secreting them. However, both types of product can readily be seen as two bands of the spectrum of chemical communication to which we refer elsewhere (p. 1). Clearly they grade into chemical signals which are metabolic products and not specific secretions, but to which other individuals are adapted to respond; and, of course, it is very possible that specific pheromones evolved out of such products.

We shall consider later some examples of them in invertebrates (p. 259).

As regards mammalian reproduction, pheromones are produced in both sexes. Those produced by females enable the male to identify receptive individuals. In sheep, for example, the ram detects by odour those ewes which are in oestrus, and are therefore receptive, and its ability to do this is abolished if its olfactory lobes are destroyed. Pheromones produced by males serve mainly as aphrodisiacs, but they may also influence the course of the reproductive cycle. For example, male sheep or goats, if introduced to females shortly before the breeding season, bring them rapidly from anoestrus into ovulation and heat. It is essential, however, that the male shall be a new partner. If females are already adapted to its presence, this effect is not shown.

The control of the sexual cycle by male pheromones is a widespread phenomenon, shown in many different patterns of reproduction. It is well seen in the mouse, *Mus musculus*, where the introduction of a male into an all-female group initiates synchronous oestrous cycles in all the individuals, regardless of their previous condition. Another example, known as the 'Whiffen effect', after its discoverer, is given by wind-tunnel experiments in which groups of female mice are placed either upwind or downwind of a group of male mice, the three groups being separated by distances of 2 m. The proportion of individuals in oestrus is found to be greater in the downwind group than in the upwind one, an indication of the diffusion of a sex pheromone from the males. Primates are less dependent than other mammals on olfaction, but, even so, olfactory pheromones can play some part in the reproduction of non-human species. For example, pheromones produced by the female rhesus monkey have an aphrodisiac effect on the male. And the profitability of the scent industry suggests that man is not immune from the action of artificial ones.

8.2. Sexual periodicity in birds

Gonadotropins are secreted by the pituitary of birds, but it is uncertain whether they are identical to those of mammals or whether two separate hormones are present, although there is evidence that the effects of mammalian FSH differ from those of LH. Treatment of a hypophysectomized capon with the former results in considerable enlargement of the testes but does not affect the comb, the development of which is known to be dependent upon male hormone; LH treatment, however, results in enlargement of both testes and comb. Experiments upon other birds have also provided evidence that the two gonadotropins differ in their effects, but much remains to be learned regarding the details of pituitary functioning in these animals.

Androgens are secreted by the testes (presumably by the interstitial tissue), and oestrogens, progestins, and androgens by the ovaries. The oestrogens are secreted by the follicles; progestins are perhaps produced by the interstitial tissue, or by the postovulatory follicles, although these latter rapidly disappear. Direct chemical evidence of the nature of the secretions is sparse, but testicular tissue can synthesize testosterone and androstenedione *in vitro* from progesterone, while 17β-oestradiol has been identified in the faeces of the fowl. However, the influence of gonadal steroids upon the sexual characters of birds is well enough established, although the relationship is not always the same as in mammals.

For example, the sexual dimorphism in the plumage of the English sparrow is determined by the direct action of genes, without the intervention of hormones at all, while the situation in certain finches is curiously varied. In *Steganura* the blackening of the feathers and beak in the breeding male is under the direct control of the pituitary (gonadotropic) secretion, while in *Euplectes* the feather colour is determined in the same way but the beak colour by the secretion of the testes. The domestic fowl provides other familiar examples of these interrelationships. The capon (castrated cock) retains the male type of plumage, but implantation of an ovary will result in the development of feathers of female type. In this respect, then, the male characterization is essentially the neutral one, while the female characterization is hormone dependent. This principle is not, however, applicable to all characters, even in this one species, for the exaggerated comb and wattles of the cock undergo atrophy in the capon and can only be brought to full development by the action of male hormone (Fig. 7.14).

Particularly interesting differences between birds and mammals are seen in the ways in which their hormonal equipment is deployed in accordance with their different modes of reproduction. The most striking contrast (leaving the Monotremata out of consideration) lies in the serial production by birds of large and yolky eggs which are physiologically expensive to produce and which require the addition of an elaborate set of egg membranes. In connection with this, we find that oestrogens, in addition to promoting the development of the Müllerian duct system, also bring about the increased absorption of food material and the mobilization of food reserves which are needed to facilitate the manufacture of yolk by the liver; these biochemical effects presumably underlaid the use of stilboestrol by the poultry industry (p. 114). Other examples of the adaptive organization of this system are the control of yolk deposition in the ovum by the gonadotropins, the part played by progesterone in evoking ovulation by stimulating (apparently through a hypothalamic neural mechanism) the release of gonadotropins from the pituitary, and the combined action of oestrogen and progesterone (and, probably, androgen) in promoting the secretion of albumen by the oviduct.

The seasonal onset of reproductive behaviour in birds, often accompanied by remarkable migrations to areas suitable for the rearing of the young, are matters of common knowledge, and current interpretations of this agree in ascribing the regulation of it to an interplay of exogenous and endogenous factors, although there are differences of opinion as to the relative importance that should be attached to these. The significance of photoperiod in this connection was first clearly demonstrated in the classical studies of Rowan who, from 1925 onwards, showed that the gonads of the migratory Canadian bunting, *Junco hyemalis*, which normally comes into breeding condition in the spring, could be made to grow and mature during the winter if the animal was subjected to periods of increasing illumination. These results are applicable to other species, so that the role of exogenous factors in the sexual periodicity of birds is thoroughly well established.

The gonads of birds undergo remarkable fluctuations in size during the year (Fig. 8.4). In the temperate zone they are typically at their minimal size during the winter, and start to enlarge when day-length increases. Intense spermatogenesis begins shortly before the breeding season, and the testes may finally increase in weight by as much as five hundred times. This growth is accompanied by increasing hormone output which, in its turn, influences the development of sexual behaviour; manifested, for example, in the selection of territory and in the use of song to assert territorial rights. It is characteristic of birds that the female lags behind in sexual maturation, and that ovulation is not rigorously determined by the onset of an oestrus-like phase. Instead, special stimulation is required, peculiar to each species, before the completion of the final stages of oocyte development can be achieved. The song and display of the male are important factors in this stimulation, and provide one of the clearest demonstrations that secondary sexual

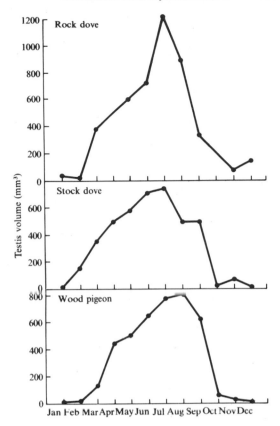

FIG. 8.4. The annual cycle in testicular size of three species of British birds. (From Lofts (1970). *Animal photoperiodism.* Edward Arnold, London.)

characters are as essential for successful insemination as are the genital ducts. No useful distinction can be made between them and the accessory sexual factors from this point of view (p. 112).

After breeding, the gonads of most birds in the temperate zone undergo regression. Sexual behavior diminishes, and those birds which have been living in pairs usually form flocks. The testis tubules become reduced, and cholesterol-rich lipid appears in large amounts in the Sertoli cells. These regressive changes result from the cessation of secretion of gonadotropins, and, in consequence, of androgens. Evidence for this is that gonadal regression can be terminated by injections of FSH, which lead to loss of lipid and onset of spermatogenesis. Conversely, regression can be induced at any time by hypophysectomy. Many birds, in Britain and elsewhere, show signs of sexual activity during the autumn. This, however, is checked by winter conditions, such as low temperature; photostimulation early in the new year then promotes a renewal of the activity in time to permit reproduction in the favourable months of spring and early summer.

Birds will not respond to artificial increase in photoperiod during the regression phase, which, for this reason, is called the refractory period. It may last for weeks, or even for months. The time is a reflection of the circumstances to which the species is adapted, for the refractory period is an adaptation to prevent the production of young when feeding conditions may be adverse. The point is well illustrated by the rook, *Corvus frugilegus*. This bird produces young in April and May, and then passes into a refractory phase which lasts until the autumn. Thus the birds cannot be stimulated into further reproductive activity by the long days of summer. This is probably an adaptation to the difficulty of obtaining earthworms during the (hopefully) dry summer weather; they are essential food for the young, and there could be wasteful mortality if young were produced during that period.

The influence of temperature, already noted, shows that photoperiod, while certainly a common modulating agent in avian reproduction, is not the only one. Indeed, the concentration of endocrinologists in temperate regions has probably resulted in undue importance being attached to the value of day-length as predictive information. Some birds (e.g. the domestic duck) will show sexual cycles in complete darkness. In other birds, the influence of light has become lessened as a result of adaptation to artificial conditions resulting from association with man (cf. p. 132). Thus the town pigeon breeds throughout the year, although the rock dove (*Columba livia*), from which it is descended, shows a seasonal reproductive behaviour like that of the wood-pigeon (Fig. 8.5). This is presumably a result of food for the pigeon being plentiful throughout the year, for, as we have seen, the natural breeding cycles are largely adaptations to seasonal food supplies. Similar effects have been produced in the domestic fowl by human selection for maximum egg production. Even in natural photoperiods this bird maintains an active ovary throughout the year, and seasonal fluctuations in egg production can be further reduced by artificial lighting.

Natural selection has also operated to adapt particular species to special features of their environment. An example is the red-billed weaver-finch, *Quelea quelea*, which is adapted for reproduction in an arid environment where dependence upon photoperiod might prove fatal. These birds are adapted to make an immediate response to rainfall, upon which

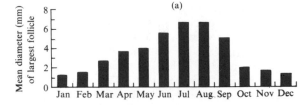

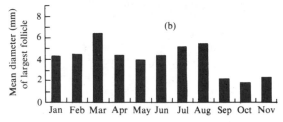

FIG. 8.5. (a) Seasonal variation in the mean diameter of the largest ovarian follicle in the wood-pigeon. A follicle diameter of over 5 mm indicates an ovary close to egg-laying. (b) Seasonal variation in the mean diameter of the largest ovarian follicle in a population of feral town pigeons. The seasonal trend noted in the wood-pigeon (Fig. 8.5(a)) has been eliminated. (From Lofts (1970). *Animal photoperiodism*. Edward Arnold, London.)

they depend for the provision of nesting material and of insect food for the young. Once favourable conditions are available, nest-building and courtship are rapidly completed, so that individuals are able to ovulate within eleven days of the arrival of rain.

We can mention only one other example from the many fascinating ones which could be used to illustrate the principle of the interaction of endogenous and exogenous factors in birds. The mutton-bird, or short-tailed shearwater (*Puffinus tenuirostris*), leaves South Australia in flocks during autumn (April) to undertake a circum-Pacific migration, through Japan and western North America, which brings them back with remarkable regularity to breed at their starting point during a period of twelve days in November. Captive birds maintained under abnormal conditions of lighting, food, and temperature have been found to come into breeding condition at much the same time as that at which they would have done had they been able to complete a normal migration, which suggests that an endogenous rhythm exists, and can operate without being stimulated by exogenous factors. Nevertheless, the condition of the reproductive system is not wholly normal in these experimental animals, and there is a marked retardation of spermatogenesis, which again suggests that such endogenous rhythms must be modulated by external stimulating factors.

It seems likely that migratory behaviour itself must be influenced by hormones, but the factors involved are obscure. The gonadal steroids might be expected to play a part, yet the characteristic restlessness which occurs in captive birds at the time of their normal migration is seen also in birds that have been castrated. Photoperiod might also be thought a likely factor, but, if it is so, the birds must be responding to an increasing photoperiod in the spring and to a decreasing one in the autumn. This is not an impossibility, but the causal chain is not understood.

8.3. Sexual periodicity in the lower vertebrates

The fact that pituitary gonadotropins are essential for reproduction in Amphibia has been amply demonstrated. Thus, hypophysectomy of male *Rana esculenta* in autumn leads to degeneration of the primary spermatocytes, so that in the next summer only primary spermatogonia are present in the testis tubules, although spermatogenesis is normally proceeding actively at that time (Fig. 8.6). Administration of extracts of frog pituitaries will restore

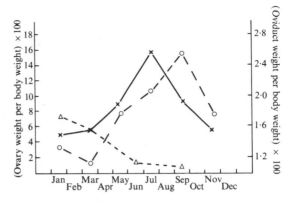

FIG. 8.7. Seasonal variation in weight of the ovaries and oviducts of *Xenopus laevis* and the effect of hypophysectomy. ($\times$———$\times$) ovaries and (o———o) oviducts of free-living animals; ($\triangle$————$\triangle$) ovaries from animals hypophysectomized in February. (From Smith (1955). *Mem. Soc. Endocrin.* **4.**)

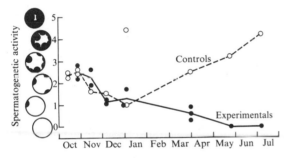

FIG. 8.6. Spermatogenetic activity from October to July in hypophysectomized *Rana esculenta* (*experimentals*) and in unoperated animals (*controls*) living under laboratory conditions. The circles to the left indicate six stages of spermatogenetic activity, from 0 (testis tubules with only a few primary spermatogonia) to 5 (testis tubules almost filled with nests of spermatogenetic cells). (From Sluiter *et al.* (1950). *Q. Jl microsp. Sci.* **91.**)

spermatogenesis in hypophysectomized males, and will similarly restore the size of the ovaries in hypophysectomized females, which normally suffer ovarian degeneration after this treatment (Fig. 8.7). Another illustration is the fact that ovulation can be induced in *Xenopus laevis* at any time of the year by the introduction of pituitaries from the same species, or by the administration of extracts of the pituitaries of cattle, while the induction of ovulation in this and other species by treatment with human urine constitutes a well-established diagnosis of pregnancy.

As an illustration of the interplay of endogenous and exogenous factors in these animals we may consider briefly the reproductive cycle of the male frog,

which has been extensively studied by many workers. Often it is markedly seasonal, as it is in *Rana temporaria*. In this species, the cycle can be divided into three phases, the first being the reproductive phase, which typically occurs during the first two weeks of March. This phase, immediately following hibernation, comprises ovulation, spawning, and fertilization. It is succeeded by a resumption of gonadal activity, extending from April to October, during which time spermatogenesis and oogenesis take place and lead to the establishment of mature testes and ovaries. The third phase, hibernation, is necessarily one of sexual inactivity, but the animals are throughout in a condition that enables them to respond immediately to the onset of spring, and thus to reproduce sufficiently early to permit the tadpoles to grow and metamorphose under favourable circumstances. Interstitial tissue giving positive responses to tests for steroids is well defined in anuran testes; in urodeles, the equivalent tissue has the form of boundary cells, similar to those of teleosts (p. 138). These tissues, regardless of their position, doubtless secrete androgens which promote the development of such sexual characters as the thumb-pad in frogs and the crest in the male newt, for these atrophy after castration. Moreover, the interstitial tissue shows a well-defined seasonal cycle. During the winter the testis is inactive, with little sudanophilia. As the breeding season approaches, there is accumulation of lipid droplets and of 3β-HSDH. Cholesterol-positive lipid is conspicuous after breeding, but there is no 3β-HSDH, and the interstitial cells in *Rana temporaria* regress. The Sertoli cells, as in amniotes, give evidence of steroid-secreting capacity.

They have a well-developed endoplasmic reticulum, and contain 3β-HSDH. Lipid is plentiful in them after breeding, but 3β-HSDH disappears, and the cells slowly regress.

The restriction of spermatogenesis in *Rana temporaria* to the late spring and the summer is an example of the discontinuous type of reproductive cycle which is characteristic of the Anura in temperate zones. In many anurans, however, sperm can be formed throughout the year, the cycle thus being of the continuous type. Both types may occur in the same species, as they do in *R. esculenta*, which has a continuous cycle in Mediterranean regions, but a discontinuous one in temperate regions. The difference suggests an adaptation of populations to their environments. It has been suggested that the onset of spermatogenesis in *R. temporaria* is determined by an exogenous stimulus, the environmental temperature, but that its termination at the onset of hibernation is brought about by an endogenous rhythm. Raising the temperature during the first part of the hibernation period does not, however, increase the activity of the testis, which suggests that the termination of spermatogenesis at hibernation is brought about by an endogenous rhythm. On the other hand, spermatogenesis can be induced at any time in *R. esculenta* by raising the temperature, so that in this species the exogenous factor predominates throughout. The cycle of *R. esculenta* is therefore potentially continuous, even in those populations in which it is actually discontinuous, whereas the discontinuous cycle of *R. temporaria* is innate and, as far as is known, cannot become continuous.

The importance of the endogenous rhythm in *R. temporaria* was noted by Witschi in his pioneer studies of its geographical races in Europe. In one of these, the 'early race', reproduction occurs in March and spermatogenesis from May until September, while in the other, the 'late race', reproduction is delayed until May, with spermatogenesis extending from April to August. These differences are clearly adaptations to the conditions of the Western lowlands and to those of the Alpine and Northern regions in which the 'early races' and 'late races' respectively live; they seem to be largely innate, for they are not modified when, for example, the 'late race' is transferred to lowland conditions.

Finally, we can draw some examples from teleost fish. It is generally supposed that the development of the sexual characters of these animals is determined by the secretion of gonadal hormones, and there is probably justification for this view since, for example, testosterone has been identified in the blood of spawned Pacific salmon, and oestrogens in the blood of spawning Atlantic salmon. Moreover, experiments involving gonadectomy or treatment with steroid sex hormones in certain species have given results in accordance with this view, although castration is difficult to carry out in fish without high mortality, and, as in all animals with a limited reproductive season, the results will be influenced by the time at which the experiments are performed. In *Gasterosteus*, amongst others, there is a relationship between the breeding dress of the male and the presence of testes, while the treatment of both sexes of Poeciliidae and Cyprinodontidae (such as *Lebistes* and *Xiphophorus*) with male hormone, either by injection or by immersion of the fish in a solution of methyl testosterone, will promote the transformation of the anal fin into the characteristic male gonopodium. It is hardly necessary to emphasize that such experiments require the closest control of all conditions, including particularly the strength of the hormone dosage.

Leydig cells are readily seen in male *Gasterosteus*, but it is difficult to find them in many species of teleosts, and it was once assumed that they lacked androgen-secreting cells. This, however, is not so. They are present in such species as boundary cells, so called because they are not in the interstitial position typical of vertebrates. Instead, they are represented by cells containing lipids and cholesterol which are situated in the walls of the testis lobules, and which are derived from fibroblasts. One example is given by the pike, in which the testis undergoes a seasonal cycle very similar to that of birds, including the breaking down of the lobules into cholesterol-positive lipid material after spawning, and the disappearance of the lobule boundary cells; a new generation of these begins to become lipoidal in September (Fig. 8.8).

The production of gonadotropins by the pituitary gland is well established for fish, and probably occurs also in the cyclostomes. Hypophysectomy of the river lamprey, *Lampetra fluviatilis*, prevents the prespawning growth of the eggs, while amongst the effects which have been reported in elasmobranch fish are a breakdown in the early stages of spermatogenesis and atretic degeneration in the ovaries. In hypophysectomized teleosts the oocytes can begin their growth phase but undergo degeneration at the start of vitellogenesis; there appears, then, in these animals, as in mammals, to be a critical stage beyond which the ovarian function is dependent upon the presence of pituitary gonadotropin secretion (p. 118). Whether the latter comprises one or more hormones

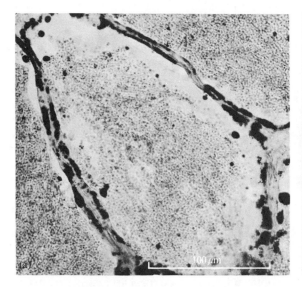 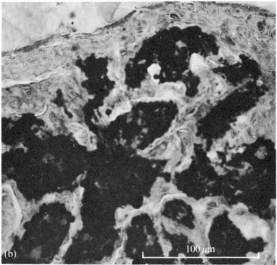

FIG. 8.8. (a) Testis of the pike (*Esox lucius*) in March, just prior to spawning; the lobules are full of sperm and the boundary cells of the lobule walls are charged with cholesterol-positive lipids (formaldehyde–calcium fixation; Sudan black and haemalum. (b) Testis in May, immediately after spawning; dense cholesterol-positive lipid is now found in the lumina of the lobules. (From Lofts and Marshall (1957). *Q. J. microsp. Sci.* **98**.)

is at present uncertain, as it is for all of the lower vertebrates, since the necessary chemical studies are lacking; nor can we be sure that the gonadal steroids react upon the pars distalis as they are known to do in mammals.

The reproductive cycles of fish are known to be closely linked with annual seasonal changes in their environment, and there is much evidence to suggest that their mode of regulation is similar in principle to that found in higher forms, as we might expect from the nature of the hormonal equipment which we have just outlined. Thus the breeding behaviour of the viviparous South American fish, *Jenynsia lineata*, closely resembles that of the sheep, in that when it is moved from the southern to the northern hemisphere it readily adapts its reproductive cycle to the shift in the seasons (p. 132). These animals are influenced both by temperature and photoperiod; by suitable experimental manipulation of these factors it is possible to induce the same fish to breed twice in a year, once under conditions of Argentinian day-length (from October to February) and again under conditions of North American day-length (during May, June, and July).

It is impossible to do more than glance briefly here at one or two other examples of reproductive cycles in fish. The minnow, *Phoxinus phoxinus*, breeds in Windermere from May to July, the length of this period resulting from the fact that different indi-viduals mature at different times. Immediately following this there is an initiation of gametogenesis in both sexes and this process continues throughout the autumn but virtually ceases during the winter. With the arrival of spring there is then a rapid completion of maturation in both sexes, with considerable enlargement of the gonads. Spermatogenesis and oocyte growth can be accelerated by subjecting the fish during the winter months to an artificially increased photoperiod of seventeen hours, provided that the temperature is maintained above a certain threshold value (Fig. 8.9). Presumably, light and temperature are exogenous factors controlling the reproductive cycle in this species. On the other hand, if the fish are kept in continuous darkness during the early months of the year, they still show gonadal development during the summer, although with some delay. This suggests an internal reproductive rhythm which can operate independently of these external factors, but which is normally modulated by them.

A cycle similar to that of *Phoxinus*, but one that illustrates the differences in detail between different species, is found in *Gasterosteus aculeatus*, the three-spined stickleback. Here again reproduction occurs in April and May, and maturation of the gonads sets in during the summer, but in this species the development of the germ cells can continue during the winter, although its rate is influenced by the water temperature. It is supposed that light is not an

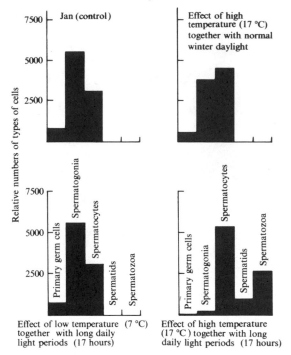

FIG. 8.9. Histograms showing the relative numbers of cell types in the testes of minnows subjected to various experimental conditions. (From Bullough (1940). *Proc. zool. Soc. Lond.* A**109**.)

important factor, and that the final stages of maturation are evoked by the rise in water temperature during the early months of the year.

For fish, as for birds, there is thus much evidence to show that environmental signals determine in broad terms the time of reproduction, but that finer details of the environment provide the final synchronization, just as in the female bird. This is well-known to fish breeders. Goldfish require green plants to evoke breeding, while the Japanese bitterling (*Rhodeus ocellatus*) is said to need the company of a particular fresh-water mussel. Equally important is the presence of other individuals of the species, without which spawning may be restricted or non-existent. We may feel confident that in these matters a fundamental uniformity of principle operates throughout the vertebrates, and that we all have our problems. It would be surprising if this were not so, for the capacity to bring internal reproductive rhythms into relationship with a fluctuating environment must have been of prime importance at all stages of vertebrate evolution.

8.4. Hormones and behaviour

Our analysis of reproductive cycles has implied a far-reaching influence of hormones upon behaviour.

This is particularly well seen in the female mammal, where the mating responses of oestrus contrast sharply with the maternal activity which develops at the end of pregnancy, and where there is usually a close correlation between high secretory activity of the gonads and the attaining of a complete pattern of mating behaviour. In males the correlation may appear less obvious, but this is merely because both sexual and secretory activity tend to be continuous in those species that are polyoestrous all the year round; in those that have only a limited breeding period, the activity of the male does, in fact, coincide with the recrudescence of the interstitial tissue as, for example, in the deer. Because of this correlation, it is not surprising to find that the mating behaviour of the female cat is completely eliminated by the removal of both ovaries, and this in itself is a striking illustration of the dependence of that behaviour upon the ovarian hormone. A castrated female responds aggressively to any male that attempts to mount her, but a normal sexual response can readily be restored by an injection of oestrogen. Another illustration is provided by the treatment of immature female mammals with gonadotropins; the result of this may be to evoke secretory activity in the ovaries, and this will then bring about precocious sexual activity. Under such circumstances, female rats may show the typical behaviour of oestrus when they are only twenty-two days old, and when they are so small that adult males cannot copulate with them. It would appear, then, that the neuromuscular basis of sexual behaviour is organized well in advance of the attainment of sexual maturity, but that the activation of the physiological mechanisms awaits the presence of a sufficiently high level of circulating sex hormone.

The means by which such activation is achieved are difficult to analyse because of the inherent complexity of the situation, but a number of possibilities have been formulated. It may be that hormones influence behaviour indirectly by their influence upon the growth and metabolism of the whole organism, or upon the maturation of specific structures which are required for effecting a particular response. On the other hand, they may exert a more direct influence by some form of action upon the nervous system, by promoting its development, for example, or by sensitizing peripheral receptor mechanisms, or by facilitating its integrative functions in some way. Beach has developed on this basis the concept of the sexual arousal mechanism. According to this, sexual behaviour is activated by a variety of sensory stimuli, and it is a function of the gonadal

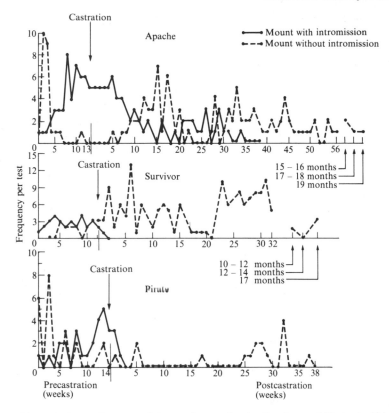

F IG. 8.10. Comparisons of intromissions and mounts of three male cats, Apache, Survivor, and Pirate, typifying the three modes of decline of sexual behaviour after castration. (From Rosenblatt and Aronson (1958). *Behaviour* **12.**)

hormones to lower the threshold of this arousal mechanism by exerting a sensitizing action upon the nervous system. To such possibilities we must add that sexual behaviour may be affected by other hormones than those which are regarded as sex hormones in the strict use of that term. The situation here is closely analogous to the control of growth and metabolism which we considered earlier, and which we found to be influenced not only by pituitary growth hormone and insulin but by other hormones with interrelated actions. The thyroid hormones, for example, may be expected to have some effect upon reproduction in mammals simply by virtue of their profound influence on metabolism (Chapter 10).

The castration of male cats, however, illustrates the complexities of these problems, for the effects of this operation, as estimated from the subsequent sexual behaviour of the operated animals, prove to be curiously variable. Some will continue to mount females almost indefinitely, and will achieve successful intromission for several years, others will continue mounting for a year or more but quickly lose the capacity for intromission, while others quickly lose the capacity for both of these components of successful mating (Fig. 8.10). It has sometimes been suggested that in these circumstances the adrenocortical secretions (Chapter 12) may be substituting for the sex steroids, but satisfactory evidence for this seems to be lacking. The differences are certainly influenced by the previous sexual experience of the animals, and are probably determined also by differing characteristics of the nervous system. For example, castrated guinea-pigs, belonging to two strains that differ in their level of sexual activity, can have their sexual behaviour restored by testosterone injections, but retain their different levels of activity, regardless of the amount of hormone administered.

An important factor in all aspects of the behaviour of mammals is the importance assumed in its regulation by the higher centres, and especially by the cerebral cortex. As a result, although various reflex elements of sexual behaviour can be elicited by experimental stimulation of the spinal cord, the higher centres seem to be needed for the achievement of the complete integration of an effective behaviour pattern; both hypothalamus and cortex, in fact, have their parts to play, and it would appear that while a totally decorticate male cat loses all sexual responses, a decorticate female is capable of fertile mating provided that her hypothalamus is intact.

An illustration of a direct action of an oestrogen upon the nervous system is that the implantation of stilboestrol or oestradiol into the brain of ovariectomized cats will restore sexual behaviour to an extent amounting sometimes to nymphomania. A particularly interesting feature of this response is that the genital tracts of the excited animals remain in a completely anoestrous condition, so that the hormones must be assumed to be acting directly upon the nervous system without exerting any more generalized effect upon other parts of the body.

Arising from this, it has sometimes been suggested that there is an evolutionary trend in mammals which leads to a more or less complete domination of the sex hormones by the cerebral cortex in man. It is highly doubtful, however, whether there is any evidence for such a trend, and it is certain that the situation in the human is sufficiently remarkable to justify its inclusion amongst the unique features of our species. The essential peculiarity lies in the fact that structurally the human being appears to be capable of sexual behaviour from perhaps five or six years of age, but that the full release of this behaviour through the mediation of the sex hormones is delayed during a prolonged juvenile phase, this being one special aspect of the extended period of development and maturation which is an important characteristic of man. This period of sexual latency, which has been aptly referred to as an odd example of 'brinkmanship', creates psychological tensions which are thought possibly to be the origin of the Oedipus complex. Thus it is by no means surprising to find that when the sexual functions have fully matured, they are subservient to cortical control rather than to gonadal hormones. It is perhaps partly because of this that both sexes may continue to show a high level of sexual capacity after removal of the gonads, although, as we have seen, this phenomenon is not peculiar to the human species, even though it may there be exceptional in its degree of development. Indeed, it is arguable that the most important influence of hormones upon sex behaviour in the mammals is their effect in securing the appropriate degree of structural development and the initial integration of the behaviour patterns. Even in the lower mammals, there is some evidence that animals which have been gonadectomized prior to puberty may subsequently show fewer signs of effective sexual behaviour than those which have been gonadectomized after they have had some adult sexual experience.

The considerations which we have outlined seem to be applicable in broad terms throught the vertebrates, although relevant information is sometimes very limited and, in the case of cyclostomes and elasmobranchs, virtually non-existent. Even in teleosts, which have received considerable attention, there is little direct evidence for an action of sex steroids on behaviour, although, as we have seen, they certainly affect other aspects of the secondary sexual characters. The sexual colouration of the male stickleback is associated with a complex and well-studied chain of behaviour, involving nest-building, mating, parental care, and territorial defence. Castration results in a loss of sexual colouration, but its effects upon behaviour depend on the photoperiod operating at the time of the experiment, and on the particular phase of behaviour that is dominant at the time. Other complications are the existence of the inevitable species differences, and also the difficulty of ensuring that the gonads have been completely removed and that there has been no regeneration. However, when allowance has been made for these factors, it still appears that some elements of the behaviour pattern are affected more than others, and that some males may retain parts of the pattern for a long time after castration. Thus, males of *Xiphophorus* may continue to show thrusting and swinging movements of the gonopodium, and sidling movements alongside the female, for up to nine months after the operation. It may be, then, that reflex responses to sexual situations can still be evoked in gonadectomized animals by the stimuli provided by other members of the group.

In any case, the gonadal hormones are unlikely to be the only endocrine factors involved in the regulation of sexual behaviour in fish. We shall see later evidence of some involvement of the thyroid hormones in the reproductive migration of sticklebacks (p. 177) from sea water to fresh water, while in several species these hormones produce an increase in general locomotor activity.

Two other examples will illustrate this point. The salmon (*Salmo salar*), in addition to its upstream spawning migration, also has a downstream migration at the smolt stage. The smolt is sexually immature, which suggests that migratory movements are not dependent upon gonadal hormones, and that this may also be true of sexually mature ones. Again, populations of the cod, *Gadus callarias*, which feed during the summer on the Bear Island–Spitzbergen Banks, undertake in the autumn, at the onset of sexual maturation, a migration of hundreds of miles to their spawning grounds off the north Norwegian coast. It would seem reasonable to ascribe this to some stimulatory effect exerted by the sex hormones, were it not for the fact that immature fish undergo a similar migration, known as the 'dummy run'; this takes them in the same direction, and sometimes over very much the same distance. The most obvious endocrine factor that the immature and mature animals have in common is a high level of activity of the thyroid gland. This suggests that the thyroid hormones rather than the gonadal ones may be the significant endogenous factor (p. 183).

This is exactly the field in which hormonal interaction is much to be expected, and it is well exemplified in the paradise fish, *Macropodus opercularis*. Here androgen increases building activity, but prolactin is needed to ensure the secretion of the mucus that is used in building the bubble nests. One possibility in these and other cases is that the gonadal hormones may influence the timing of the elements of reproductive behaviour, and perhaps potentiate the action of the other hormones involved. We are here confronted with the fundamental principle that the endocrine glands constitute an interacting and integrated system. Each element of the system has its contribution to make to the execution of a complex response. The problem facing the experimenter is to interpret, in the context of the total behaviour of his animals, the results obtained with individual hormones.

8.5. Hormones and viviparity

The reproductive cycle of the female eutherian mammal comprises two phases: a follicular phase, concerned with the production of the ova and ensuring of internal fertilization, and a luteal phase, concerned with the safeguarding of the foetus. The first of these is the more primitive. Evidence of a functional relationship between the pituitary gland and the ovary in cyclostomes and fish shows that it is one of the primary elements of the endocrine organization of vertebrates, and that its establishment must have antedate the evolution of viviparity.

As regards the second (luteal) phase, the situation is less clear. In all the vertebrate classes, with the exception of birds, corpora lutea develop from the post-ovulatory follicles. Often they look gland-like, and contain cholesterol-positive lipid; 3β-HSDH activity may also be present, most clearly in reptiles, but only doubtfully in teleosts. Progestins are often

identifiable in non-mammalian ovaries, but there is no convincing evidence that these are secreted by the corpora lutea, or, indeed, that these have any secretory function at all. Because of this, it has been suggested that they are a device for tidying-up the discharged follicle and, where necessary, for the ingestion of moribund ova. Only in mammals do they have a clearly defined endocrine role, but it is not difficult to visualize the evolution of this from the corpora lutea of lower groups, perhaps by utilization of the biosynthetic capacity of the degenerating follicle. In some such way they must have been drawn upon to make an essential contribution to the endocrine regulation of pregnancy.

What is surprising is that this has not happened in other vertebrate classes, all of which (with the exception of cyclostomes and birds) have evolved, in at least a few species, various patterns of viviparity. Perhaps the reptiles have come nearest to achieving a true luteal phase, for ovariectomy terminates pregnancy in certain snakes, if carried out during the early stages of pregnancy, while progestin secretion by the ovary is more pronounced in pregnant snakes than in non-pregnant ones. Nevertheless, the uptake of labelled amino acid into the amniotic fluid and body of the early embryo of a lizard, *Xantusia vigilis*, is not affected by either ovariectomy or removal of the corpora lutea (Fig. 8.11), which suggests that placental absorption in this animal is not under endocrine control.

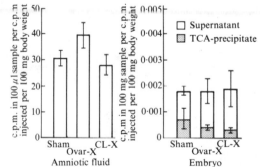

FIG. 8.11. Transfer of [³H]leucine into embryonic compartments of the lizard, *Xantusia vigilis*. Operations were made on pregnant females within the first two weeks of gestation. After one month, labelled amino acid was injected into the thigh muscles of the female. The embryo was sampled 4 hours later. *Left*, total protein plus labelled amino acid in amniotic fluid. *Right*, labelled amino acid (supernatant) plus protein (trichloroacetic acid (TCA) precipitate) in embryo. (Ovar-X, ovariectomized; CL-X, deluteinized). (From Yaron (1972). *Gen. comp. Endocrin.*, Suppl. 3 (eds W. S. Hoar and H. A. Bern).)

The modification of the reproductive cycle in adaptation to mammalian viviparity is seen in a simple form in marsupials. In this group (with only

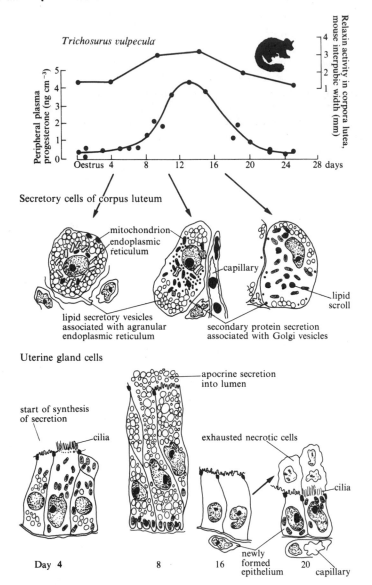

FIG. 8.12. Oestrous cycle of the brush possum, *Trichosurus vulpecula*. The lipid vesicles probably contain cholesterol and subsequently pregnenolone, which is converted to progesterone on the mitochondria at day 8–12, before being secreted into the adjacent capillaries. The small dense secretion, which appears later and is associated with the Golgi region, is released between day 12 and 16, and may be relaxin. The uterine gland cells begin to synthesize secretion by day 4; maximum release occurs between day 8 and 12; the exhausted cells are then replaced by an underlying epithelium, newly formed from stromal cells. (From Tyndale-Biscoe (1973). *Life of marsupials*. Edward Arnold, London.)

two exceptions), gestation is completed in a shorter time than the length of the oestrous cycle. For example, in the brush possum, *Trichosurus vulpecula* (Fig. 8.12), which is seasonally polyoestrous, a cycle extends over 28 days, while gestation lasts for about 18 days. Ovulation, therefore, could theoretically occur at the end of gestation without disturbing the

regularity of the oestrous cycle, and this is what does occur if the young are prevented from entering the pouch. Normally, however, ovulation is delayed by their entry, and the consequent stimulation of suckling; it is then resumed when suckling ends.

In this pattern of events, the corpora lutea have a more limited role than in eutherian reproduction.

They are needed for the initiation of uterine secretion, through the mediation of the progesterone which they secrete, but this phase, once initiated, can continue without them. They inhibit ovulation during the first part of the oestrous cycle, although it is not clear whether this effect, too, is mediated by progesterone. They also secrete, in addition to progesterone, a polypeptide product which is believed to be another hormone, relaxin, that has been identified in the ovary. This hormone is referred to again later (p. 146). Its function in marsupials is obscure, but it is likely to be concerned, in conjunction with progesterone, in facilitating parturition by action on the pubic region. What is particularly characteristic of marsupial reproduction, however, is that the corpora lutea are not responsible for the maintenance of gestation.

Eutherians are fundamentally different in this respect, for in these animals the maintenance of gestation depends upon the continued action of progesterone, and hence requires a prolongation of the luteal phase of the cycle. This is achieved in one or other of two ways. One of these is the continued secretion of progesterone by the corpus luteum; this requires an additional source of luteinizing or luteotropic hormone in order to maintain luteal activity. The other involves the development of an additional source of progesterone, so that the corpora lutea are no longer required to be present throughout gestation. Unfortunately, too little is known of the endocrinology of the various placental groups for it to be possible to organize the facts into any evolutionary series, and in any case it may well be that there has been much independent and parallel evolution within this field. We shall therefore merely consider one or two examples in which the facts have been clearly determined.

The rat is one of a number of mammals (the opossum, rabbit, goat, and cow are others) in which the ovary must be present for at least the greater part of pregnancy in order to ensure the maintenance of gestation; resorption or abortion will occur if the ovaries are removed, particularly if the operation is carried out during the first half of pregnancy. The pars distalis is also essential for the establishment of pregnancy and its presence is needed up to the eleventh day, but from then onwards it can be removed without interrupting gestation. This is because by that time another source of prolactin has become available for the maintenance of the corpora lutea (p. 130). The placenta is the additional source of this hormone; in consequence, pregnancy can be maintained in rats that have been hypophysectomized

on the sixth day of gestation, provided that placental tissue is implanted into them. Moreover, if extracts of rat placentae are administered to hypophysectomized rats, they will continue to be able to develop uterine deciduomata. It follows that the extracts contain a tropic hormone which is capable of maintaining the activity of the corpora lutea in the absence of the prolactin (luteotropin) of the pituitary.

We find, therefore, in the rat an illustration of the first of the two methods suggested above for the prolongation of the activity of the corpus luteum, but it cannot be assumed that an exactly similar method will be found in other groups, nor is it clear that the luteotropic action of prolactin is at all widespread. The mouse does, in fact, seem to be very much the same as the rat in this regard, but in the hypophysectomized rabbit it has been possible to maintain luteal function by treatment with oestrogens as well as with gonadotropins. This suggests that in the rabbit, the gonadotropins act only indirectly on the corpora lutea by promoting the secretion of oestrogen by the ovary. Such differences are, of course, to be expected if, as suggested above, some degree of independent evolution has occurred in the various groups.

Another illustration of this is the fact, first demonstrated by Aschheim and Zondek in 1927, that pregnancy in the human female is characterized by the appearance in the urine of a gonadotropin (human chorionic gonadotropin, HCG) which reaches its maximum concentration between the sixtieth and eightieth days of pregnancy. Similar hormones have been found in the rhesus monkey and the chimpanzee, although with marked differences in the amounts excreted and the lengths of time during which they are pregnant. These three hormones are very like LH in action, for they will not stimulate follicular growth in hypophysectomized rats, but will luteinize follicles that are already present. In the intact animal, however, they react synergistically with the pituitary gonadotropins, and in the immature mouse will produce both follicle stimulation and luteinization; a reaction which is the basis of the Aschheim–Zondek pregnancy test. Injected into mature non-pregnant rabbits, they will produce ovulation and luteinization, reactions which, as we have seen, would not normally occur unless the animals had copulated. This is the basis of the Friedman test for pregnancy. Chorionic villi are known to be able to synthesize a hormone of this type in tissue culture, and, since under these conditions the villi give rise to cytotrophoblast but not to syncitiotrophoblast, the hormone must arise from the former tissue. This is why it is known as chorionic gonadotropin. It will be noted that it is being secreted by the embryo and not by the mother.

Another illustration of independent evolution in the promotion of the activity of the corpora lutea is provided by the appearance in the serum of the pregnant mare of a gonadotropin, known as pregnant mare serum gonadotropin, which reaches a maximum concentration at about the eightieth day of pregnancy. This differs from chorionic gonadotropin both in its origin and in its mode of functioning. As regards the former, it is believed to originate not in the chorion but in the specialized uterine tissue known as the endometrial cups. Functionally, the effect of this hormone on hypophysectomized animals is to bring about follicular growth with considerable increase in ovarian weight, stimulation of the interstitial cells, and an increased output of oestrogens, while ovulation and corpus luteum formation may also occur. It thus differs from the chorionic gonadotropin of primates in its marked capacity for stimulating follicular development, and its particular significance in pregnancy may be associated with the presence in the mare of many accessory corpora lutea.

We have so far considered the endocrinology of pregnancy in terms of the production of progesterone, but oestrogen is also necessary for the maintenance of gestation, for the administration of both hormones is needed to ensure this in the ovariectomized pregnant rat or hamster. On the other hand, the ovariectomized mouse and rabbit require only progesterone alone, while neither hormone is needed by the ovariectomized mare, monkey, or human, once a certain state of pregnancy has been reached. These facts suggest that the placenta has gradually become a source of these steroid hormones, so that eventually complete independence of the ovaries is achieved. The assumption is that neither hormone is secreted by the placenta of the rat and hamster, that oestrogen is secreted by it in the mouse and rabbit, and that in the other three mentioned it secretes both oestrogen and progesterone.

The evidence for steroid secretion by the placenta is, in fact, very convincing. In the human there is an increase in oestrogen excretion during pregnancy, and an abundance of oestrogen is found in the placenta, while oestradiol, oestriol, and progesterone have been extracted from the placenta of the rhesus monkey. In the horse, the oestrogens secreted by the placenta are chiefly equilenin and equilin (Fig.

7.5, p. 112), which are only present in the pregnant animal. It is of great interest that this trend towards the independent action of the placenta is accompanied by its independence of the pituitary gland, for the presence of the pars distalis is not necessary for the maintenance of placental secretory activity. Thus pregnancy in the monkey will continue without interruption after hypophysectomy at the thirty-second day, and a woman has been successfully delivered at the end of the thirty-fifth week after having been hypophysectomized nine weeks previously. In the words of one writer, the embryo is registering a very early vote of no-confidence in its parent!

It must be emphasized once again that these data refer to only a very few mammalian species, and that they cannot possibly be regarded as indicative of a phylogenetic series. However, the general principle of the involvement of the placenta in prolonging the life of the corpora lutea and, probably later, coming to substitute for them, seems to be very well founded, and we must hope that future work will see this amplified with more detail.

It remains to mention the hormone relaxin, a polypeptide (molecular weight 9000) which is found in the corpora lutea, uterus, and placenta of various eutherians, including pregnant women, the amount being low during early gestation, increasing later, and then rapidly falling again after parturition. As we have already seen, it is present also in marsupials. Its actions in eutherians, which are dependent upon the previous sensitizing or 'priming' of the connective tissue by oestrogen, are varied, but are particularly associated with parturition, the best-known one, and the one from which its name is derived, being the relaxation of the symphysis pubis and sacro-iliac joints. These effects result from the breaking-down of the cartilage and collagen fibres, and depolymerization of the matrix of the connective tissues. It is believed to be involved also in other functional changes associated with pregnancy and parturition, including, for example, the inhibition of spontaneous contractions in the uterine myometrium and increase in the distensibility of the cervix uteri, but the exact nature of its actions vary a good deal from species to species, as also does the actual amount of the hormone produced. It would seem, therefore, that here, as with the placental gonadotropins, the physiological adaptations of pregnancy have been achieved by routes which have resulted in the establishment of much interspecific variability.

9

The endocrine glands of the pharynx

The stomach and intestine are not the only regions of the vertebrate alimentary tract that have contributed to the endocrine system. The pharynx has also played an important role, perhaps because of its primitive secretory capacity, its inherent tendency to proliferation, and the changes in function which have accompanied its evolution.

9.1. The thymus

The thymus, present in fish as well as in tetrapods, develops by proliferation from certain of the visceral

pouches. In frogs, for example, it forms as a single pair of rudiments from the dorsal walls of the second pair of pouches, and in salamanders (Fig. 9.1) as three pairs arising respectively from each of the third, fourth, and fifth pouches (the first, in this nomenclature, being the homologue of the spiracle of fish). In birds, it arises from the posterior faces of the third and fourth pouches, and in mammals (Figs 9.2 and 9.3) from the ventro-lateral regions of the third and fourth pouches. Regardless of these differences in detail, the organ always develops a lymphoid

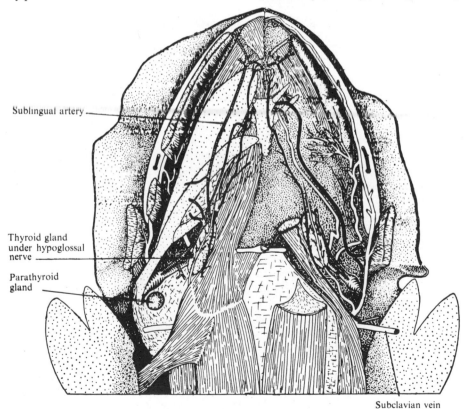

Sublingual artery

Thyroid gland under hypoglossal nerve

Parathyroid gland

Subclavian vein

FIG. 9.1. Dissection of the ventral side of the head of *Salamandra salamandra*. (From Francis (1934). *The anatomy of the salamander*. Clarendon Press, Oxford.)

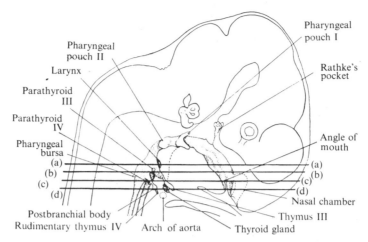

FIG. 9.2. Pharynx of 15 mm pig embryo, schematically represented in relation to the outline of other cephalic structures. The heavy horizontal lines indicate the levels of the correspondingly lettered sections in Fig. 9.3. (From Patten (1948). *Embryology of the pig.* Blakiston, Philadelphia.)

structure. The reason for this was long unknown, but it is now clear that the mammalian thymus plays an important role in securing full expression of host immunity.

The lymphocytes which are concerned with immune responses arise in the embryo in the yolk sac and foetal liver, but in the adult they are replenished from the bone marrow. Two populations of these cells are recognized. Those of one population are processed by the thymus, and then reappear in the blood stream as recirculating lymphocytes. These are responsible for the cell-mediated immunity which is manifested in the rejection of tissue grafts, for example, and in the responses to viruses and invasive bacteria. The cells of the other population, which are supposedly not processed by the thymus, are responsible for antibody-mediated immunity. It is, of course largely with their activities that we have been dealing in our analysis of the immunological properties of the polypeptide hormones.

Evidence for the involvement of the thymus comes from experiments in which the thymus is removed from newly born rats (neonatal thymectomy), or from clinical studies of thymic deficiency in man. In the absence of the organ, the cell-mediated immune responses are virtually absent, there is extreme lymphopenia, and consequent susceptibility to a wide range of infections. There is little effect, however, on the production of the blood-circulating antibodies. The means by which the thymus acts is not fully understood, but one factor is held to be a protein called thymosin, present in a fraction obtained from calf thymic tissue. The supposition is

that this substance acts upon lymphoid cells that enter the thymus, and endows them with immunological competence. There is evidence that cell-free thymic extracts also have this effect, and that thymosin can diffuse from porous chambers that are impermeable to cells. It is thus thought that the thymus, through the mediation of circulating thymosin, may be able to influence lymphocytes peripherally, as well as within the substance of the organ. Some workers have therefore felt justified in regarding thymosin as a thymus hormone, but there is no general agreement on this, and it remains uncertain whether or not the thymus can justly be regarded as an endocrine gland.

9.2. Calcium metabolism and the parathyroid hormone

The level of calcium in the body fluids of mammals is controlled with great precision. It has to be, for ionic calcium influences, amongst other things, membrane permeability, muscular contraction, neural transmission, and the activity of certain enzyme systems. Normal fasting plasma levels of calcium in man range from around 10 mg per 100 ml, with diurnal fluctuations of less than $\pm$ 0·3 mg per 100 ml, and departures from this cannot go unnoticed. Hypercalcaemia leads to many symptoms, including skeletal weakness, nausea, cardiac disturbances, and deposition of calcium in the kidney. Hypocalcaemia, at levels below 4–5 mg per 100 ml, causes neuromuscular excitability, tetanic convulsions and death.

Calcium levels in mammals depend on three main

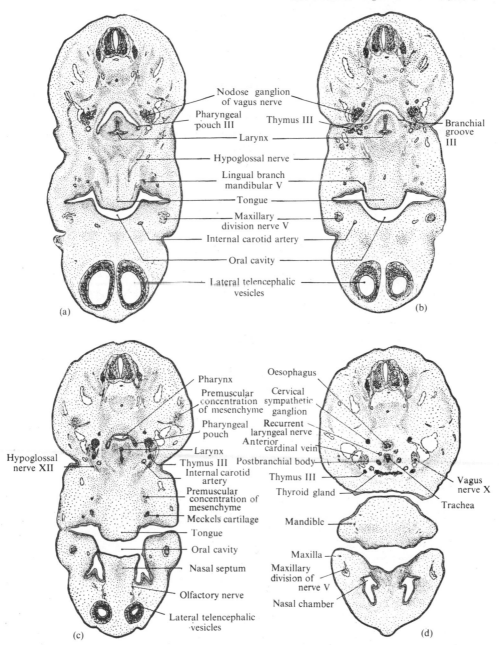

FIG. 9.3. Transverse sections through the pharyngeal region of a 15 mm pig embryo at the levels indicated in Fig. 9.2. (From Patten (1948). *Embryology of the pig*. Blakiston, Philadelphia.)

centres of action (Fig. 9.6). One of these is the small intestine, which is responsible for the active uptake of ingested calcium, while some loss occurs in the intestinal secretions. A second centre is the kidney. Much of the calcium which passes from the blood into the glomerular filtrate is normally reabsorbed in the tubule, and the kidney is an important path for the removal of excess calcium during hypercalcaemia. As much as 70 per cent of an injected calcium load may be removed by this route in man during the first twenty-four hours after the injection.

The third centre of action is the calcium store in the bony skeleton, which may contain up to 99 per cent of the total amount of calcium in the body.

Indeed, it has been suggested that the value of the skeleton as a calcium store may account for the early appearance of bone in the history of vertebrates, and it is likely enough that ready availability of the ion would indeed have facilitated the physiological organization of their actively pelagic life. Continuous exchange takes place between the plasma and the skeleton. This exchange, in conjunction with dietary intake, maintains a plasma level in man of 7–8 mg per 100 ml; hormonal action is responsible for the raising of this to the normal level.

The activities of these three centres are regulated by two hormones (parathyroid hormone and calcitonin), working in conjunction with vitamin D. This vitamin, which facilitates intestinal absorption of calcium, and is probably an essential requirement for it, is a steroid that can be obtained from oily foods, and that can also be formed in the skin, as vitamin D_3, from the precursor 7-dehydrocholesterol. Vitamin D is metabolized by the kidney into 1,25-dihydroxycholecalciferol, and it is probably this metabolite that is active in the intestine. It is believed to bind specifically to the nuclear membranes of the epithelial cells, and presumably influences the synthesis of the enzyme systems required for calcium transport. It will be obvious that the distinction between a vitamin and a hormone has here become a very narrow one.

Parathyroid hormone (parathormone, PTH) is secreted by the parathyroid glands (epithelial bodies), which develop as paired outgrowths from the ventral region of certain of the visceral pouches. Appearing first in the amphibians (Fig. 9.1), they seem to be a product of the reduction of the gills which results from the assumption of terrestrial life. In mammals (Figs 9.2 and 9.3), as in amphibians, they develop from the third and fourth pair of pouches, but there is some variation in this respect in other groups. They are often four in number in mammals, in correspondence with the four outgrowths from which they are derived, but there is variation in this also, both between individuals and species. They take their name from their close association with the thyroid gland; the single pair of the rat, for example, is embedded in the surface of the thyroid, while the four glands in man lie against its posterior surface. (It is this association which was the cause of the fatal results which followed early operations for total thyroidectomy.) Histologically, however, the parathyroids remain sharply differentiated from the thyroid gland. Their cells are smaller than is usual for endocrine cells, with granules that are difficult to see with routine staining methods, but which are

visible as membrane-bound bodies in electron micrographs.

It was shown in 1908 and 1909 that the convulsions which followed the removal of the parathyroids from dogs were associated with a fall in blood calcium, and that the condition could be relieved by injecting calcium salts. However, it was not until 1925 that the endocrine nature of the parathyroids became well defined as a result of the preparation of a parathyroid extract which raised the level of blood calcium in parathyroidectomized animals. It thereby abolished the convulsions which are a consequence of the increased neuromuscular irritability resulting from the induced hypocalcaemia.

The hormone has now been purified and fully characterized as a polypeptide with 84 residues. Amino-acid sequences have been determined for the bovine and porcine hormones (Fig. 9.4), and also for

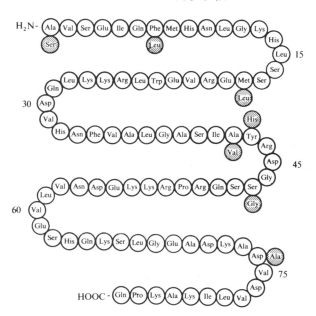

Fig. 9.4. Parathyroid hormone of cattle and pig. The main structure represents the bovine hormone; the shaded residues represent the differences in amino-acid sequence found in the pig's hormone. (From Aurbach *et al.* (1972). *Rec. Prog. Hormone Res.* **28**.)

two minor variants of the bovine hormone (BPTH-II and BPTH-III) which have been found in extracts. These and the human hormone are similar in physical properties, but with amino-acid substitutions (Fig. 9.4) that can be accounted for by single base substitutions (p. 100). A polypeptide comprising residues 1–29 (a nonacosapeptide), which has been isolated from the native hormone by hydrolysis, is the shortest sequence known to be biologically active.

Sequence 1–34 has been synthesized; this polypeptide has biological activity which is qualitatively identical with that of the native hormone, while its immunological activity is virtually identical with that of the 1–29 native sequence. It remains to be determined whether the hormone actually circulates as one or more fragments of the complete polypeptide.

The secretory activity of the mammalian parathyroid, unlike that of the thyroid gland, is not controlled by the pituitary gland, but is directly regulated by the level of calcium in the blood, a fall in this level evoking an increased output of parathyroid hormone. This response, which is a linear one (Fig. 9.5), provides a very sensitive control mechanism,

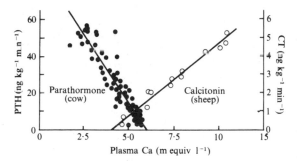

FIG. 9.5. Effect of the plasma calcium concentration on the rate of secretion of parathyroid hormone (PTH) in the cow and of calcitonin (CT) in an adult sheep. (From Copp (1969). *J. Endocrin.* 43.)

for the biological half-life of the hormone in the blood stream is only 20 minutes. The effect of the hormone is also shown by the rise in blood calcium which ensues when parathyroid hormone is injected into dogs, or into parathyroidectomized rats.

The action of the hormone is exerted on all three of the centres mentioned above (Fig. 9.6). It promotes mobilization of skeletal calcium, primarily by an action on the osteoclasts; this is accompanied by a rise in intracellular cyclic AMP (p. 46), which can be used as a basis for *in vitro* assay. The hormone also acts upon the kidney, where it increases calcium reabsorption, this being mediated by an activation of renal adenylate cyclase, which is the basis of another *in vitro* assay. There is also an increased excretion of cyclic AMP, followed by an increased excretion of phosphate; the latter is thought to be a secondary result of the increased utilization of high-energy phosphate. The receptor cells are probably in the proximal (cortical) kidney tubules. They are thus anatomically separate from the receptors for vasopressin, which are within the

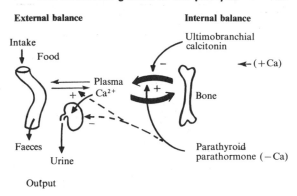

FIG. 9.6. Factors involved in calcium regulation. (From Copp (1969). *J. Endocrin.* 43.)

cells of the medullary tubules. Finally, the hormone enhances the intestinal absorption of calcium, a response which depends upon the presence of vitamin D, as also does the skeletal response. The effect on the kidney, however, is not dependent upon the vitamin.

9.3. Calcium metabolism and calcitonin

It was supposed for a long time that the parathyroid hormone provided a fully adequate basis for the regulation of blood-calcium levels in mammals, with falling plasma levels of calcium evoking an increased output of the hormone, and vice versa. In 1961/1962, however, it was shown that this could not be so. The experiment that demonstrated this, illustrated in Fig. 9.7, involved the perfusion of the thyroid–parathyroid complex of dogs for successive periods of 2 hours with hypercalcaemic and hypocalcaemic fluid. This produced the expected fall and rise, respectively, in the systemic plasma calcium levels.

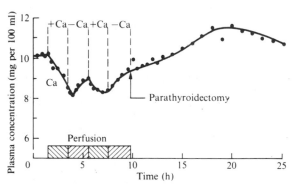

FIG. 9.7. Changes in plasma calcium during successive perfusions of thyroid/parathyroid glands in a fasted dog with blood alternately high and low in calcium. Glands were removed as indicated at the end of the last perfusion. (From Copp *et al.* (1962). *Endocrinology* 70.)

When, however, the animals were thyroid–parathyroidectomized at the end of a period of low-calcium perfusion, the plasma calcium levels continued to rise for 10 hours, instead of falling, as would be expected if the operation had completely removed the parathyroid hormone. This must have been due to the continuing action of the parathyroid hormone which had been secreted during the period of hypocalcaemic perfusion, and which had not yet been removed from the circulation. But this meant that the rapid fall in blood calcium level which set in promptly upon the perfusion with hypercalcaemic fluid (Fig. 9.7) could not have been due to the immediate cessation of the secretion of parathyroid hormone, but must instead have been due to a previously unrecognized hypocalcaemic factor. This, it was postulated, was another calcium-regulating hormone, and it was name calcitonin. Its existence was then rapidly and amply confirmed, but its exact source proved much more difficult to determine.

At first it was supposed that it was secreted by the parathyroid gland, but doubt was cast on this when it was found that a potent hypocalcaemic factor could be extracted from the thyroid gland of rats. Conclusive evidence came from experiments on the goat, in which animal the superior pair of parathyroid glands are separate from the thyroid, and can therefore be separately perfused (Fig. 9.8). Hypocalcaemia

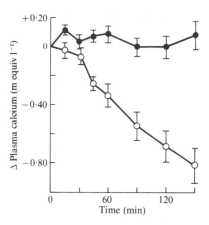

FIG. 9.9. Hypercalcaemic perfusion of the isolated external parathyroid (●——●) and total thyroparathyroid apparatus (○——○) in goats. Curves represent mean values with standard errors of changes in systemic plasma Ca from the control values. Five goats were used in each group. (From Foster *et al.* (1964) quoted in MacIntyre (1968). *Proc. R. Soc. Lond.* B**170**.)

followed hypercalcaemic perfusion of the thyroid, whereas no effect resulted from separate perfusion of the parathyroids (Fig. 9.9); this implied that the hypocalcaemic factor must originate in the thyroid. By this time the name 'thyrocalcitonin' had been independently suggested for this postulated thyroid principle, but it now appeared that it and calcitonin must be one and the same hormone. It then remained only to determine its source.

Within the thyroid gland there are distinctive cells, separate from the follicular epithelium, and long known as the parafollicular cells. These cells were found to show cytochemical and morphological changes in correlation with changes in blood calcium levels, and this suggested that they might be the source of 'thyrocalcitonin'. Proof that they were indeed secreting the hormone came with the availability of a calcitonin preparation which was sufficiently pure to permit the raising of antibody to the porcine hormone. Immunofluorescent studies clearly showed a positive response in the parafollicular cells (Fig. 9.10), with no response at all in the follicular cells that secrete thyroglobulin (p. 158).

At this stage in the analysis, 'thyrocalcitonin' seemed an appropriate term for the hormone, but the situation was changed by the discovery that the parafollicular cells are derived from the ultimobranchial tissue. This tissue forms the ultimobranchial glands, which are found throughout the non-mammalian gnathostomes (including fish), but which have not yet been identified in cyclostomes. They appear in

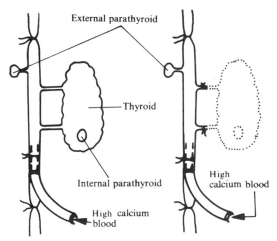

FIG. 9.8. Schematic diagram of areas perfused in goats. In each instance all contralateral thyroid and parathyroid tissue was removed before the control period. (a) Isolated, perfused segment of the common carotid artery. The internal parathyroid is not visible to the naked eye. (b) Isolated, perfused carotid artery segment after removal of the thyroid. The thyroid was removed at the same time as the glands on the other side. (From Foster *et al.* (1964) quoted in MacIntyre (1968). *Proc. R. Soc. Lond.* B**170**.)

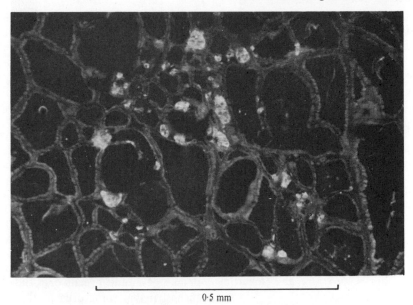

FIG. 9.10. C cells in thyroid of dog, revealed by immunofluorescent reaction to anti-pig calcitonin. (Photograph by courtesy of
A. G. E. Pearse.)

the embryo as outgrowths of the epithelium of the
last branchial pouch; often paired, but sometimes
(e.g. elasmobranchs, reptiles) on one side only. In
clasmobranchs, the ultimobranchial gland is separate
from the thyroid, lying between the pharynx and
pericardium, on the left side, just anterior to the
oesophagus. In teleosts, where it is median or paired,
it lies in the transverse septum below the oesophagus.
In tetrapods it lies close to the thyroid, but separate
from it (Fig. 9.11), except in mammals. In this group,
by an accident of development, which has been
decisively demonstrated by histochemical studies,
the ultimobranchial cells move into the thyroid (the
scaly anteater is said to be an exception) and give rise
to the parafollicular cells (which are now called C
cells, because they secrete calcitonin). These resemble the ultimobranchial cells of non-mammalian
forms in their general cytological features, and the
homology has been confirmed by the extraction of
calcitonin from the ultimobranchial gland of one or
more species of each of the non-mammalian groups;
in fish, as in mammals, it is a polypeptide (p. 154).
It follows that the hypocalcaemic hormone is not
truly a thyroid product at all; calcitonin thus proves
to be the more suitable name for it, and this has
been internationally agreed.

This complicated story is an outstanding tribute
to the power of the comparative method in endocrinology. But yet another surprising matter remains

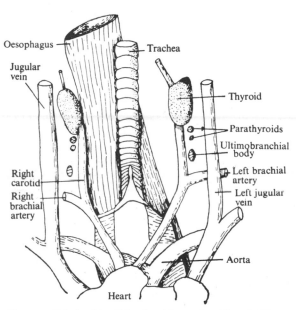

FIG. 9.11. Relationship of the thyroid, parathyroid, and ultimobranchial bodies to the blood vessels in the region of the heart in
the domestic fowl. (From Adams and Eddy (1949). *Comparative
anatomy*. Wiley, New York.)

to be discussed. Embryological studies of the rat show
that cells with the histochemical features of calcitonin-
secreting cells cannot be identified in the region of
the last branchial pouch until the twelfth day of

gestation. Where, then, do they come from? To answer this question it is necessary first to examine more closely the cytochemical features of the calcitonin-secreting cells. These features are not re-restricted to the C cells, but are found to a greater or less extent in some other endocrine cell types as well, all of which have in common the function of secreting polypeptides. Included in these characters are the following.

(1) Uptake of amine precursors (especially 3,4-dihydroxyphenylalanine (DOPA) and 5-hydroxytryptophan (5-HTP), which can be demonstrated by using [^{14}C] or [^{3}H]labelled compounds.

(2) Appearance of fluorescence in the cells after freeze-drying and the application of formaldehyde vapour. This demonstrates the presence of 5-hydroxytryptamine (5-HT), either endogenous, or by uptake after injection. Catecholamines and other biogenic amines also give this formalin-induced fluorescence.

(3) A presumed content of amino-acid decarboxylase, although there sometimes may be no direct evidence of this.

(4) A high content of non-specific esterase or cholinesterase, or both; this may be related to phospholipid synthesis.

Pearse refers to cells with these characters as cells of the APUD series, the term being an acronym for 'Amine and Precursor Uptake and Decarboxylation'. Those which are thought to fall into this series include the corticotropin and melanocyte-simulating hormone cells of the adenohypophysis, certain of the gastro-intestinal endocrine cells (Chapter 2), the A$_1$, A$_2$, and B cells of the pancreatic islets, and the calcitonin cells. This concept of APUD cells raises questions that cannot yet be answered. For example, are the common features of these cells a consequence of convergence resulting from the evolution of similar functions in cells of diverse origin, or do they indicate that these cells have had a common ancestry? There might, of course, be a combination of common origin and convergence, just as, on present evidence, polypeptide hormones fall into a small number of types, each of which has shown diversification from a presumed common ancestry

One major complication is that the ultimobranchial (calcitonin) cells are now thought to originate in the neural crest, and to migrate from there to the pharynx before taking up their position within (in mammals) the thyroid gland. This is why they cannot be identified in the pharynx during the earliest days of development. The evidence for this unexpected conclusion is in part cytochemical. After injection of DOPA into pregnant mice, cells with formaldehyde-induced fluorescence can be identified within the crest; some of them later invade the pharynx to form the future C cells, while others give rise to melanoblasts (p. 207) and to the future chromaffin cells of the adrenal medulla (p. 193). Additional and very elegant evidence comes from heterospecific grafts of the neural tube of the embryos of the quail (*Coturnix coturnix japonica*) and the chick. The quail cells can be distinguished from those of a chick host by the large size of their nucleoli, and cells with this clearly marked feature can be followed from a quail neural implant into the branchial pouch and ultimobranchial tissue of a host chick (Fig. 9.12).

Thus the calcitonin-secreting cells of vertebrates share a common embryological origin with the chromaffin cells of the adrenal gland. This could account for their rich amine content, and for their uptake of amine precursors. Indeed, it has been suggested that some cells of the neural crest (the future chromaffin and pigment cells) retain the ancestral biogenic amines as their secretion product, while in others the amine-storing proteins (p. 190) of the ancestral cells have evolved into polypeptide hormones. This argument is most readily applicable to the C cells, but the possibility lies open that other polypeptide-secreting cells of the postulated APUD series may also originate in the neural crest, which would thus be the source of peripherally distributed components of the endocrine system. This is a hypothesis that merits close attention in the future.

Calcitonin has been isolated in homogeneous form from cattle, the sheep, the pig, man, and the salmon (*Oncorhynchus*). Peptide sequences have been determined for some species (Fig. 9.13), and have been confirmed by total synthesis. In all the above cases the molecule is a single chain of thirty-two amino acids, with a proline amide at the carboxyl terminus, and a disulphide bridge at the amino end, at positions 1–7. There are, however, interspecific differences involving a number of amino-acid substitutions (Fig. 9.13), and these certainly influence the biological properties of the molecules. Pacific salmon elaborate the hormone in three molecular variants, two of which may be present in one species. All the calcitonin variants are active in the rat, but they differ in the duration of their actions, in their potencies as determined by laboratory assay (calcitonin of the salmon is twenty-five times as active as that of the pig), and in the influence upon their action of the route by which they are administered. Despite these substitutions, however, biological activity remains

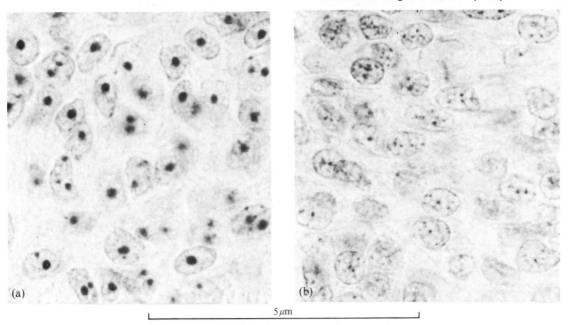

5 µm

FIG. 9.12. Demonstration of the origin of the ultimobranchial (calcitonin) cells from the neural crest. (a) Feulgen-stained quail embryonic neural cells; much of the chromatin is condensed in a mass in the centre of the nucleus. (b) Feulgen-stained chick embryonic neural cells; the chromatin forms a network homogeneously scattered in the nucleus.

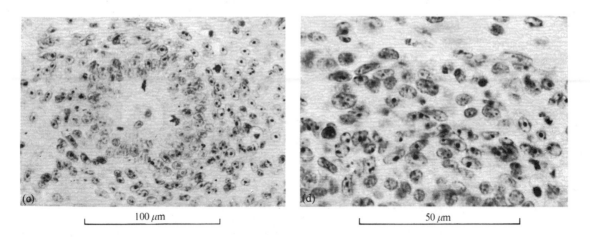

100 µm   50 µm

(c) Ultimobranchial pouch of a 5-day-old chick embryo in which a quail rhombencephalic rudiment has been orthotopically grafted. The ultimobranchial vesicle is formed by an epithelium of chick cells, surrounded by quail cells derived from the grafted neural primordium. Feulgen. (d) The same experiment as in the preceding figure. Ultimobranchial body of an 11-day-old chick embryo, showing its invasion by numerous quail cells. (Photographs by courtesy of Mme. Nicole Le Douarin.)

high; yet, in contrast to parathyroid hormone, removal of the COOH-terminal proline amide leaves the remaining 1–31 sequence almost totally inactive.

The physiology of the calcitonin-secreting cells, and the mode of action of the hormone, are best understood in mammals. The cells respond directly

to elevation of blood calcium levels, for injection into rats of 10 mg per kg calcium results in depletion of the secretory granules within a few hours. Perfusion experiments in the pig show that the output of calcitonin is directly proportional to changes in the level of calcium in the perfusing fluid. In this

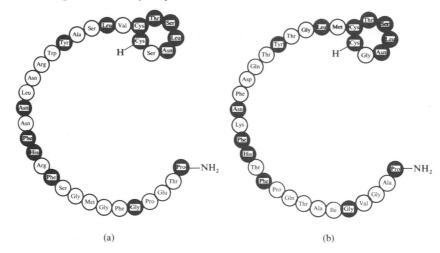

FIG. 9.13. Diagrammatic representations of the sequences of (a) pig calcitonin and (b) human calcitonin. The residues which are in the same position are indicated by dark circles. (From MacIntyre (1972). *Modern trends in endocrinology*, Vol. 4 (eds F. G. Prunty and H. Gardiner-Hill). Butterworth, London.)

respect calcitonin secretion resembles the secretion of parathyroid hormone, but, of course, in the inverse sense (Fig. 9.5).

The action of the hormone, which is more rapid than that of parathyroid hormone, is demonstrable by injecting it either intravenously or subcutaneously. The effect (which is the basis for bioassay) is a fall in plasma calcium within a few minutes, the level reaching a minimum after about 1 hour. The fall, which is a result of inhibition of calcium resorption from the bone, is independent of any action of the parathyroid gland, and can occur in the absence of parathyroid hormone; nevertheless, resorption induced by that hormone is inhibited by calcitonin. The effect is exerted on the osteoclasts, as can be demonstrated by *in vivo* and *in vitro* isotope studies, and is not due to any influence on excretion; this conclusion follows from the same result being found in preparations from which the alimentary tract and kidneys have been removed. However, calcitonin does have an effect upon the kidney, where it increases renal excretion of phosphate, but this action is a minor one, and is not actually responsible for the lower blood phosphate which is a characteristic of calcitonin action.

No direct action of the hormone upon the intestine has been detected. Nevertheless, the release of calcitonin is stimulated by gastrin, cholecystokinin, and glucagon. One consequence of this is that it can then act to reduce any rise in plasma calcium which result from the absorption of digestive products. The action of the hormone upon bone and kidney involves activation of adenylate cyclase in both cases, but there is no competitive inhibition by parathyroid hormone. Presumably, therefore, the two hormones have distinct receptors.

The effects of calcitonin are thus reasonably clear, but the same cannot be said for its physiological significance, which is difficult to assess. Clearly its action upon bone gives protection against high calcium levels; thyroidectomized rats can no longer resist hypercalcaemia. But this protection will be most effective in younger animals, where there is a rapid turnover in the skeletal calcium store. In older animals, the alimentary tract and the kidney are likely to be more important, and here, as we have seen, other hormones are operative, including especially parathyroid hormone. Perhaps, therefore, calcitonin is primarily of value in conserving the skeleton by protecting it from excessive resorption. The matter is one on which much light may eventually be shed by studies of the lower vertebrates; this, indeed, is already indicated by certain facts relating to amphibians and fish.

As regards amphibians, a relation between the ultimobranchial glands and blood calcium levels in *Rana pipiens* is show by the depletion of secretion granules and hypertrophy of the gland that occurs in response to experimentally maintained hypercalcaemia; the condition is reversible when levels are allowed to return to normal. However, the results of removing the glands from this animal are surprising, for there is initially a slow rise in calcium levels, to 10 mg per 100 ml from the normal value of 9.4 mg per 100 ml.

This hypercalcaemia is maintained for some six weeks, after which the level falls until, after 12 weeks, the animals become hypocalcaemic with levels of 7·8 mg per 100 ml.

The explanation of this sequence of events is related to a well-known feature of anuran anatomy: the paravertebral lime sacs. These structures are out-growths of the endolymphatic sacs of the inner ear, which extend along the vertebral canal, and emerge between successive vertebrae. They provide a store of calcium, which increases in animals receiving calcium chloride and vitamin D. X-ray examination shows that the period of hypercalcaemia which immediately follows removal of the ultimobranchial glands is the result of a steady loss of calcium from the sacs. The phase of hypocalcaemia sets in when depletion of this calcium store has become far ad-vanced; at this stage, calcium deprivation begins to affect the skeleton, which suffers from demineraliza-tion, shown in X-rays by less dense shadows. The response in these later stages is accompanied by decrease in number of osteoblasts and increase of osteoclasts; a particularly striking effect, because osteoclasts are only rarely seen in amphibians.

These observations suggest that calcitonin in *Rana* inhibits the mobilization of calcium, by depressing the formation of osteoblasts, and by reducing the flux of sodium from the lime sacs into the blood stream. This may help to account for a puzzling feature of the comparative endocrinology of the ultimobranchial glands: their presence as well-developed structures in elasmobranchs, which have no bone (although, of course, they do have calcified cartilage), and in teleosts, many of which have a very characteristic acellular bone that does not undergo the resorption that is common in other vertebrate groups. That the ultimobranchial glands of teleosts have some function relative to the skeleton is indi-cated by the fact that the Mexican cave-fish (*Astyanax mexicanus*) develops bone deformities when main-tained in completed darkness for long periods, and that there is also marked hyperplasia of the glands. It is worth noting also that calcitonin lowers blood calcium levels in the eel, which has no cellular bone, but not in *Fundulus hetereoclitus*, which has acellular bone. These facts are too meagre to permit useful generalizations (particularly in view of what occurs in *Rana*), but it is at least possible that calcitonin in fish may act primarily to regulate calcium transport across membranes, including particularly those of the gills, the intestine, and the kidney tubules, all of which are important in other aspects of ionic regulation in these animals.

The most thoroughly studied endocrine derivative of the pharynx is the thyroid gland. This was first described anatomically in 1656 by a London physician, Thomas Wharton, who also gave to it its accepted name, deriving this from the Greek (*thureos*, a shield, and *eidos*, form). It lies in man and other mammals on either side of the larynx, with a median isthmus connecting the two main lateral portions. Noting this, and also its follicles with their contained colloid, Wharton concluded that it served in human beings to smooth the contours of the neck, a supposition which conveniently accounted for it being larger in females, whose necks were thereby made more even and more beautiful.

The thyroid gland is one of the few endocrine organs of which something of the evolutionary history is known, for there is convincing evidence that it is homologous (p. 5) with the endostyle of the protochordates (e.g. ascidians, amphioxus) and the larval lamprey. This organ (Fig. 9.14), which is

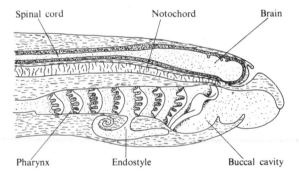

FIG. 9.14. Diagrammatic longitudinal section of the anterior end of the larva of the lamprey.

a glandular structure lying in the floor of the pharynx, and which is part of the feeding mechanism, gives rise to the thyroid gland of the adult lamprey at metamorphosis. The transformation, which must reflect evolutionary history, explains why, in all higher vertebrates, the thyroid gland develops as a median downgrowth from the floor of the pharynx of the early embryo. Remnants of its connection with the pharynx may sometimes persist as acces-sory thyroids in man, but normally in all verte-brates it separates off as a quite independent organ which is usually compact and median, but sometimes paired, as in amphibians (Fig. 9.1, p. 147) and birds (Fig. 9.11, p. 153). In cyclostomes, and usually in teleost fish, it forms a loosely organized gland which extends along the ventral aorta (Fig. 9.15) and often into the branchial

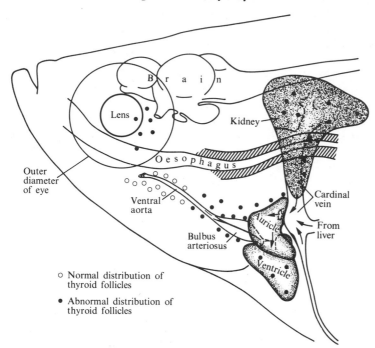

FIG. 9.15. Diagram of the anterior part of a platyfish showing the normal and abnormal distribution of thyroid follicles. (From Baker *et al.* (1955). *Cancer Res.* **15**.)

○ Normal distribution of
thyroid follicles

● Abnormal distribution of
thyroid follicles

arches; this is thought to result from the tendency of thyroid cells in these animals to migrate during development, a tendency which in extreme cases results in the establishment of thyroid tissue in unusual parts of the body (heterotopic), more particularly in the kidneys. This migration, and the possibility of its occurrence in other animals, needs to be borne in mind in assessing the results of experimental studies on thyroid function.

The histological structure of the gland is very characteristic (Fig. 9.16), for its colloid-like secretory product is stored in hollow follicles, the walls of which are formed by the secretory epithelium. This varies in its appearance according to the condition of the cells, which may range from a very flattened and almost squamous shape to a cubical or even columnar form. This variation reflects the activity of the gland, the cells being at their most flattened when the activity is least, although the relationship may not be an entirely simple one. The gland is richly vascularized, networks of capillaries closely surrounding the follicles and carrying with them a delicate investment of connective tissue cells and fibres. The vessels are accompanied by non-medullated nerve fibres, which take their origin from the cervical sympathetic ganglia. They are vasomotor in function, the secretory cells having no secretomotor innervation. As with the gonads, then, we shall have to

examine in due course how the activity of this gland is regulated.

The material which fills the follicles, and which is also visible as small droplets within the cells, stains brilliantly with acidic dyes such as eosin or phloxin, while with the Azan procedure it may be coloured either by the azocarmine and orange G or by the aniline blue; the difference is said to depend upon the viscosity of the material. Numerous vacuoles are seen around the edge of the colloid mass when the gland has been fixed with one of the standard reagents. These have been thought to arise from the breaking-down of the colloid, and to be an index of the amount of secretion which is being discharged into the blood, but if the gland is prepared by freeze-drying, or for electron microscopy, they are usually not visible at all. It has therefore been argued that they are merely an artifact of fixation. Probably, however, their existence reflects, in at least some degree, the condition of the colloid, even though they may not be present in that form in the unfixed material.

The main component of the colloid is a glycoprotein, thyroglobulin, with a molecular weight of 650 000–700 000. Density gradient centrifugation of thyroid extracts shows that 75–80 per cent of the macromolecular content has a sedimentation coefficient of 19 Svedberg units (19S), and this value

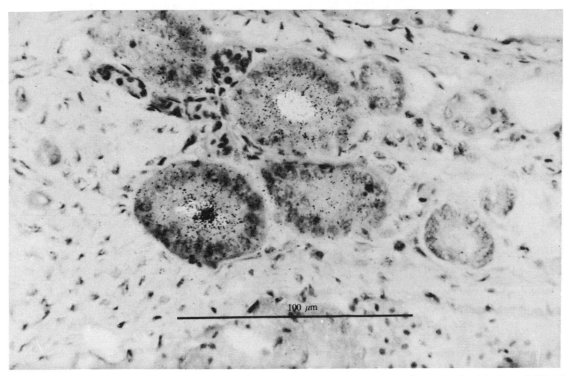

FIG. 9.16. Autoradiograph of thyroid follicles of the river lamprey, *Lampetra fluviatilis*, 14 days after the injection of [131]I. The concentration of radio-iodine in the follicular lumen indicates storage in the colloid. The presence of labelled iodine within the cells probably indicates the reabsorption of hormones from the lumen prior to their release into the blood stream. (From Larsen and Rosenkilde (1971). *Gen. comp. Endocrin.* 17.)

is regarded as a diagnostic property of thyroglobulin. Because of its carbohydrate content, the colloid gives a strong positive reaction with the periodic acid/Schiff (PAS) procedure (see p. 66).

In some species, the follicular epithelial cells are said to bear cilia, perhaps a consequence of the pharyngeal derivation of the gland. More significant for the functioning of the cells, however, are micro-villi, revealed by electron microscopy as projecting from the cell surfaces into the follicular colloid. There are numerous mitochondria, and a well-developed endoplasmic reticulum, which is in part agranular, and in part a rough endoplasmic reticulum with abundant ribosomes. Autoradiography with labelled tracers shows that the protein component of the thyroglobulin arises in the rough endoplasmic reticulum, carbohydrate being added there and in the well-developed Golgi zone. Small vesicles break away from this region and pass to the cell apex, where they are thought to fuse with the cell border and discharge their contents into the follicular lumen. The vesicles of electron microscopy do not necessarily correspond with the colloid droplets seen in light microscopical preparations, for these droplets are a heterogeneous population. The larger ones, readily visible as PAS-positive material by light microscopy, are not the initial secretory product, but consist of material that has been reabsorbed from the follicular contents, either by micropinocytosis in the microvilli, or through pseudopodia-like processes of the cell surface. They are closely associated with lysosomes, from which are derived the enzymes required (as we shall see later) for the hydrolysis of the resorbed colloid and the release of its stored hormones, and for the de-iodination of the iodotyros-ines. It will be apparent, when the course of thyroidal biosynthesis has been reviewed, that the functioning of these cells is remarkably complex.

9.5. The clinical approach to the problems of thyroid function

As with some of the other endocrine glands, it is the study of disturbances of function in human beings which has provided the foundation of our understanding of the thyroid. By far the commonest of those disturbances, and they are by no means restricted to man, are the 'non-toxic' or endemic goitres which occur in all parts of the world, but especially in those regions (not necessarily mountainous) where the iodine of the soil has been reduced by flooding or by glacial action. As a result of this iodine shortage, and for a reason which we shall examine later, the thyroid enlarges to form a simple or diffuse goitre (Fig. 9.17(a)). The prevalence of this may be judged from the fact that in 1944 the goitre Subcommittee of the Medical Research Council estimated that in England and Wales, amongst young people of ages ranging from five to twenty years, there were perhaps as many as 500 000 cases showing some degree of thyroid enlargement. Nodules may sometimes appear in enlarged thyroids, apparently as a result of alternating phases of hyperplasia and involution, and this gives rise to adenomatous or nodular goitre, but both this and the diffuse form are fundamentally different from the 'toxic' goitres, which are characterized by an increased output of thyroid secretion.

The ashes of marine sponges are said to have been used by the Chinese as long ago as 1500 B.C. for the treatment of goitre and, although some doubt has been cast upon the correctness of this statement, the remedy, with the use of sea water as a variant, has been widely recommended by European medical writers in the past and must presumably have been based upon some degree of success. The explanation of this did not become apparent until the nineteenth century, the first step towards it being the isolation of iodine from the seaweed *Fucus vesiculosus* by the French chemist Courtois in 1811, and the identification of this as a new element by Gay-Lussac. Fyfe's demonstration in 1819 that iodine was present in sponges (a discovery from which he himself drew the unhappy conclusion that these organisms must be plants) suggested that this element might account for their value in the treatment of goitre, and it was particularly the Swiss physician Coindet who drew public attention to this possibility. By the middle of the century Chatin, in France, had strengthened the argument by bringing forward evidence that endemic goitre was associated with the use of water of low iodine content, but his conclusion was rejected by the French Academy of Sciences. This setback seems to have resulted partly from certain weaknesses in the medical procedures which were then being brought into use. But in any case, as Harington has pointed out, 'the notion that a disease could be caused, not by an actively noxious agent, but by the mere deficiency of an element which in any case was never present except in minute quantities, was one for which medical and scientific opinion was quite unprepared'. In other words, the successful exploitation of new ideas in science needs a proper climate of opinion, and this was not available either for Coindet or for Chatin.

During the early years of the present century, however, the relationship between goitre and iodine shortage became clearly established. Of particular interest to the comparative endocrinologist was Marine's study of goitre in the American brook-trout, *Salvelinus fontinalis*. This condition, which was marked by a conspicuous swelling or reddening of the pharyngeal floor, had arisen in fish which were being reared in a hatchery, and he was able to show that it resulted from a deficiency of iodine in the food, and that it could be alleviated by the addition of whole sea-fish to the diet.

Meanwhile, clinical observations had been leading to the recognition that a disorder of the thyroid underlay the condition long known as cretinism (Fig. 9.17(b)), in which a variety of characteristics, including stunted growth and feeble-mindedness, are associated with thyroid deficiency in infancy. Comparable deficiencies in adults were first defined in 1873, when Gull presented to the Clinical Society of London an account of *A cretinoid state supervening in adult life in women*. Shortly afterwards, two more cases of this adult type were described by Ord who, in 1877, named the condition myxoedema. This is characterized by thickening of the subcutaneous tissue, sensitivity to cold, lethargy, and progressive loss of the mental faculties, features which had suggested to Gull the comparison with cretinism. Ord made the very important observation that in one of his patients the thyroid had become atrophied. This suggested a direct relationship between the condition and a lack of thyroid tissue, and a striking confirmation came from Swiss surgeons who, as a result of the discrediting of iodine medication, had been treating goitre by removal of the thyroid gland. They found that in some patients from whom the whole of the gland had been removed there later supervened a condition identical with the myxoedema described by Gull and Ord; a good demonstration, incidentally, of the importance of a clear definition of the syndrome associated with a specific clinical condition.

These circumstances led after fourteen years to the use of thyroid extract by Murray for the treatment of myxoedema, the patient being a woman who in 1891, at the age of 46, showed an advanced stage of this condition. There resulted a rapid and dramatic return to health which was maintained for twenty-eight years, initially by the use of injections of

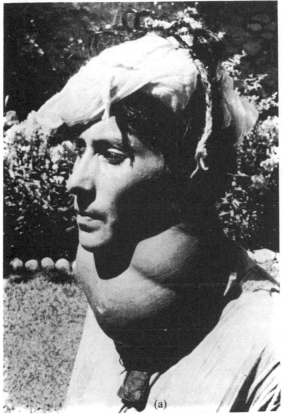

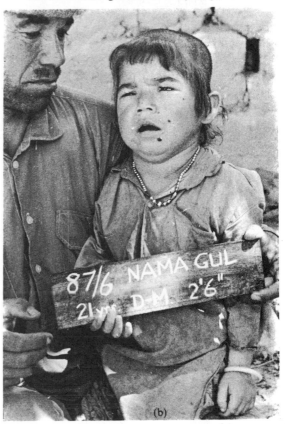

FIG. 9.17. Iodine deficiency in the north-west frontier district of West Pakistan, one of the most goitrous regions in the world.

(a) A woman with an exceptionally large goitre.

(b) A female cretin, about 20 years old, but only 2 ft 6 in high. (From Chapman *et al.* (1972). *Phil. Trans. R. Soc. Lond.* B**263**, 459–91.)

thyroid extracts and subsequently by oral administration of these. The patient finally died at the age of 74, having during the course of her treatment made use of the thyroids of over 870 sheep. She provides a famous and classical example of the employment of replacement therapy, and the work of Gull, Ord, and Murray must be reckoned as providing one of the major steps in the development of endocrinology.

9.6. The thyroid hormones and thyroidal biosynthesis

The comparatively leisurely rate of scientific advance in these fields at that time is illustrated by the fact that not until 1895–6 did Baumann demonstrate that iodine was actually present in the thyroid, and in organic combination, while another twenty years was to elapse before Kendall, working at the Mayo Clinic, succeeded in isolating an iodine-containing hormone from the gland on Christmas Day 1914. He named it thyroxin (thyroxine in conventional English usage)

and obtained 33 g of it from about three tons of pig thyroid. This achievement made clear the nature of the association of the element with the gland, and at the same time paved the way for the elucidation of the structure of thyroxine by Harington and Barger in England, and its synthesis by these same workers in 1927. As a result of their work it was established that it is an iodinated amino acid, tetraiodothyronine (T_4; Fig. 9.18), formed in the thyroid gland by the iodination of tyrosine in a way which we shall consider below. The L-isomer, which can be obtained by synthesis from L-tyrosine, is the natural form of the hormone, and is three times as active as the D-isomer.

For many years it was supposed that the sole hormonal product of the gland was thyroxine, but the use of radioactive iodine, and the introduction of paper chromatography, which made possible the separation of the iodinated products of the gland in micro-quantities, led in 1951 to the discovery of an unknown iodine-containing compound in hydrolysates of the thyroid of the rat. In 1952 it was shown that this substance was also present in the blood of human patients with thyroid carcinoma, who were being treated with radio-iodide, and, after comparisons with various thyroxine derivatives, it was characterized as $3,5,3'$-triiodothyronine (T_3; Fig. 9.18). Although it may be present in the thyroid in smaller amounts than thyroxine, its importance is shown not only by its distribution throughout the vertebrates, but even more by its high biological activity, which in some respects is greater than that of thyroxine. It is, in fact, a second thyroid hormone. Its discovery, like that of aldosterone (p. 200), is a useful reminder not to expect the biosynthetic activity of endocrine glands to be confined to those substances which are most readily detectable by our laboratory procedures.

Iodine is ingested as iodide, and is absorbed into the blood stream in that form. The first step in the biosynthesis of the hormones is the trapping of this iodide by the thyroid gland, which has a remarkable capacity for doing this, being able to maintain a concentration gradient between itself and the serum of about 25:1. The action of this iodide pump can be followed by administering radioactive iodine as iodide, and measuring its uptake by the gland (p.

166). It is important that it should be given in very minute quantities called tracer doses, however, for larger amounts will disturb the normal iodide balance and may actually depress the rate of uptake.

Some capacity for concentrating iodide is not peculiar to the thyroid gland, for the iodide content of the notochord of the lamprey is 100–300 times higher than that of the plasma, and the ovaries of lampreys, trout, and frogs are other examples of organs that accumulate large amounts. Such iodine remains largely, if not entirely, inorganic. The unique properties of the thyroid depend upon the association of its iodide pump with a highly specialized biochemical mechanism which binds iodine to tyrosine. The binding is initiated by the rapid oxidation of the iodide to reactive iodine within the secretory cells, this being catalysed by peroxidase. The iodine is then combined with tyrosine. This leads first to the formation of 3-monoiodotyrosine (MIT; Fig. 9.18), which is present in the gland in only small amounts, and which was not even known to exist in it until 1948, when it was identified chromatographically in extracts of the thyroid of the rat.

The next stage is the formation of 3,5-diiodotyrosine (DIT; Fig. 9.18), a substance which was first isolated in 1895 from the gorgonid coelenterate

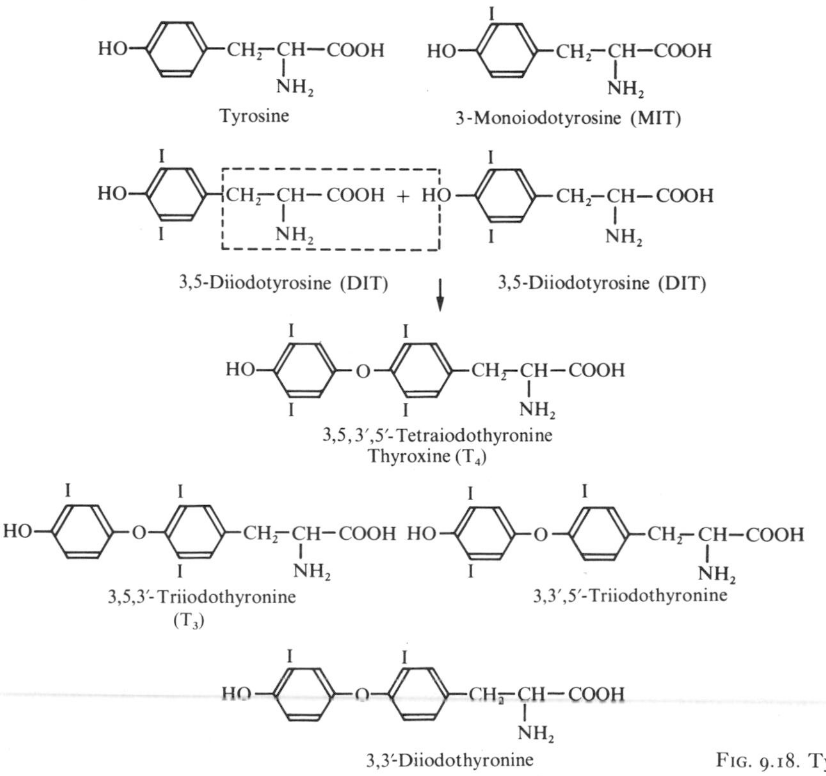

FIG. 9.18. Tyrosine and its iodination products.

Eunicella verrucosa, and which was therefore called iodogorgoic acid at that time. It was isolated from the thyroid in 1929, at which time it was supposed that it and thyroxine were the only iodinated amino acids present; a natural conclusion, for it represents a large amount of the total organically bound iodine in the gland. Neither of these iodotyrosines are biologically active; their presence in the gland is a consequence of the stepwise biosynthetic process.

Thyroxine is formed by the coupling of two molecules of diiodotyrosine with loss of an alanine side chain (Fig. 9.18). 3,5,3'-triiodothyronine could theoretically be synthesized either by the coupling of one molecule of monoiodotyrosine with one of diiodotyrosine, or by a deiodination of thyroxine, but it is probable that the former is the path actually followed. Two other thyronines are said to be present in the glands of the rat and pig. These are 3,3',5'-triiodothyronine and 3,3'-diiodothyronine, the latter having also been detected in the rat's blood. These are only present in very small amounts, however, and they do not function as hormones.

When these reactions have been completed, the hormones are firmly bound in the thyroglobulin molecule, and the tyrosine is probably bound in it during the whole of the iodination process. Autoradiographic studies show that the initial stages of binding occur at the cell border, immediately prior to the secretion of the colloid into the lumen, or perhaps at the periphery of the follicular colloid. Because of this situation, the hormones must be released from the thyroglobulin before they can be liberated into the blood. This is effected by the taking up of colloid droplets into the cells, as already indicated, and by their hydrolysis by a thyroid protease. The result is the liberation of all the iodinated amino acids, but it is a remarkable demonstration of the refinement of adaptation which has developed in these processes that only the thyronines are actually found in the blood and that monoiodotyrosine and diiodotyrosine do not normally leave the gland in significant amounts, at least in mammals. This is because the thyroid contains an enzyme that deiodinates the tyrosines with the release of iodine, which is taken up again into the biosynthetic cycle. The action of this deiodinase, which can be demonstrated *in vitro*, seems to be restricted to the free tyrosines and it is without effect upon them when they are bound in the thyroglobulin molecule.

The circulating hormones are bound to plasma proteins, as a result of which they cannot be separated by dialysis but come down with the protein on treatment of the plasma with protein precipitants. The hormones so precipitated, however, can readily be extracted with butanol and can thus be estimated. In this way it is possible to determine the concentration of the protein-bound iodine, which reflects the dynamic balance between the rate of output of secretion from the gland and the rate of its use and metabolism by the body. This binding of the hormones in the blood has nothing whatever to do with their binding to thyroglobulin in the gland. The latter is directly involved in the mechanism of biosynthesis; the former presumably provides a convenient means of transport, and may also be expected to set some limit on the rates at which the hormones can react with the cells.

The rate of metabolism of thyroidal iodine, which varies a good deal from species to species, even within the mammals, can be expressed by reference to the progressive fall in the amount of an injected dose of radio-iodine which is retained in the thyroid. The time taken for this amount to fall to 50 per cent of the maximum uptake is called the biological half-life of thyroidal iodine for that species. Some values for thyroxine are given in Fig. 9.19. It will be noticed

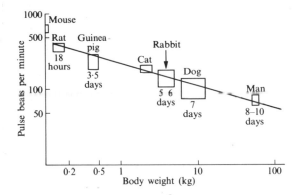

FIG. 9.19. The relationship between the rate of peripheral utilization of thyroxine, body weight, and metabolic rate (expressed in terms of pulse rate) on body weight in certain mammals. The values of 18 hours, 3.5 days, etc. are the average figures for the biological half-lives of thyroxine in the different species. (From Pitt-Rivers and Tata (1959). *The thyroid hormones*. Pergamon Press, Oxford.)

that they are smaller for the smaller animals; in other words, this hormone is used more rapidly in smaller mammals, and we can reasonably ascribe this to the part played by it in the maintenance of metabolic rate (p. 174). Owing to their relatively large surface area in relation to volume, the smaller mammals must have a relatively higher heat production, weight for weight, in order to maintain their body temperature.

This evidently requires a more rapid use of thyroid secretion, although other factors will also influence this; violent exercise, for example, increases the demand for thyroid hormones in rats.

In mammals, the liver and kidney play important parts in the catabolism of the hormones, being mainly responsible for their de-iodination. Some of the iodide released in this way is excreted in the urine, but much is returned economically to the thyroid, where it can be recycled. Not all of the hormonal secretion, however, is disposed of in this way. Some of it is conjugated, mainly in the liver, with the formation of glucuronides or sulphates, which are passed into the intestine with the bile. From here, some of the thyronines are taken up again into the blood, the rest being lost with the faeces.

Iodine binding is not confined to vertebrates. One example of this is its occurrence in the endostyle of protochordates (ascidians and amphioxus), where also iodotyrosines and thyroxine have been identified. Its function in these animals is unknown, but its occurrence is not surprising, for the protochordates, as members of the phylum Chordata, are closely related to the vertebrates, and, as already mentioned, their endostyle is homologous with the thyroid gland. Moreover, the endostyle of the larval lamprey (Fig. 9.20) also binds iodine (Fig. 9.21), and carries out thyroidal biosynthesis throughout larval life. Evidently, thyroidal biosynthetic pathways were estab-

lished in the endostyle before its transformation into a typical endocrine gland.

Iodine binding also occurs in many invertebrates that are not closely related to vertebrates. Commonly it is associated with the laying down of structural proteins, as, for example, in the chaetae of annelids or in the formation of the byssus of molluscs (Fig. 9.22). It is supposed that it is facilitated by the presence of oxidase systems, or by the quinones, that are associated with the quinone tanning of some structural proteins, for these promote the oxidation of iodide to reactive iodine. It is uncertain whether iodine binding in these conditions is of any physiological significance, or whether it is perhaps a metabolic by-product. Moreover, while iodotyrosines are commonly formed, it is doubtful whether these often give rise to significant amounts of iodothyronines, although triiodothyronine has been identified in nemertine mucus.

However, it certainly seems that vertebrates have turned to endocrine advantage a process that antedated their own emergence. Evidence from other parts of the vertebrate endocrine system suggests that hormones may sometimes have been evolved out of metabolic products (pp. 29, 182), but the exact circumstances in which this occurred are difficult to determine. In the particular case of the endostyle, however, the secretion of this organ is a protein-rich filtering membrane, so that it is at least possible

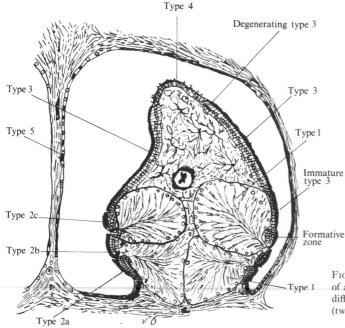

FIG. 9.20. Transverse section of the right half of the endostyle of a lamprey larva anterior to its opening into the pharynx. The different types of epithelium are indicated, the glandular tracts (two pairs) constituting type 1 (cf. Fig. 9.21). (From Barrington and Franchi (1956). *Q. Jl microsp. Sci.* **97**.)

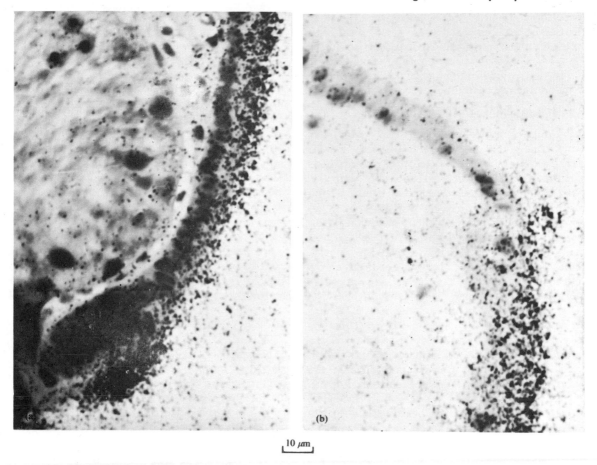

(b)

⌊10 μm⌋

FIG. 9.21. Autoradiographs of the endostylar epithelium of a lamprey larva which had been immersed for 48 h in water containing 200 μCi of ^{131}I per litre (cf. Fig. 9.20). (a) The outline of the dorsal glandular tract is faintly seen in the centre. Radio-iodine is present in the type 2 cells, below left, and in the type 3 cells above right. (b) Radio-iodine is present in the type 3 cells below right, but absent from the type 4 cells above left. (From (Barrington and Franchi (1956). *Q. Jl microsp. Sci.* **97**.)

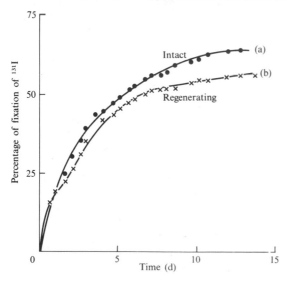

FIG. 9.22. Fixation of ^{131}I from the surrounding sea water by groups of nine mussels (*Mytilus galloprovincialis*), measured by direct counts of radioactivity. (a) Intact animals; (b) animals with byssus regeneration; prior section of the byssus has no significant effect upon the rate of uptake. (From Roche *et al.* (1960). *C.r. Soc. Biol. Paris,* **154**.)

that iodine binding became established in it in correlation with specialized protein metabolism. This seems the more likely because it also occurs in the tunic of ascidians, associated with quinone tanning and the formation of the proteins that give strength to that protective covering.

9.7. The measurement of thyroid activity

The course of thyroidal biosynthesis is qualitatively similar throughout the vertebrates from the ammocoete larva upwards, but there are great variations in the speed and in the maximal values of ^{131}I uptake. For example, uptake is very low in lampreys, and has been said not to exceed 0·53 per cent of an injected dose at 13–15 °C, while in teleosts it ranges from 10 per cent in *Fundulus majalis* at 22 °C to less than 1 per cent in *Cyprinus carpio*. Low uptake values, however, do not necessarily indicate an inactive gland; thus in the lamprey the actual turnover of iodine is very rapid, the maximal uptake level being reached in 6 hours, by which time labelled hormone is identifiable in the blood. Great importance therefore attaches in comparative studies to the measurement of the activity of the thyroid gland, which may be thought of as the rate at which it is releasing its hormones into the circulation. For this purpose several types of procedure are available, each of which has its value provided that it is carefully related to the known course of biosynthesis in the gland and that due attention is given to its limitations and to the particular sources of error that may be associated with it.

(a) Histological methods

A much favoured method has been the measurement of the heights of the secretory cells, it being assumed that increased height is indicative of greater secretory activity. This assumption has some justification, inasmuch as greater cell height is certainly associated with the greater activity which results from stimulation of the gland by thyrotropin (p. 170). The method needs to be handled with care, however, for there is much variation amongst the cells, and it is necessary to avoid any subjective element in selecting those which are to be measured. Another and more fundamental difficulty is our ignorance of the precise mode of functioning of the thyroid cells, which means that we cannot feel certain that cell height is always related in a simple way to cell activity. Moreover, the method is relatively insensitive, so that minor, but possibly important, fluctuations in activity are likely to pass unnoticed. These difficulties are to some extent reduced in a variant of this method,

in which account is taken of the amount of colloid present, by expressing the activity of the gland as a percentage ratio of epithelial area to colloid area.

(b) Measurement of protein-bound iodine content

It is possible to carry out direct chemical estimations of the protein-bound iodine content of the gland, but unfortunately the significance of the data is difficult to judge, since it is impossible to decide whether an increased content is indicative of diminished demand and increased storage, or of increased demand and increased production.

Some importance has been attached to measurements of the protein-bound iodine content of the plasma as an index of thyroidal activity, for clinical studies are said to show a good correlation between the two, a high plasma content being associated with a hyperthyroid state and vice versa. This correlation, however, remains to be established in the lower vertebrates.

(c) Measurement of the radio-iodine turnover of the gland

The activity of the thyroid will, in general, be reflected in its iodine turnover, and a number of procedures have been used for measuring this, the introduction of radio-iodine making it possible to work with very small quantities of material. Such methods are probably the most useful and reliable of all.

One approach is to inject a standard dose of radio-iodide into a series of animals, and then to measure the radioactivity of aliquots of their thyroids by sacrificing individuals at predetermined intervals. This may require the use of a large number of specimens, but an alternative possibility is to make a series of readings on single individuals by external application of a Geiger counter to the thyroid region (Figs 9.23 and 9.24). With such *in vivo* counting it is necessary to pay attention to various sources of error such as the correct and consistent placing of the counter (technically known as the geometry of the apparatus), variations in the exact location of the gland, and (in teleosts, for example) the distribution of heterotopic thyroid tissue. It must be remembered, too, that in the first few hours after an injection a considerable proportion of the dose will still be in the body fluids, and this will introduce a further source of error. Thus in the rabbit (Fig. 9.25) more than 30 per cent of the total count in the thyroid region may be due to this source at four hours, although this will have fallen to less than 5 per cent after twenty-four hours, at which time the radio-iodine

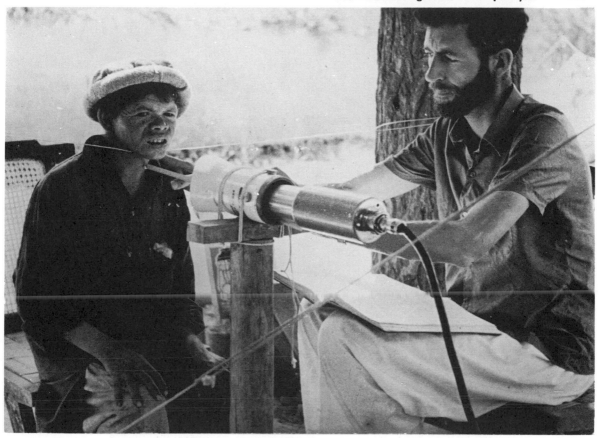

FIG. 9.23. *In vivo* measurement of iodine uptake. The counter is tied to a post, and a villager (West Pakistan) sits with his chin resting on a stiff wire. (From Chapman *et al.* (1972). *Phil. Trans. R. Soc. Lond.* B **263**, 459–91.)

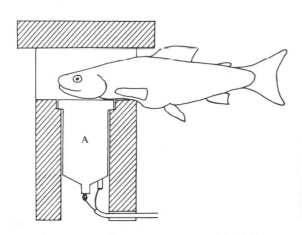

FIG. 9.24. Diagram to show a procedure for *in vivo* counting of the thyroidal radioactivity of a teleost fish. The animal is anaesthetized with urethane and placed with its thyroid area over a lead-shielded end-window-type Geiger–Muller tube (a). (From Swift (1955). *J. exp. Biol.* **32**.)

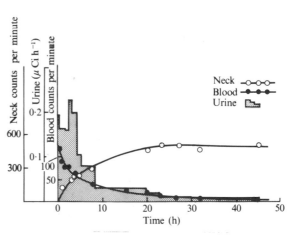

FIG. 9.25. The distribution of ^{131}I in the thyroid region, blood, and urine of a rabbit following the intravenous injection of 3 μCi of ^{131}I at 0 hours. (From Brown-Grant *et al.* (1954). *J. Physiol.* **126**.)

content of the animal's thyroid may be expected to have reached a maximum. This is also the case in the trout, where there is a high background count from the body during the first few days after an injection into the body cavity. This count drops rapidly, however, falling by some 50 per cent during the first two and a half days, so that it is particularly during this early phase that it is important to make corrections for background count when measuring thyroidal activity. A comparable situation is seen in the lizard, *Agama stellio*; following an injection of radio-iodine, there is early accumulation of ^{131}I in the stomach, prior to maximum build-up in the thyroid gland (Figs 9.26 and 9.27).

Data obtained in these ways need to be interpreted with caution. As we have remarked, the rate of uptake of iodide is not necessarily a measure of the rate at which the products of biosynthesis are released; this is well seen in a study of *Fundulus heteroclitus* (Fig.

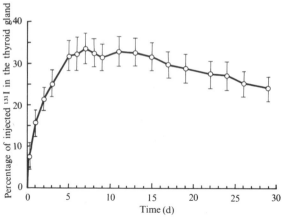

FIG. 9.26. Whole-body scannings of a lizard (outline superimposed) at specified times following intraperitoneal administration of $8\cdot5\,\mu$Ci ^{131}I. Early accumulation in the stomach and later in the thyroid are seen. (From Shaham and Lewitus (1971). *Gen. comp. Endocrin.* **17**.)

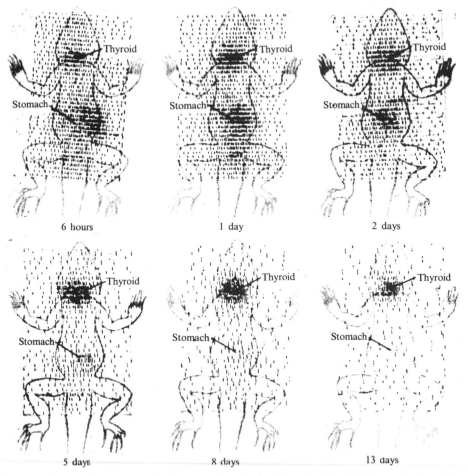

FIG. 9.27. The accumulation and disappearance of radio-iodine from the thyroid gland of lizards following injection of $8\cdot5\,\mu$Ci ^{131}I. The curve is the mean of values $\pm$ standard errors from nine animals. (From Shaham and Lewitus (1971). *Gen. comp. Endocrin.* **17**.)

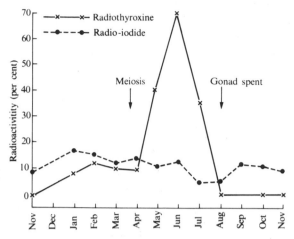

FIG. 9.28. Radio-iodide uptake and radiothyroxine production in *Fundulus heteroclitus* during 11 months of the year. (From Berg *et al.* (1959). *Comparative Endocrinology* (ed. A. Gorbman). Wiley, New York.)

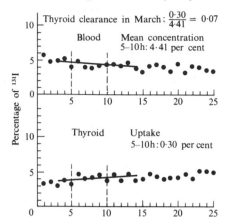

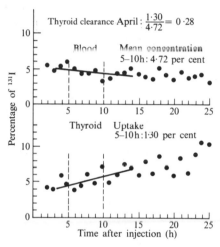

FIG. 9.29. Uptake of radio-iodine by the thyroid gland, and levels of ^{131}I in the blood of coho parr caught in March and at the beginning of April shortly before the onset of migration. Thyroid clearance was determined between 5 hours and 10 hours after injection of the tracer dose. (From Baggerman (1960). *J. Fish. Res. Bd. Can.* **17**.)

9.28), in which animal the production of radio-thyroxine was found to reach in June a sharp peak, which was not reflected at all in the radio-iodide uptake measurements. Another difficulty is that the level of radio-iodine in the gland at any one time is a resultant of uptake and of secretion, so that in effect two different phases of thyroidal metabolism are being measured at the same moment. Further, the amount of iodide trapped by the thyroid will depend upon the amount brought to it in the body fluids, and this will be influenced by factors determining the rates of metabolic and excretory processes. It is not surprising, therefore, to find that in practice such uptake measurements show a good deal of variation both from animal to animal and even in the same animal at different times. This difficulty can, however, be dealt with by relating the radio-iodide uptake during a given period of time to the mean concentration of iodide in blood samples taken during the same period. This gives a measure of what is called the thyroidal iodine clearance. In the parr of the coho salmon (*Oncorhynchus kisutch*), the curves for thyroid uptake and for disappearance of isotope from the blood follow straight lines during the period extending from 5 to 10 hours after injection, and the thyroidal iodine clearance can be readily calculated from them. The data illustrated (Fig. 9.29) show that the clearance is higher in April than in March. It is therefore assumed that the gland is more active in the former month, although this cannot be proved from such data.

Another approach to the problem, and one which has been used with success in both mammals and

fish, is to determine the rate at which iodine is released from the gland, the procedure being to inject a dose of radio-iodide and then to start regular *in vivo* counts after a suitable interval. Ideally, this would be selected so that the curve of uptake would have reached its peak while the radio-iodine content of the body fluids would have fallen to a negligible value. We have seen that in the rabbit this interval is reached within twenty-four hours, and it has been shown that from this point onwards the radio-iodine content of the thyroid falls exponentially, so that semi-logarithmic plotting of the counts against time gives a straight line (Fig. 9.30, p. 171). The slope of this line, or its regression coefficient, can then be taken as a very reliable index of thyroid secretory activity, for the loss of radio-iodine from the gland is a consequence of the loss of labelled hormone.

9.8. Thyrotropin and the regulation of thyroid activity

The thyroid gland resembles the endocrine tissue of the gonads not only in its lack of a secretomotor nerve supply, but also in the system of control by which its secretory activity is regulated. One factor in this system is its negative feedback relationship with the pars distalis, a relationship to which the term thyro-pituitary axis is often applied, and which is essentially similar in principle to that existing between the gonads and the pituitary gland.

Evidence indicative of this relationship was available in the last century, although it was not possible at that time to present a satisfactory interpretation of it. For example, it was recognized that the human pituitary might become greatly enlarged, to a weight as much as four times the normal, in goitrous cretins and in thyroidectomized individuals. The first comprehensive experimental demonstration came, however, from studies of the metamorphosis of frog tadpoles. We shall see later that the thyroid gland is essential for this, but so also is the pars distalis of the pituitary gland, a fact first established in 1914, when it was shown that the removal of the 'anterior lobe' from tadpoles retarded the growth of the thyroid; no colloid was deposited in it, and, as a result, metamorphosis did not occur. It was later found that if the 'anterior lobe' was implanted into a hypophysectomized tadpole, or if extracts of it were injected into the body cavity, the animal would metamorphose. For a time this was thought to indicate that the pituitary was itself exerting a direct control over metamorphosis. It was soon apparent, however, that this could not be so, for a thyroid-ectomized tadpole, which would not, of course, metamorphose, could not be induced to do so even if additional 'anterior lobe' material were implanted into it, despite the fact that the implant maintained itself in what seemed to be good functional condition. The only reasonable explanation was that the thyroid was dependent upon the 'anterior lobe' for the maintenance of its normal functioning, and that the effect of the latter gland upon metamorphosis was an indirect one, exerted through its effect upon the thyroid.

It now has been thoroughly established that the maintenance of the activity of the thyroid gland throughout the vertebrates, at least from fish upwards, is dependent upon a hormone secreted by the pars distalis, and that this activity is reduced as a result of hypophysectomy (Fig. 9.30). The hormone is termed thyrotropin, thyrotrophin, or TSH (for thyroid-stimulating hormone). Its molecular weight is about 28 000, and, like FSH and LH, it is a glycoprotein. This accounts for the PAS-positive response of the follicular colloid in which it is contained.

The similarity with FSH and LH, however, goes much further than this, as we have already seen (p. 119), for TSH, like the other two glycoprotein hormones, can be separated into two subunits. It will be recalled that TSH-α and LH-α are virtually identical (Fig. 7.17, p. 119), with 96 residues, and with carbohydrate moieties linked at positions 56 and 82 to asparagine residues. TSH-β differs considerably from TSH-α, in amino-acid and carbohydrate content, and it differs also from LH-β. However, there are resemblances between TSH-β and LH-β (Fig. 7.18, p. 120), with areas of similar structure that amount to about 50 per cent structural homology.

In LH and TSH it is the β-subunit that is specific to the particular hormone, and the β designation is the convention for representing this. The α-subunits are essentially common to the two hormones, and the α designation represents this. The isolated subunits are largely inactive. Activity can be restored by recombining them, and in this recombination the α-subunit of either hormone can substitute for the other. TSH-α and LH-β will combine to give LH activity, while TSH-β and LH-α will combine to give TSH activity. The facts suggest a close evolutionary relationship between the pituitary glycoprotein hormones, but the full implications of this will only appear when more information is available, particularly from the lower forms.

The simplest demonstration of the existence of thyrotropin is secured by injecting into a test animal a suitable adenohypophysial extract; the result is an enlargement of the follicle cells of the thyroid, which can then be measured in terms of cell height. In this way the thyroid of the guinea-pig, for example, has been found to respond to pituitary extracts of mammals, chick, and amphibians; and that of the goldfish to extracts of fish, amphibians, chick, and mammals. The effects depend upon the strength of the injected extracts. With larger doses, or with sufficiently frequent injections, the gland becomes hyperplastic (with increased numbers of cells) as well as hypertrophied; this, together with its increased vascularization, results in a marked increase in volume and weight. The adaptively significant result of an increased supply of thyrotropin is, of course,

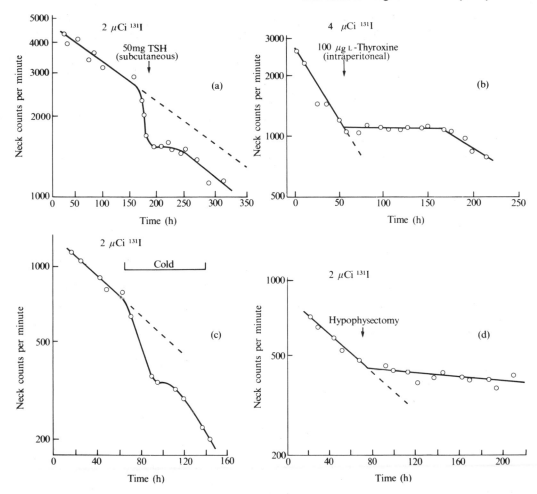

FIG. 9.30 The influence of various experimental treatments on the release of ^{131}I from the thyroid gland of the rabbit after injection of amount shown. The data are plotted semi-logarithmically, the slope of the line representing the ratio of hormone secreted per unit time to the total amount in the gland. (a) subcutaneous injection of thyrotropin; (b) injection of thyroxine; (c) removal to colder environment; (d) hypophysectomy. (From Brown-Grant et al. (1954). J. Physiol. 126.)

an increase in the output of thyroid hormones into the circulation. The first step is an increased blood flow through the gland, and an acceleration in the proteolysis of the colloid and in the release of the stored secretion (Fig. 9.30). This is succeeded by an increased rate of synthesis, marked by an increased rate of iodide uptake and cell hypertrophy, while later, the cells and follicles may increase in number.

These facts explain why a goitrous enlargement of the thyroid results from iodine deficiency. It is a consequence of stimulation of the gland by an increased output of thyrotropin, which is itself a reaction to a low level of circulating thyroid hormones. Conversely, a high level of these will depress the output of thyrotropin. This results in a reduction

of output from the thyroid gland, as can readily be shown by injecting thyroxine into an experimental animal (Fig. 9.30). Here, then, is another example of a feedback mechanism in operation.

An excellent demonstration of this under experimental conditions is seen in the action of certain so-called anti-thyroid compounds, the administration of which (in the food or drink, by injection, or, in the case of aquatic animals, by solution in the surrounding medium) causes a blockage of one or other of the steps of thyroidal biosynthesis. As a result, there is a fall in the level of the circulating thyroid hormones; this brings about the usual response of an increased output of thyrotropin, and this leads in its turn to a goitrous enlargement of the thyroid. The administration of these compounds to the rat, for example, results in heightened epithelium and loss of colloid appearing within twenty-four to forty-eight hours of the beginning of the treatment; after two weeks there is extensive hypertrophy and hyperplasia, with almost complete loss of colloid and greatly increased vascularization. With discontinuation of treatment, there is a rapid reversion to the normal functioning of the gland, with a reaccumulation of colloid, although it may be some time before a normal size is regained. The reaction, which gives to these compounds the name of goitrogens, is in effect a form of compensatory hypertrophy, but it brings no benefit to the animal, since biosynthesis will continue to be inhibited for as long as the goitrogens are administered. The conclusion that it is mediated by thyrotropin rests not only on its similarity to the response induced by direct administration of that hormone, but also on the fact that it does not occur in hypophysectomized animals. Further, the pars distalis of intact animals treated with goitrogens shows characteristic changes in certain secretory cells which can be directly correlated with the discharge of the hormone (p. 67).

The study of anti-thyroid compounds arose in part out of the investigation of the goitrogenic action of certain food materials. From 1928 onwards it became apparent that the leaves of *Brassica* plants contained a goitrogen which was believed to be an organic cyanide, and it was shown that the effect of this could be overcome by the administration of iodine to the affected animal. Later, it was found that certain *Brassica* seeds, including rape, were also goitrogenic, but that their influence, believed to be due to a derivative of thiourea, differed from that of the leaves in that it could not be overcome by iodine treatment. The intensive modern study of the phenomenon dates, however, from 1941, in which year an investigation of the action of sulphaguanidine upon intestinal bacteria brought unexpectedly to light the fact that this substance was goitrogenic, while another group of investigators then showed that thiouracil also possessed this property.

Anti-thyroid compounds fall into two main categories. The action of one of these depends upon the presence of certain monovalent anions, including thiocyanate and perchlorate, which block the iodide-trapping activity of the thyroid and at the same time cause a discharge of stored iodine from the gland. Their effect can be alleviated by the administration of iodide in amounts sufficient to overcome the blockage, in which respect such substances differ from those of the second group. These inhibit

thyroidal activity by blocking the enzymic oxidation of iodide to iodine, so that their effect can be alleviated only by the administration of the thyroid hormones which the animal is unable to synthesize for itself. Included in this second group are thiocarbamide derivatives such as thiourea, thiouracil, propylthiouracil, and carbimazole (Fig. 9.31), and aniline derivatives such as *p*-aminobenzoic acid,

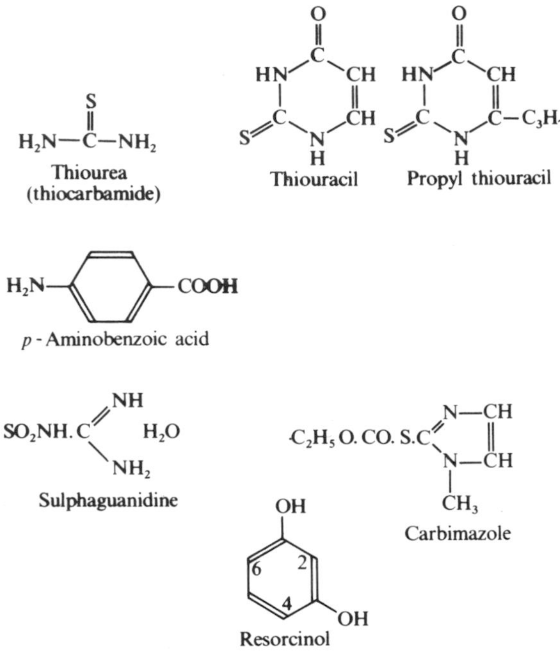

FIG. 9.31. Goitrogenic substances.

sulphaguanidine, and sulphadiazine. The recognition of symptoms of myxoedema in a patient whose varicose ulcers were being treated with resorcinol led to the further discovery that this substance was also included in this category, together with a number of its derivatives, although its isomers, quinol and catechol, are inactive.

Results of goitrogen action similar to those found in the mammals have been reported for all groups of vertebrates from fish upwards. The effect is particularly striking in frog tadpoles, since thyroid hormones are essential for their metamorphosis (p. 178). This can be indefinitely postponed by the immersion of tadpoles in solutions of thiourea or thiouracil, the thyroid showing a reduction in colloid, a heightened epithelium, and an increased vascularization.

The effects of goitrogens on fish, administered by immersion of the animals, have been studied particularly in teleosts because they provide a means of carrying out 'chemical thyroidectomy' in a group which, apart from exceptional forms such as the parrot-fish, *Scarus*, which have a compact thyroid, does not lend itself to surgical thyroidectomy because the gland is diffuse. Thiourea and its derivatives evoke a goitrous response throughout the scattered follicles, and they will presumably affect also any heterotopic tissue which may be present, but it cannot be assumed that they constitute a perfect substitute for the surgical approach. It would be easier to judge this if the mode of action of these substances was entirely clear, but it is at least known that thiourea and its derivative are anti-oxidants, and it seems likely that prolonged immersion of aquatic vertebrates in solutions of such compounds must have deleterious effects. It is prudent, therefore, to interpret studies of goitrogen-treated fish with caution (p. 178).

The role of the pars distalis in the regulation of thyroid secretion is thus very clearly demonstrated, but the thyroid is also influenced by the nervous system. One example of this is seen in (Fig. 9.30, p. 171), which shows how the rate of output of radio-iodine from the rabbit's gland is increased when the animal is removed from its constant temperature room to a lower temperature. The explanation is that the release of thyrotropin, like that of the gonadotropins, is regulated by chemical transmission from the hypothalamus, with the median eminence again acting as the neurohaemal relay centre.

The evidence for this is exactly similar in principle to that obtained from the gonadotropic studies already discussed. For example, localized hypothalamic lesions, placed mid-ventrally from the anterior region of the median eminence to the optic chiasma, prevent rats developing goitrous enlargements in response to thiouracil treatment. Further, electrical stimulation of localized regions of the hypothalamus by remote control (p. 124) can evoke increased thyroid activity, a result analogous to the evoking of ovulation in rabbits.

The conclusion has been satisfactorily confirmed by the isolation of thyrotropin-releasing hormone (TRH) from the mammalian median eminence (7 mg from 200 000 pig hypothalami, and 1 mg from 25 kg of lyophilized sheep hypothalami) and by its synthesis. This hormone, in contrast to the FSH/LH-releasing hormone, is a tripeptide (Fig. 9.32). Administration, either by mouth or injection, results in increased thyrotropin output in experimental animals or human volunteers (Fig. 9.33). Increased output also follows when the hormone is infused into the vessels

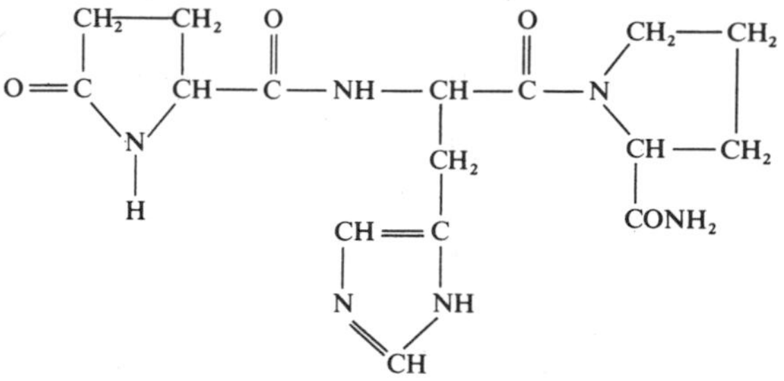

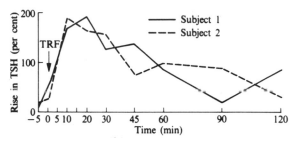

FIG. 9.32. Structure of ovine hypothalamic thyrotropin-releasing factor (TRF). (From Schally and Kastin (1972). *Gen. comp. Endocrin.*, Suppl. 3.)

FIG. 9.33. The effect of an intravenous injection of 50 μg of synthetic TRF (thyrotropin-releasing hormone) on blood thyrotropin levels in two human subjects. (From Hall *et al.* (1970). *Br. Med. Jl* quoted in El Kabir (1972). *Modern trends in endocrinology*, Vol. 4. (eds F. G. Prunty and H. Gardiner-Hill). Butterworth, London.)

of the hypophysial portal system of experimental animals, or when it is applied to pituitaries *in vitro*.

The use of TRH that has been radioactively labelled with tritium or ^{14}C has shown that it accumulates preferentially in the pituitary gland, some also accumulating in the kidney and liver because these organs are involved in the inactivation and excretion of the hormone. It is likely that the action of the hormone is mediated by cyclic AMP, for TRH stimulates adenylate cyclase activity, while the labelled hormone can be shown to be bound to membrane receptors of the pituitary cells. All of these studies are of clinical as well as theoretical importance, for the hormone has great potential for the treatment of human cretinism, which sometimes results from a deficient output of thyrotropin. Treatment with the releasing hormone might well rectify this condition.

Given, then, that the hypothalamus is involved in the regulation of thyrotropin secretion, it becomes possible to examine what paths of communication are actually involved in the feedback mechanism. It was thought at one time that reduction of circulating thyroid hormones acted directly upon the pars distalis to bring about an increased output of thyro-tropin, but this simple concept is no longer adequate. We must conclude, from what has been outlined above, that the thyro-pituitary axis is also mediated by neural pathways involving the hypothalamus. However, this does not exclude the possibility of a direct action of the thyroid secretion upon the pars distalis, and, indeed, there is good evidence that this does occur. Thus, the temporary inhibition of radio-iodine release from the thyroid, which we have seen to be produced by the injection of thyroxine into rabbits, can be evoked even in hypophysectomized animals if these have functional implants of pituitary tissue in their eyes. This implies that the thyroxine must be acting directly upon the implants. More-over, inhibition of release can also be produced by direct injection of thyroxine into the pars distalis of the rabbit in doses that would be too small to produce any effect if they were injected into the general circulation. It would seem, however, that the thyro-tropin-controlling region of the hypothalamus may also be sensitive to direct stimulation by thyroxine, for an inhibition of thyroid secretion in rats can be produced by the injection of as little as 0·05 μg either into that area or into the pars distalis itself. Further, injections of thyroxine into the hypothalamus of rats that are under treatment with propylthiouracil have been shown to inhibit the goitrous response that would normally be evoked by the latter.

It appears likely, then, that both the hypothalamus

and the pars distalis are capable of responding to changes in the concentration of circulating thyroid hormones, so that the feedback can operate through either path. Superimposed on this, however, will be the reflex neural control arising from environmental stimulation. Perhaps this takes functional priority, the feedback relationship serving to ensure the maintenance of an optimal level of circulating thyroid hormones under basal conditions (Fig. 9.34).

9.9. Effects of thyroid hormones in mammals and birds

The thyroid hormones have a profound influence on metabolism in mammals. This is exemplified in the depressed oxygen consumption in patients suffer-ing from myxoedema, and in the elevation of consumption in those with Grave's disease, which is associated with an excessive output of thyroid secretion. The relationship is characteristic of mam-mals in general, and also of birds. In both groups the hypothyroid condition is marked by a low basal metabolic rate; thyroidectomy of pigeons, for ex-ample, reduces this rate by more than 20 per cent. Conversely, the hyperthyroid condition is marked by a high rate. Injections of thyroid hormones produce a marked rise in oxygen consumption (Fig. 9.35), of as much as 60 per cent in rats and mice,

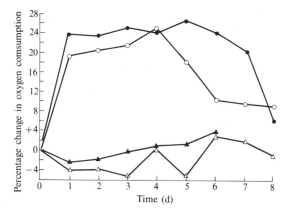

FIG. 9.35. Effect of thyroid extracts upon the percentage change in oxygen consumption of rats. $\triangle$, normal controls; $\blacktriangle$, injected with 2·0 ml 0·9% saline; $\bullet$, injected with 100 mg mammalian thyroid powder; $\bigcirc$, injected with 95 mg dogfish (*Scyliorhinus canicula*) thyroid powder. (From Matty (1954). *J. mar. biol. Assoc. U.K.* **33**.)

and 50 per cent in the house-sparrow. A fall in liver glycogen and a rise in blood sugar accompany this response.

After these injections there is a latent period, ranging from several hours to as much as two days

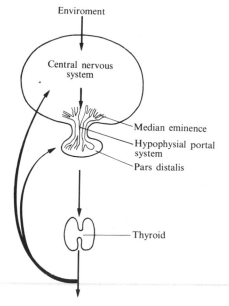

FIG. 9.34. Regulation of thyroid activity by negative feedback loops.

(Fig. 9.35), before the metabolic effect is seen. In this respect, the thyroid hormones differ from adrenaline, which evokes its metabolic response without a latent period. Associated with the difference is the fact that adrenaline will produce its effect on excised tissues as well as in the intact animal, whereas the thyroid hormones will not usually do this. Their stimulatory action upon the oxygen consumption of tissues can only be demonstrated if these are removed from animals that have previously been treated with the hormones. Tissues from such animals will have an oxygen consumption higher than that of identical tissues from untreated control animals, but no response is obtained if the hormones are added to tissues after they have been removed from untreated animals.

In any case, only certain tissues show this metabolic response. Amongst these are heart, diaphragm, liver, and skeletal muscle, all of which have metabolic rates that parallel those of the intact host, with increased oxygen consumption in the hyperthyroid state and decreased consumption in the hypothyroid one. Amongst the tissues which do not respond in this way are the gonads, brain, and smooth muscle of the alimentary tract. The reason for the difference between the two categories of tissue is not known, and it certainly cannot be accounted for by any qualitative difference in their enzyme complement. This is an illustration of the action of a hormone being determined by target specialization, and we shall see other examples in our analysis of thyroid function.

The metabolic action of the thyroid hormones is directly related to the regulation of body temperature in birds and mammals, and for this reason it is commonly referred to as the calorigenic effect of the hormones. Myxoedematous patients often complain of feeling cold, while thyroidectomy lowers the resistance of experimental mammals to low temperatures. Thyroidectomized rats, for example, show a smaller degree of increase in metabolic rate in the cold than do unoperated control animals. Another aspect of this is seen in Fig. 9.30 (p. 191), which shows the increase in the rate of output of the thyroid gland, provoked, through the mediation of thyrotropin, by removal of a rabbit from its constant temperature room to a lower temperature. The thyroid, of course, is only one of the factors involved in this chemical thermoregulation. The sympathetico-chromaffin system (p. 194) also plays an important part, for exposure of mammals to low temperature brings about an increased output of catechol hormones; this results in vasoconstriction,

cardiac acceleration, a rise in blood-sugar level, and an increase in the metabolic rate.

It is to be expected, from what we have already learned of the endocrine regulation of intermediary metabolism, that the calorigenic action of the thyroid hormones will be associated with wide-ranging metabolic effects, and this proves to be so. For example, hyperthyroidism results in loss of weight and reduced fat content, because of the increased caloric demands, while hypothyroidism in man is accompanied by increased plasma cholesterol, which is a common feature of myxoedema. So also in birds, where thyroidectomy causes an increase in plasma cholesterol in drakes, while thyroxine treatment of pigeons results in hyperglycaemia, together with reduced liver glycogen. Hyperthyroidism in general, because of the increased caloric demand for carbohydrate, and the consequent depletion of hepatic glycogen stores, may be associated with increased blood-glucose levels, and with a shift of the glucose tolerance curve towards a mildly diabetic condition. It leads also, and for the same reason, to increased gluconeogenesis, loss of weight, and increased nitrogen wastage.

These effects, however, are not necessarily specific effects of the thyroid hormones themselves; they may be mediated through the action of other hormones, including somatotropin and the glucocorticoids, which become drawn into the calorigenic response. Much more specific is an anabolic action of the thyroid hormones, particularly apparent in young animals, where these hormones interact with somatotropin in the synthesis of new protein. This anabolic action is part of a spectrum of thyroid effects referred to as the growth and maturation action of these hormones. In birds and mammals, it is not always easy to separate this action from the calorigenic one, but the distinction is a real one, and this is very evident in poikilotherms (see later).

We have already noted the importance of somatotropin and insulin in the regulation of growth. The importance of the thyroid hormones is no less well defined, being particularly evident in the new-born mammals, and to some extent also in the foetus. Growth during early pregnancy is probably not thyroid dependent. This follows from the fact that it is not affected by goitrogen treatment, which represses the supply of the maternal hormones as well as of any that the foetus would normally manufacture for itself. Some thyroid hormone is necessary in later pregnancy, but the amount needed is difficult to define, since a supply is obtained from the mother as well as from the foetal gland. Human babies without thyroids are of normal size at birth, although bones that normally begin to ossify shortly before birth show delayed ossification, and growth ceases within a few months. Probably, therefore, the foetal needs can be met by only very small quantities of the hormones.

The neo-natal requirement for thyroid hormones is, of course, well substantiated, notably in human cretinism (p. 160), where thyroid deprivation results in reduced skeletal and somatic growth, arrested sexual development, mental deficiency, a low basal metabolic rate (perhaps as low as 55 per cent of the normal), and increased risk of infection. Comparable results, some of which have already been mentioned, are obtained by thyroidectomy of new-born laboratory and domestic mammals, and they are also well documented in birds, although in this group they have been less closely studied. Hypothyroidism in birds, established at an early stage by treatment with goitrogen or with radio-iodine, results, just as in mammals, in defective skeletal growth and sexual development. These effects can be corrected by thyroid treatment.

The growth-promoting action of the thyroid hormones, which is distinct from their calorigenic action, must necessarily involve interaction with other hormones, notably somatotropin. The effects of these various hormones are not easy to disentangle. However, both thyroxine and somatotropin enhance the growth of dwarf mice, whether administered together or whether administered separately, and the effect of the one hormone is not an exact replica of the effect of the other. It may therefore be concluded that the thyroid hormones do have some independent action, and are not functioning solely in a supporting role. Further analysis of their effects has tended to concentrate on the nervous system, because of its critical importance in human cretins.

Their effect upon this system is quite clear. For example, if rats are made thyroid-deficient at birth, the cerebral cortex fails to develop normally. Its RNA content is reduced (Fig. 9.36), its cell bodies and axons are smaller than normal, and the dendrites are few, with the important consequence that dendritic connections are fewer than normal. Not surprisingly, there are effects on behaviour. Such rats are sluggish, they perform poorly in learning experiments, and they are defective in exploratory behaviour. The defects in the cerebral cortex can be corrected by thyroxine treatment, but only if the rats are treated within a critical period of about 15 days after birth (cf. Fig. 9.36). If the treatment is delayed, the defects are irreversible, as they are also in the

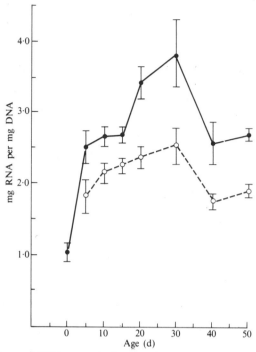

Fig. 9.36. RNA content in the cerebral cortex from normal control and hypothyroid rats, using litters of eight animals as either control or experimental groups. Results are expressed as mg RNA per mg DNA. ●——● normal controls; ○———○ hypothyroid. P values are indicated where they are significant. Vertical bars indicate standard errors. (From Gomez (1971). In *Hormones and development* (eds M. Hamburgh and E. J. W. Barrington). Appleton–Century–Crofts, New York.)

human. This is in line with current interpretations of the nature of differentiation, which assume that certain genes are active during only limited periods of development. Once their period of activity has passed, defects of gene expression, resulting from defects in the internal environment, are beyond the possibility of correction.

9.10. Effects of thyroid hormones in fish

The calorigenic action of the thyroid hormones in birds and mammals is clearly part of the complex of adaptations associated with homeothermy. It is thus not surprising that attempts to establish the existence of a similar action in poikilotherms, with their different metabolic organization, have led to somewhat confusing results. On the whole, the findings are predominantly negative, and particularly so in fish; a group which effectively illustrates some of the problems facing investigators of the lower vertebrates.

Negative results have been obtained in studies of

the dogfish *Scyliorhinus canicula* and the parrot-fish *Scarus guacamaia*. Thyroidectomy in both of these has no detectable effect upon oxygen uptake, despite the fact that extracts of the dogfish thyroid increase the oxygen consumption of rats (Fig. 9.35, p. 174). As might be expected from these results, thyroxine injections into various species of fish have usually produced no effect on oxygen consumption. Yet thyroid powder administered to the guppy, *Lebistes reticulatus*, produced a rise of 15 per cent. There are many difficulties in these experiments, which account for such inconsistencies in the results. Among these difficulties may be mentioned the low metabolic rate of fish, their great individual variability (especially under laboratory conditions), the possibility of the existence of ectopic thyroid tissue, and the risk of exaggerated doses producing results that are merely pharmacological. The stimulation of oxygen consumption in goldfish with doses of 0·5–1·0 mg of thyroxine is of little physiological significance when the animal probably produces less than 1 μg of the hormone per day.

In any case, it remains possible that the thyroid hormones do influence the oxygen consumption of fish, or of individual tissues, but only when internal or external factors are making increased metabolic demands. As an illustration of this, thyroidal activity in the starry flounder, *Platichthys stellatus*, as measured by thyroidal clearance (p. 169), is greater when the animal is in salt water than when it is in fresh (Table 9.1). The standard metabolic rate, as indicated by oxygen consumption, is also greater in salt water, so that there is a correlation between this and the activity of the thyroid gland in circumstances in which the osmoregulatory mechanism is presumably making substantial metabolic demands. This could mean that the thyroid hormones were merely supporting this mechanism indirectly, perhaps by facilitating some generalized aspect of cell metabolism, but the possibility that they have a direct relationship with osmoregulation is certainly not excluded.

An example suggestive of this last possibility is provided by the three-spined stickleback, *Gasterosteus aculeatus*. This animal may winter in the sea, and then undergo a pre-spawning migration into fresh water during the early months of the year, with a reverse post-spawning migration occurring later in the year and lasting until November. These migrations are associated with changes in salinity preference, which are determined not by the gonads but by the thyroid gland. Removal of the gonads does not eliminate the seasonal change in preference,

TABLE 9.1

Activity of thyroid gland of the starry flounder, Platichthys stellatus, *expressed as thyroid clearance of radioiodine from the blood at stated intervals after the injection of a standard tracer dose of* ^{131}I *into the body cavity. The clearance rates are expressed as the volume of blood (as percentage of body weight) cleared of radioiodine by the thyroid per hour. Note that thyroids of salt-water animals are more active than those of freshwater ones.* (From Hickman (1959). *Can. J. Zool.* **37**.)

Hours after injection	Mean blood concentration of ^{131}I (% of dose per g of blood × body weight/100)	Thyroid uptake (% of dose accumulated by whole gland)	Clearance
	Freshwater flounder		
3–4	1·500	0·02	0·0133
4–5	1·485	0·02	0·0135
5–6	1·470	0·02	0·0136
	Saltwater flounder		
2–3	1·6	0·27	0·169
3–4	1·38	0·28	0·202
4–5	1·32	0·29	0·22

although it may delay its onset. Immersion of the animals in thyroxine, however, evokes a fresh-water preference within a few days in fish that were initially showing a preference for salt water. It is typical of the difficulties encountered in attempting to generalize from such data that thyroxine treatment of *Gasterosteus* evokes a fresh-water preference, whereas in the flounder, as we have just seen, it is the salt-water phase that is marked by increased thyroid activity. The situation is further complicated by the corticosteroids being probably involved in water and salt electrolyte metabolism in fish, as also is prolactin. The thyroid hormones can hardly be acting in isolation, therefore, and much of the earlier data that appear to implicate the thyroid in osmoregulation need to be re-evaluated from this point of view.

An involvement of the thyroid hormones in the growth of fish, and in aspects of metabolism associated with this, is reasonably well substantiated; as with mammals, however, the precise role of the thyroid is difficult to define. No doubt the balance between the anabolic and catabolic effects of thyroid treatment must be affected by the size of the administered dose, so that some of the experiments are not truly physiological; this is probably a major factor in the contradictory results that have been reported. Thyroxine treatment is said to increase ammonia excretion in goldfish, and to increase also the incorporation of labelled amino acid into muscle protein, but the best-attested effect on nitrogen metabolism is the silvering that results when salmonids are treated with the hormone. Unfortunately, however, the effect, which is due to increased guanine deposition, is difficult to interpret because the precise source of this material is obscure, although it has been assumed to be a product of nucleic-acid metabolism.

Thyroxine treatment also promotes growth in length and weight in *Salmo gairdneri* (rainbow trout, Fig. 9.37), while immersion of teleosts in goitrogen

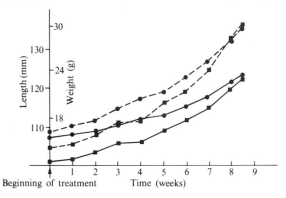

FIG. 9.37. The influence upon the growth of rainbow trout (*Salmo gairdneri*) of the addition of thyroid powder to the food. Mean weekly measurements of weight (■) and length (●) of experimental (———) and control (——) groups of fish. (From Barrington *et al.* (1961). *Gen. comp. Endocrin.* **1**.)

solution impairs growth. Goitrogen treatment, which amounts to immersing the animals in a solution of an antioxidant, is not the happiest experimental procedure, but in this instance the physiological validity of the result has been substantiated by radiothyroidectomy, in which the gland is destroyed by the accumulation within in it of injected radio-iodine. The results are similar in principle to those obtained with goitrogens. Trout show a reduced growth rate, a smaller head, reduced calcification, smaller scales, a decrease in red blood cells, increased cephalic cartilage and abdominal fat, and an arrest of sexual development. Essentially the animals are cretins; a consequence which affords an impressive demonstration of unity of action of the thyroid hormones in two groups as diverse as teleosts and mammals, and which must encourage those who are convinced of the value of the comparative approach in endocrinology. It justifies the belief that common patterns of hormonal action underly the specializations that characterize individual groups.

We have earlier seen, in our discussion of mammals, that growth is a field in which individual hormones cannot be acting in isolation. Somatotropin must also be involved, and in a way that is

different from the involvement of the thyroid hormones. This is shown by the fact that thyroxine treatment by itself cannot restore growth in hypophysectomized fish, or in individuals of *Poecilia* that are carrying ectopic pituitary transplants (p. 81). However, although the mode of action of the thyroid hormones is thus difficult to define, it is possible to show that they do have specific actions upon particular tissues. Thus, treatment of trout alevins, during the first four weeks after hatching, enhances the growth of certain dermal bones of the skull, while the treatment of sturgeons with thyroxine promotes growth of dermal bones as well as of scales. More specifically still, treatment of yearling trout with thyroxine increases the activity of the chondrocytes, which show an enhanced uptake and binding of the sulphate which they incorporate into the cartilage matrix. These are *in vivo* findings. The results of *in vitro* studies of sulphate binding by teleost chondrocytes are much less clear cut, but tend to be negative as far as thyroxine action is concerned. Perhaps this is not surprising. Hormonal action is part of a complex physiological situation, and is not necessarily repeatable after abstraction into a culture medium.

9.11. The thyroid hormones and amphibian metamorphosis

The best-known illustration of the effect of the thyroid gland upon growth and differentiation is its influence upon the metamorphosis of amphibians; this will not take place in animals that have been thyroidectomized, or which are treated with goitrogens. The first indication of this relationship was the demonstration in 1912 by Gudernatsch that administration of thyroid material to frog tadpoles would bring about precocious metamorphosis. This made a profound impression at that time, for the development of the concept of internal secretion was still in its early days, and it had been assumed that the main effects of endocrine glands were physiological, influencing, for example, blood pressure and metabolism. This new discovery showed that their effects could also be exerted in an integrated way upon the growth and differentiation of all parts of the body. Subsequently, as we have already seen, it was shown that the activity of the thyroid gland was itself under the control of the thyrotropic hormone of the pituitary gland.

The general course of amphibian metamorphosis is too well known to need detailed description here (Fig. 9.38). The first phase of larval life is termed premetamorphosis; it lasts for some 20 days in *Rana*

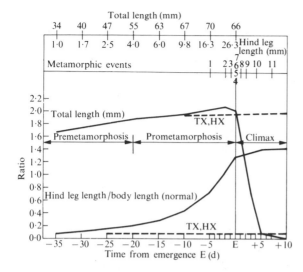

FIG. 9.38 Pattern of metamorphosis in *Rana pipiens*. Data from one batch of normal animals raised at 23 °C shown by solid line. Comparable data for thyroidectomized animals (TX) and hypophysectomized animals (HX) are shown by broken lines). The metamorphic events are: 1, anal canal piece, first definite reduction; 2, anal canal piece reduction completed; 3, skin window for forelegs clearly apparent; 4, loss of beaks; 5, emergence of first foreleg; 6, emergence of second foreleg; 7, mouth widened to level of nostril; 8, mouth widened to level between nostril and eye; 9, mouth widened to level of anterior edge of eye; 10, mouth widened past level of middle of eye; 11, tympanum definitely recognizable. (From Etkin (1968). In *Metamorphosis* (eds W. Etkin and L. I. Gilbert).)

pipiens. This is succeeded by metamorphosis, divided into prometamorphosis (extending over another 20 days), in which changes proceed slowly, and the metamorphic climax (some 10 days), in which the final changes are rapidly completed. The whole of the larval life and transformation is marked by an orderly sequence of events (Fig. 9.38), involving complex and highly specific responses of individual tissues, both morphological and biochemical. The problem, then, is to determine how this patterning is achieved, and how the thyroid hormones can evoke such a diversity of effects.

Studies with radio-iodide have shown that both thyroxine and triiodothyronine are present in the thyroid gland of tadpoles. During premetamorphosis the gland is small and, on histological criteria, looks to be relatively inactive, although it is already binding iodine and forming hormones. During prometamorphosis there is both absolute and relative growth of the gland, the cell height increases, and there is considerable uptake and binding of radio-iodide. At metamorphic climax there is extensive vacuolation and a rapid reduction in the stored colloid, accom-

panied by a decrease in the amount of bound iodine. Clearly, then, there is an orderly patterning of thyroid activity throughout larval life.

How is this patterning achieved? One interpretation is based on the assumption that it depends on the regulation of the thyroid by the hypothalamus, mediated by chemical control as in adult vertebrates. One factor is the progressive differentiation of the median eminence (Fig. 9.39), which would facilitate increased stimulation of the thyroid. The eminence is poorly differentiated in the premetamorphic larva, but becomes increasingly well vascularized during prometamorphosis, until, by the time of climax, it can provide for maximum activation of the thyroid. Its differentiation is thought to be determined by an interaction between the thyroid and the hypothalamus. The latter, on this interpretation, becomes increasingly sensitive to action by the thyroid hormones, which, by positive feedback, promote increasing differentiation of the median eminence, and hence a corresponding increase of their own output.

Further, prolactin is thought to be involved also. During the earlier stages of larval life this hormone, it is supposed, promotes growth and inhibits metamorphosis. At this time the hypothalamus is not yet fully differentiated, so that its normal inhibiting action upon prolactin output is minimal. Later, as the median eminence differentiates, this inhibition increases, with the result that prolactin output declines while thyroxine output is increasing. This interpretation, which has support from experimental studies, outlines, therefore, a subtle example of hormonal interaction, which is further complicated by the growth of the tadpole being also influenced by thyroid hormone levels. Yet another complication in the system is that mammalian somatotropin has little or no effect upon larval growth and metamorphosis, whereas in postmetamorphic amphibians it is this hormone which primarily influences growth, with prolactin having little effect.

However, quite apart from these changing patterns of hormonal interaction, there is another important factor in the ordering of metamorphosis; this is the development of differential sensitivity to thyroxine in the target tissues. The tissues of the embryo are insensitive to thyroxine, but sensitivity develops at the end of the embryonic period, although to different degrees in different tissues. In normal premetamorphic larvae the ratio of hindleg length to body length is slightly different from that in thyroidectomized ones, which shows that even at this early stage some tissues are already sensitive to the very

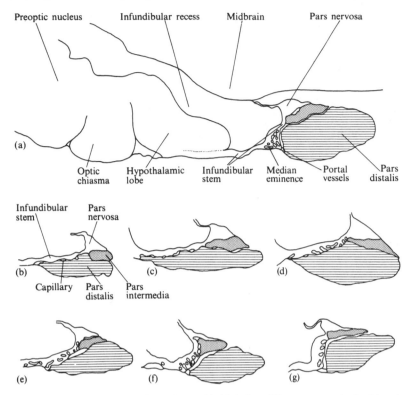

FIG. 9.39. Sagittal sections of the pituitary region of *Rana pipiens*. (a) Adult frog; (b) premetamorphosis; (c) early prometamorphosis; (d) late prometamorphosis; (e) beginning of climax; (f) mid-climax; (g) post-climax. (From Etkin (1968). In *Metamorphosis* (eds W. Etkin and L. I. Gilbert).)

small amounts of hormone which are then circulating. Later, marked differences in sensitivity appear; at the beginning of climax, for example, future adult tissues, such as the tongue, may lose their sensitivity, while those more immediately involved in the climactic changes become highly sensitive.

The importance of the relation between the patterned changes in thyroid output and the changes in target sensitivity are readily demonstrable. Treatment of young tadpoles with a concentration of thyroxine as low as one part per 1000 million is sufficient to promote slight increase in the growth rate of the hind legs. At three parts per 1000 million their growth is increased, relative to the body, to a level approaching that characteristic of early prometamorphosis. Such low levels, however, are inadequate to evoke tail reduction; this requires treatment at 243 parts per 1000 million.

In all of this we see most effectively demonstrated the exquisite refinement of relationships that can develop between a hormone and its target tissues. They are illustrated no less strikingly by the contrasting responses that may be given by individual cells, or localized tissues, that lie close together in the larva and, by the standards of light microscopy, may be indistinguishable. One example is the corneal reflex; a reaction in which the bulb of the eye is withdrawn, with raising of the nictitating membrane, when the cornea is touched. This reflex is dependent for its full development at metamorphosis upon the presence of an adequate concentration of thyroid hormones. The neural centre for it is situated in the medulla. The addition of thyroxine to the water in which frog tadpoles are being reared results in the development of the reflex being accelerated rather less than that of the body as a whole. If, however, the hormone is applied locally to the medulla, by the implantation of an agar pellet that has been soaked in thyroxine, the opposite result is obtained. The development of the reflex is now accelerated in relation to the metamorphosis of the body as a whole, in consequence of the high concentration of hormone to which the centre is now subjected.

Another illustration is given by the formation of the opercular window through which the left forelimb emerges. A thyroxine pellet inserted in this

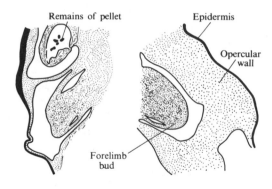

FIG. 9.40. Transverse sections through the opercular regions of larvae of *Rana pipiens*. *Right*, untreated control. *Left*, an experimental animal ten days after implantation of a cholesterol pellet containing thyroxine; there has been marked thinning of the opercular wall, but thickening of the epidermis above it. (From Kaltenbach (1953). *J. exp. Zool.* quoted in Barrington (1964). *Hormones and evolution*. English Universities Press, London.)

at the level of transcription and of translation, and this is borne out by the fact that the induced regression is impaired by actinomycin D (which inhibits transcription) and by puromycin (which inhibits translation). On this interpretation, the response of any particular cell to thyroidal stimulation will depend upon its initial genetic programming.

This concept can, of course, be generalized to apply to the whole range of thyroidal effects throughout the vertebrates. It would appear that the capacity of the iodothyronines to influence information flow in the cell has been exploited to give rise to an almost infinite diversity of responses. This has provided a reserve of potential adaptation which must have contributed a great deal to facilitate the exploitation by vertebrates of new facets of their environment. And, of course, we find here another demonstration of the power of the comparative method. We can learn much from the tadpole's tail.

region evokes a thickening of most of the epidermis, which is one of the adaptations to terrestrial life that arise at metamorphosis. Where the window is to form, however, it evokes a thinning of the epidermis (Fig. 9.40). Thus, epidermal cells that look to be identical are giving two completely contrasted responses to thyroid hormone.

The only reasonable explanation of these observations is that individual target cells or tissues are specifically programmed to give precisely adaptive responses. The hormone evokes the response; the cell programme defines what the response shall be.

Considerable clarification of the situation has been achieved by studies of tadpole tails which have been removed from the body and maintained *in vitro*. Addition of thyroid hormone (triiodothyronine in this instance) evokes regressive changes in the tail; its tissues, except the epidermis, break down, giving an epidermal vesicle with contained debris and melanophores. This is accompanied by a loss of tissue protein and an increase of lysosomal enzymes that are needed for tissue destruction. Biochemical analysis of this breakdown shows that an early event in the response of the isolated tail to the hormone is accelerated production of all species of nuclear RNA. Then, after some hours, there is an abrupt increase in the rate of protein synthesis in the cytoplasm (presumably reflecting enzyme production), an increase of ribosomes, and increased membrane phospholipid synthesis (Fig. 9.41). A reasonable conclusion is that the thyroid hormone is influencing the intracellular flow of biochemical information

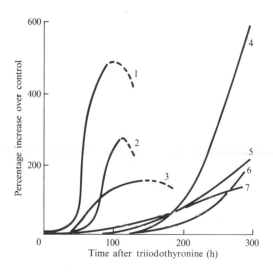

FIG. 9.41. Schematic representation of sequential stimulation of rates of RNA and phospholipid synthesis, in relation to the increases in enzymes or protein synthesized, upon the precocious induction of metamorphosis in *Rana catesbeiana* tadpoles with triiodothyronine. 1, rate of rapidly labelled nuclear RNA synthesis; 2, specific activity of RNA in cytoplasmic ribosomes; 3, rate of microsomal phospholipid synthesis; 4, carbamyl phosphate synthetase; 5, cytochrome oxidase per milligram mitochondrial protein; 6, appearance of serum albumen in the blood; 7, total liver protein per milligram wet weight. The values are expressed as percentage increases in the induced animals over those in the non-induced control tadpoles. The dashed lines in curves 1, 2, and 3 reflect the dilution of specific radioactivity in precursor molecules due to the onset of regression of tissues such as the tail and intestine. (From Tata (1969). *Gen. comp. Endocrin.*, Suppl. 2 (ed. M. R. N. Prasad).)

9.12. The thyroid hormones and vertebrate life histories

The importance of the thyroid hormones in amphibian metamorphosis raises the possibility that they may be similarly drawn upon in comparable crises in the life histories of other vertebrates, and notably in teleosts, which sometimes undergo marked metamorphosis. Such metamorphosis may be a first metamorphosis, when a larval stage assumes adult form, or a second metamorphosis, when an adult undergoes changes associated with sexual maturity. Both types may include morphological and physiological changes, which, comprising as they do a pattern of changes affecting all parts of the body, are evidently suggestive of endocrine regulation.

A well-known example of teleostean metamorphosis is the transformation (first metamorphosis) of the leptocephalus larva of the eel into the elver and, many years later, the second metamorphosis which transforms the fresh-water yellow eel into the migratory silver eel. There is no conclusive evidence regarding the regulation of these changes, although there are indications that the thyroid gland may be involved. Another well-known example, and one that has been more closely studied, is the transformation of the fresh-water salmon parr into the migratory smolt. This involves, in addition to the silvering produced by deposition of guanine (p. 178), a number of physiological changes which seem, in general, to be correlated with the requirements of the marine life

which the smolt will undertake. It develops, for example, an increased resistance to saline conditions, and the fact that this is accompanied by an increase in metabolic rate, and by histological evidence of hyperactivity of the thyroid, has been thought to imply an involvement of the thyroid hormones in the metamorphosis. Evidence that these hormones can influence locomotor activity (see later) has obvious relevance in this connection. There is fragmentary evidence that the thyroid is hyperactive during the relatively slight metamorphosis of the herring (Fig. 9.42), and during the much more drastic metamorphosis of the flounder, while thyroid treatment of the larva of the mud-skipper, *Periophthalmus*, is said to induce premature assumption of the semi-terrestrial life of the adult.

This evidence is too incomplete to carry much weight, and in any case it would be a mistake to look for a close parallel with the amphibian situation. Where a problem is solved independently in two different groups, as it must have been in these, it is to be expected that the two solutions will be different in detail, even though similar principles are involved. Natural selection will have operated upon those physiological mechanisms which were already characteristic of the groups concerned. This is well illustrated in the metamorphosis of the larval lamprey. So far it has proved impossible to influence it by thyroid treatment, and this failure is hardly surprising. The Cyclostomata are widely separated from

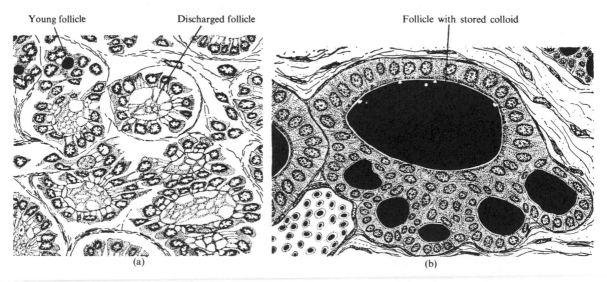

Fɪɢ. 9.42. Sections of the thyroids of herring from (a) an individual shortly after metamorphosis, with much stored colloid, and (b) a post-spawning individual, with reduced and vacuolated colloid, and with new follicles and colloid forming. (From Buchmann (1940). *Zool. Jb. Abt. Anat.* **66**.)

both teleosts and amphibians, while the thyroid is represented in the larva by the endostyle (p. 164), which itself undergoes reorganization at metamorphosis.

Another approach to this problem has been based upon studies of cyclical fluctuations in thyroid activity in fish. The data are not always completely convincing, but they have provided at least some evidence that thyroid activity may be correlated with reproductive cycles. For example, measurements of cell height (the limitations of which have earlier been noted) indicate a high level of thyroid activity in the minnow, *Phoxinus*, during the period preceding spawning. Such associations, however, even if soundly based, are not necessarily good evidence for causal relationships, and the example of the cod, quoted earlier, illustrates this. Populations of this fish, feeding near Spitzbergen, migrate in late September to spawning grounds off the north Norwegian coast, and at this time their thyroids show signs of hyperactivity (Fig. 9.43). This might easily be held to imply a correlation between thyroid activity and reproduction, were it not that immature fish make a similar run, and also possess hyperactive thyroids. This suggests that the gland may actually be involved in some way in the migratory movements (p. 143).

Another example, this time from the elasmobranchs, is given by the dogfish, *Squalus acanthias*.

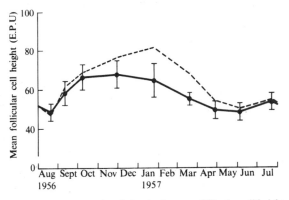

FIG. 9.43. The seasonal variation in the mean follicular cell height of the thyroid gland in immature cod. The broken line gives the seasonal variation in adult cod for comparison. The follicular cell height is expressed in eyepiece units (E.P.U.). (From Woodhead (1959). *J. mar. biol. Assoc. U.K.* **38**.)

The female shows an annual increase in thyroid secretory activity, beginning in November, with depletion of colloid and consequent loss of weight of the gland (Fig. 9.44). This, however, occurs every year, whereas gestation lasts for two years (Fig. 9.45). As with the cod, then, it is supposed that the thyroid cycle is primarily related to the annual migration. The sequence of events here is complex, but essentially the fish spend summer in the Orkney–Shetland area, and winter in Norwegian and inshore Scottish waters. However, although the thyroid is

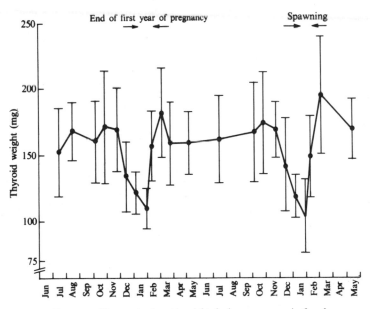

FIG. 9.44. Changes in thyroid weight during pregnancy in female dogfish (*Squalus acanthias*). The mean values and standard deviations are given. (From Woodhead (1966). *J. Zool.* **148**.)

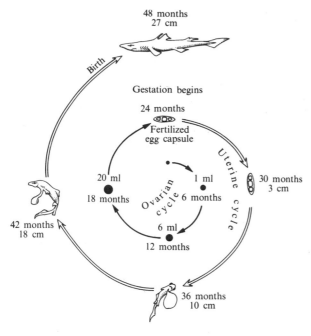

Fig. 9.45. Gestation cycle in *Squalus*. (From Woodhead (1966). *J. Zool.* **148**.)

also hyperactive in the males during the winter, it is said to be relatively more active in the females. This leaves open the possibility, therefore, that the gland may also have some relationship with reproduction or gestation.

In any case, there are good grounds for assuming at least some participation of the thyroid gland in the reproductive cycle. To mention only a few examples, there is histological evidence of hyperactivity in spawning herring (Fig. 9.42), and direct evidence of maximal output of thyroxine during the period of reproduction in *Fundulus*. Some association between the thyroid and sexual reproduction has, in fact, long been suspected, and it is curious to find that at the beginning of this century, Gaskell was using this supposed association to support his theory of the derivation of vertebrates from eurypterids. His suggestion was that the association justified a belief in the homology of the thyroid with the uterus of scorpions!

However, even if we ground our assumptions more firmly than that, it remains to reflect that reproduction covers a very wide range of activities, any one of which might conceivably be influenced by the thyroid hormones. To give only one example, there is evidence suggesting that thyroid hormones can influence both the degree and the pattern of motor activity in teleost fish, and that thyroxine treatment may affect electrical activity patterns in the central nervous system. Obviously, therefore, the suspected relationships between thyroid activity on the one hand, and reproductive and migratory activities on the other, may involve actions of the hormones upon the nervous system rather than directly upon the glands. All of which goes to explain why it is so very difficult to elucidate more precisely, at our present level of information, the evident importance of the thyroid hormones in the lives of vertebrates.

10

The chromaffin tissue of the adrenal gland

10.1. General organization of the adrenal gland

A misunderstanding of St. Jerome's translation of the Vulgate led at one time to a belief that the adrenal glands of mammals were known to Moses, but the first account of them was actually published in 1563 in a review of human anatomy by Bartolomeo Eustachius. Later authors found that they were filled with fluid, and, not realizing that this was due to post-mortem decay, referred to them as the supra-renal capsules, a term which also expresses their close association in man with the anterior end of the kidneys. This relationship, however, is not necessarily present in other mammals, where they may form a pair of organs separated from the kidneys (Fig. 10.1). Cuvier drew attention in 1805 to their differentiation into the inner and outer regions which are now known as the medulla and cortex. These constitute two distinct endocrine tissues, differing in development, organization, and mode of functioning.

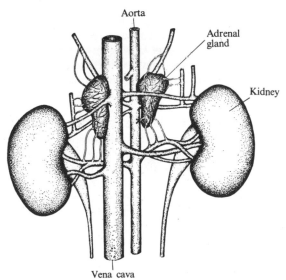

Aorta

Adrenal gland

Kidney

Vena cava

FIG. 10.1. The adrenal glands and kidney of the dog and their vascular connections. (From Hartmann and Brownell (1949). *The adrenal gland.* Lea and Febiger, Philadelphia.)

Both tissues are found throughout the vertebrates, but, since their arrangement as a medulla and cortex is peculiar to mammals, and is not always sharply defined in even them, it is convenient in comparative studies to refer to them respectively as the chromaffin and adrenocortical tissues.

In birds, the adrenal glands are present as distinct organs just anterior to the kidneys, but the two components here are intermingled to a varying degree without forming a sharply defined cortex and medulla (Fig. 10.2). In reptiles, the organs are elongated, with some variation in the arrangement of the components. Chelonians and crocodiles have the tissues disposed much as in birds, but in lizards, and in some snakes, the adrenocortical tissue may be partly encapsulated by chromaffin cells. In Amphibia, the glands are associated with the mesonephric kidneys, for the most part lying on the surface of these organs, or being embedded in them. Anurans have them organized into cords, but in urodeles and apodans they form scattered islands on the ventral surface of the kidney.

In elasmobranch fish (Figs 10.3 and 10.4), the two components are separated from each other and are not so easily identified as in the tetrapods. The chromaffin tissue forms a series of segmental glands lying immediately above the dorsal wall of the posterior cardinal sinus. Some of these can be seen by removing the ventral wall of the sinus, but the more posterior ones are embedded in the kidney, and in that region are larger in the male than in the female. They are sometimes called the suprarenal glands, but this term is better avoided; earlier writers, as we have seen, applied it to the whole gland of mammals, and the same usage still persists. The adrenocortical tissue of elasmobranchs lies in the kidney region, and is often called the interrenal gland or tissue (Fig. 10.3); it may form a compact body, or an horseshoe-shaped structure, or an elongated rod with small accessory portions at its anterior end. The arrangement in the Holocephali is similar.

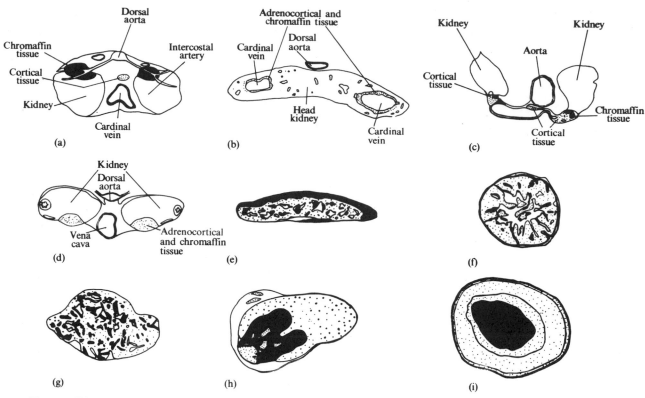

FIG. 10.2. Diagrams to show the intermingling of chromaffin tissue and adrenocortical tissue in the vertebrates. (a) Dogfish; (b) perch; (c) *Ichthyophis*; (d) frog; (e) lizard; (f) Crocodilia; (g) pigeon; (h) echidna; (i) rat. (From Chester Jones (1957). *The adrenal cortex*. Cambridge University Press, London.)

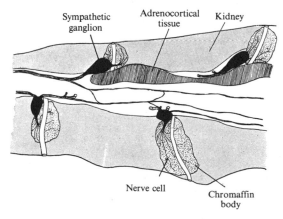

FIG. 10.3. Semi-diagrammatic representation of a horizontal section of the kidney region of *Scyliorhinus canicula* (female). (From Young (1933). *Q. Jl microsp. Sci.* **75**.)

In teleost fish, the separation of the two components is less pronounced than in elasmobranchs, and they may even be intermingled. In the lower Actinopterygii (*Polypterus, Acipenser*), the adrenocortical (interrenal) tissue is scattered throughout the kidneys, but in teleosts it is more concentrated to form groups of cells lying in close relationship with the cardinal veins in the region of the pronephros, which is usually a lymphoid organ (head kidney) in the adult. There is much variation in the amount of tissue and in its distribution between the two halves of the body, but little is known of the factors which may determine this. The chromaffin tissue is found as groups of cells in the same region, especially localized around the cardinal veins, but not necessarily intermingled with the cortical tissue.

In addition to these structures, there are also a pair of gland-like bodies, lying on, or embedded in, the mesonephric kidneys. They are called the corpuscles of Stannius, after the observer who first described them in 1839. These bodies, composed of cells with lipoprotein granules, have been regarded as adrenocortical tissue, but this view has been abandoned, for several good reasons. They differ from that tissue

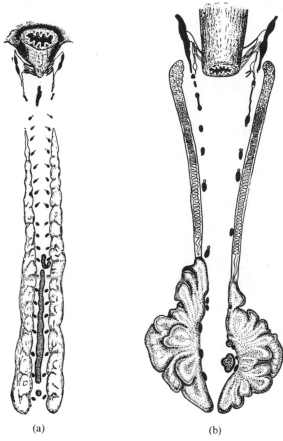

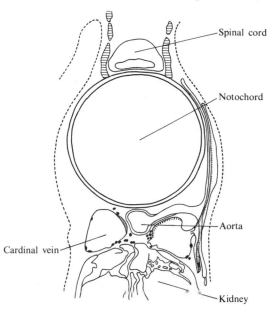

FIG. 10.5. Diagram of a section through the mid-part of the trunk of *Petromyzon marinus*. Small groups of cortical cells, black; chromaffin tissue, stippled. (From Chester Jones (1957). *The adrenal cortex*. Cambridge University Press, London.)

(a)   (b)

FIG. 10.4. Diagrams of the arrangement of the adrenal homologues in (a) *Mustelus* and (b) *Raja diaphanes*. Chromaffin tissue: double row of black bodies; adrenocortical tissue: stippled. The kidneys have been turned outwards to uncover these. The adrenocortical and the more caudal chromaffin bodies are within the kidneys, the more anterior chromaffin bodies are dorsal to them. (From Hartman and Brownell (1949). *The adrenal gland*. Lea and Febiger, Philadelphia.)

in arising as evaginations from the wall of the pronephric duct. They are not influenced by corticotropin, they lack a clearly-defined steroidogenic capacity, and it has not been possible to demonstrate 3β-HSD in their cells. Their function remains in doubt, but there is some evidence that they may be involved in osmoregulation, and that they form a renin-like substance.

The organization of the two adrenal components in the Cyclostomata (Fig. 10.5) is not well understood. Chromaffin cells are plentiful, partly in the walls of the larger blood vessels, but a remarkable feature is that many more are also found, both in lampreys and in hagfish, in the wall of the heart. Those in the blood vessels are believed to be inner-

vated by preganglionic fibres from the roots of the spinal nerves, but those in the heart are said not to be innervated at all. It has been suggested that the latter cells may be a primitive type of adrenergic nerve cell, but it is not easy to incorporate this view into the generally accepted interpretation of the adrenal chromaffin cells as originating from postganglionic sympathetic neurons (p. 193).

Supposedly adrenocortical (interrenal) cells are found in larval and adult lampreys, mainly in the region of the pronephros, although they also extend backwards throughout the trunk. These cells, which may be closely associated with chromaffin cells, originate from the mesoderm in much the same way as the adrenocortical tissue of higher forms, they contain lipid material and cholesteol, and have an ultra-structure resembling that of adrenocortical cells. Probably, then, these cells are true adrenocortical tissue, although it has not yet been possible to secure a convincing demonstration of the presence in them of 3β-HSDH activity.

10.2. The catecholamine hormones

One of the outstanding landmarks in the development of endocrinology was the publication in 1896 by Oliver and Schäfer of their classical study of the physiological effects (Fig. 10.6) of extracts of the mammalian adrenal gland. The study began with that

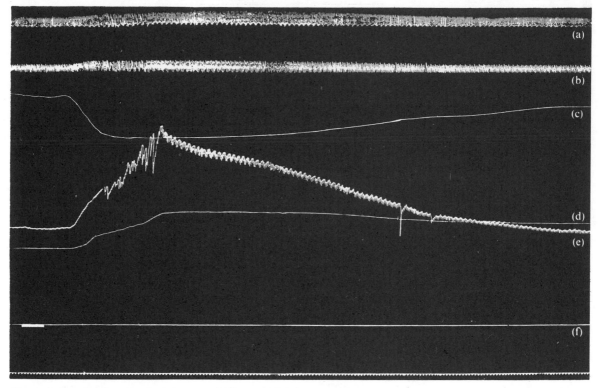

FIG. 10.6. A tracing from the classical paper of Oliver and Schäfer, illustrating the effect of an intravenous injection of an extract of the adrenal gland of the calf into a dog which had previously received morphine and atropine. Note the rise of blood pressure (vasopressor effect). The spleen decreases in volume as a result of the contraction of the arterioles, while the arm increases in volume because of the concomitant passive expansion of the larger vessels. (a) Auricle; (b) ventricle; (c) spleen; (d) arm volume; (e) blood pressure; (f) abscissa signal. The base line shows the time in seconds. (From Oliver and Schäfer (1895). *J. Physiol.* **18.**)

element of the accidental which is so often a component of successful research. Dale has told the story of how Dr. George Oliver, a Harrogate physician, discovered while experimenting upon his young son that injections of these extracts affected the radial artery. Proceeding to London to inform Schäfer of this, and finding him engaged upon an experiment which involved recording the blood pressure of a dog, he urged him to inject some of the extract which he had brought with him. This was done, and Schäfer 'stood amazed to see the mercury mounting in the arterial manometer till the recording float was lifted almost out of the distal limb'.

As a result of their subsequent investigations, they concluded that the adrenals were ductless secreting glands, and an analogy was drawn with the thyroid gland for which, as we have seen, a similar conclusion had by then been developed. Oliver and Schäfer found that the secretion which they were studying was restricted to the medulla; its effects included an increase in muscular tone, constriction of arterioles, and an increase in the blood pressure, with a consequential shrinkage of the kidney and spleen. A tracing prepared in the course of one of their experiments, and illustrating some of these effects, is seen in Fig. 10.6.

Developments rapidly followed these discoveries, aided by the fortunate circumstance that large amounts of the secretion are stored within the gland, and are readily extractable. An *N*-benzoyl derivative was isolated by Abel under the name of epinephrine (*epi*, upon; *nephros*, kidney), and by 1901 the active principle had been isolated in pure form and called by the Latin equivalent, adrenalin. This substance, the first hormone to be isolated in crystalline form, was then synthesized in 1904. It is now known in the United Kingdom as adrenaline, the terminal 'e' indicating by convention a basic substance, but the Greek form (epinephrine) is commonly used in the United States.

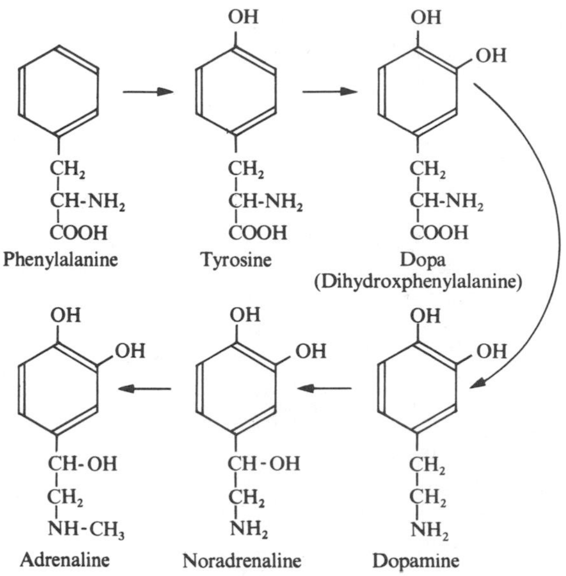

FIG. 10.7. The catechol hormones and related compounds.

Adrenaline (Fig. 10.7) is a catecholamine which exists in two optically active forms owing to the presence of one asymmetrical carbon atom. In its naturally occurring form it is laevo-rotatory, this isomer being some twelve to fifteen times as active as the dextro-rotatory form. The synthetic material is also available in the L-form. It has been suggested that the rapid progress in the isolation and characterization of the hormone was a discouragement to further exploration of this particular field, and it is certainly remarkable that although Stolz, who had synthesized adrenaline, also synthesized the non-methylated homologue noradrenaline (Fig. 10.7), it was not until 1946 that the physiological importance of the latter became appreciated.

Noradrenaline is a chemical transmitter at sympathetic nerve endings and in the central nervous system (p. 59), but is also present in the adrenal medulla, both as a hormone in its own right, and also as a precursor of adrenaline (Fig. 10.7). The catecholamines of the human medulla, for example, comprise about 80 per cent adrenaline and 20 per cent noradrenaline. Both are discharged into the venous effluent of the gland, and must therefore be regarded as joint hormonal products, just as are thyroxine and triiodothyronine. Like adrenaline, the naturally occurring form of noradrenaline is laevo-rotatory, and this is 25–30 times more active than the D-isomer.

10.3. Functional organization of chromaffin tissue

The cells of the chromaffin tissue of mammals are arranged in a closely packed network of cords, between which extend capillary vessels. The characteristic feature of these cells (Fig. 10.8) is the presence of a very large number of membrane-bound granules, with a wide range of size (50–350 nm in the rat). These granules, which contain the catecholamines, react with potassium dichromate or chromic acid to give an oxidation product with a yellowish or brown colour. This is called the chromaffin reaction, and it is because of this reaction that the catecholamine-secreting cells are called chromaffin cells. The reaction is given also by phenolic complexes in other cells as well, but yields a different reaction production. These cells (the enterochromaffin cells of the alimentary tract, for example) should not, therefore, be confused with the 'true' chromaffin cells which are the diagnostic feature of chromaffin tissue throughout the vertebrates. In any case, an adequate biological definition of these cells must take account of other parameters mentioned elsewhere, including their embryological origin from the neural crest, and their innervation by preganglionic nerve fibres. This is the more important because cells containing biogenic amines, and giving a chromaffin reaction, are not restricted to vertebrates. They occur also, for example, in the ventral nerve cord of annelid worms, extracts of which may contain both adrenaline and noradrenaline, while groups of cells in the nervous systems of *Anodonta* and of *Helix pomatia* contain either 5-hydroxytryptamine or dopamine.

The characteristics of true chromaffin cells can be further clarified in ways additional to those so far mentioned. Their biogenic amine content can be revealed by the formaldehyde-induced fluorescence reaction of Falck, mentioned earlier (p. 72), and which can be made both qualitative and quantitative by the use of microspectrophotometry. Moreover, the chromaffin reaction itself has potentialities which were not at first appreciated. After the discovery of adrenaline, this reaction was at first ascribed to the reducing properties of the catecholamine, which were thought to bring about a reduction of the dichromate to a yellowish-brown compound. Later, however, when it was shown that an identical effect could be produced by fixing chromaffin tissue in a fluid containing potassium iodate, it became apparent that the reaction was in fact due to the oxidation of the granule substance by the dichromate or iodate as the case might be.

The earlier view implied that any reducing substance might give a chromaffin reaction. The later

Endothelium   Noradrenaline cell

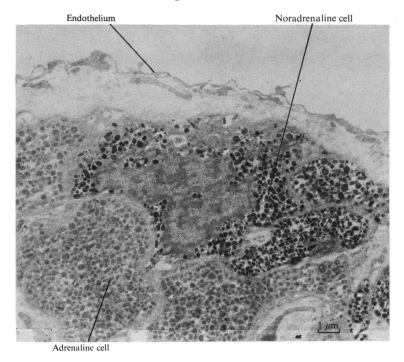

Adrenaline cell

FIG. 10.8. Electron micrograph of adrenaline- and noradrenaline-storing cells in the adrenal gland of the frog, lying adjacent to a blood capillary. See text for explanation. (Courtesy of R. E. Coupland.)

interpretation indicates a much greater degree of histochemical specificity in the reaction, and this is why it is possible, by controlled and differential oxidation, to demonstrate in the chromaffin tissue two kinds of cell, one of which is believed to secrete adrenaline, the other secreting noradrenaline. For example, both substances can be demonstrated simultaneously in thin slices of fresh tissue by using a reaction mixture consisting of 5% potassium di-chromate containing sufficient 5% potassium chromate to give a pH of between 5 and 6. In these circumstances the two cell types appear distributed as irregular patches, those containing adrenaline being darker. Clearly this provides an acceptable histological basis for the selective release of adrenaline and noradrenaline (p. 194), a response which would be more difficult to account for in the absence of two distinct types of secretory cell.

This differentiation of two cell types can also be demonstrated in all groups of vertebrates by electron microscopy. If chromaffin tissue is fixed in buffered (pH 7·4) aqueous glutaraldehyde, the adrenaline diffuses out into the fixative, which may eventually contain as much as 90 per cent of the original hormone. The noradrenaline, however, is precipitated as a result of the formation within the cell of an insoluble polymer. After subsequent treatment with osmic acid, the noradrenaline-containing cells have highly electron-dense granules, while those of the adrenaline-containing cells are much less dense (Fig. 10.8). A further difference between the two is that the noradrenaline-containing cells possess a localized Golgi region which is relatively free of granules, while the adrenaline-containing ones have their granules and organelles uniformly distributed.

The implication of the above is that the catecholamines are located within the granules of the medullary cells, and there is confirmation from differential centrifugation studies that they do, in fact, contain the bulk of the hormones, associated as a storage complex with protein (chromogranin) and ATP. (A similar complex is found in adrenergic nerve endings.) Discharge of the secretion to the outside of the cells is probably effected by the membranes of the granules fusing with the plasma membrane.

These granules are essential not only for the storage of the catecholamines, but also for their biosynthesis. Tyrosine, which is their precursor, is first hydroxylated to dihydroxyphenylalanine (dopa) by tyrosine hydrolase within the granules. Dopa is then transformed into dopamine by dopa decarboxylase, the dopamine is hydroxylated to noradrenaline, and some of this is then methylated to form adrenaline (Fig. 10.7). This last reaction takes place in the cytoplasm, and it may be that the decarboxylation of dopa takes place there as well.

Associated with this biosynthetic pathway is the cortico-medullary relationship which is such a remarkable feature in many vertebrate groups. Comparison of the catecholamine content of the chromaffin tissue in vertebrates showing different patterns of relationship (e.g. the dogfish, frog, and mammal), suggests that a close association of chromaffin tissue with cortical secretion may favour methylation of noradrenaline. However, the presence of considerable amounts of adrenaline in the elasmobranch chromaffin tissue (34 per cent in *Scyliorhinus canicula*, for example), which is widely separate from the cortical (interrenal) tissue, shows that association with cortical secretion is not essential for methylation.

10.4. Functions of the sympathetico-chromaffin complex in mammals

The main physiological actions of the catecholamines are shown in Table 10.1. Adrenaline reduces vascular tone in skeletal muscles, but, as would be expected from the observations of Oliver and Schäfer, it also has a powerful vasopressor action. This results from an increase in the volume and frequency of the heartbeat, and by an accompanying splanchnic vasoconstriction. Adrenaline also relaxes the smooth muscle of the bronchi and of the alimentary tract, thus inhibiting passage of food through the latter. It also appears to evoke the release of corticotropin, although this may be a parallel response rather than a causally mediated one. Amongst its metabolic effects are the increase of lipolysis in adipose tissue, through the mediation of cyclic AMP, and of hepatic glycogenolysis by the activation of phosphorylase (p. 55), again with cyclic AMP participating. This hepatic effect, with the consequential rise in blood-sugar levels, makes an important contribution to metabolic homeostasis (p. 56). Finally, adrenaline evokes some unpleasant subjective symptoms of expectancy and anxiety when injected into man.

It is apparent from Table 10.1 that the effects of noradrenaline do not exactly parallel those of adrenaline. Like adrenaline, it increases lipolysis in adipose tissue, but it has less effect on glycogenolysis, on the heart, and on corticotropin release. On the other hand, it is a major factor in the control of vascular tone in mammals, and it evokes vasoconstriction in most parts of the body, although this vascular action

TABLE 10.1

Comparison of the effects of adrenaline and noradrenaline. (From Bell *et al.* (1972). *Textbook of physiology and biochemistry* (8th edn). Livingstone, Edinburgh and London).

	L-adrenaline	L-noradrenaline
Heart rate	Increase	Decrease†
Cardiac output	Increase	Variable
Total peripheral resistance	Decrease	Increase
Blood pressure	Rise	Greater rise
Respiration	Stimulation	Stimulation
Skin vessels	Constriction	Constriction
Muscle vessels	Dilatation	Constriction
Bronchus	Dilatation	Less dilatation
Eosinophil count	Increase	No effect
Metabolism	Increase	Slight increase
Oxygen consumption	Increase	No effect
Blood sugar	Increase	Slight increase
Central nervous system	Anxiety	No effect
Uterus *in vivo* in late pregnancy	Inhibition	Stimulation
Kidney	Vasoconstriction	Vasoconstriction

† Increases rate of isolated heart

tends to be unremarked in man because it is not accompanied by subjective symptoms. Such differences make possible the quantitative determination of both hormones in a single extract by bioassay procedures. One method makes use of the fact that noradrenaline has the stronger effect upon the blood pressure of the cat, while adrenaline has the greater relaxing action upon the rectal caecum of the fowl.

These differences between the physiological actions of the two catecholamines is ascribed to the existence of two types of receptor site in the target tissues; one of these (the α type) responding to noradrenaline, while the other (the β type) responds to adrenaline. They can be distinguished by the use of drugs, some of which are α-adrenergic blocking agents; these block, for example, the vasoconstriction which would otherwise be produced by noradrenaline. Other drugs are β-adrenergic blocking agents; these block the vasodilatation which would otherwise be produced by adrenaline. In general, the α-adrenergic responses tend to be inhibitory, and to be mediated by a reduced synthesis of cyclic AMP, while the β-adrenergic responses tend to be stimulatory, and to be mediated by increased synthesis of cyclic AMP. The distinction is not, however, a simple and invariable one. Adrenaline and noradrenaline may sometimes both be blocked by a β blocking agent, while adrenaline may sometimes act as both an α and a β stimulator.

Probably there is a continuous spontaneous secretion from the chromaffin tissue of mammals, but

Schwann cell   Nerve ending

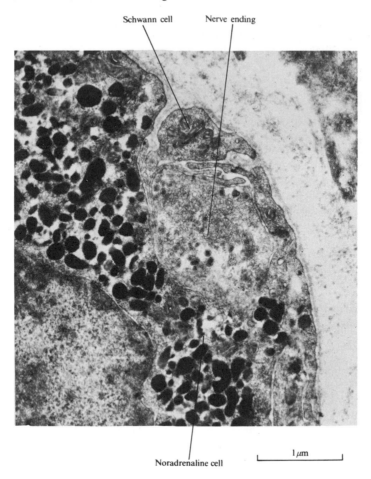

Noradrenaline cell   1 μm

FIG. 10.9. Electron micrograph of nerve ending on a noradrenaline-storing chromaffin cell of the adrenal gland of the frog. A basement membrane separates the cell from the adjacent connective tissue. (Courtesy of R. E. Coupland.)

it will be obvious from what has already been said that it must also be regulated by the nervous system. In this respect the chromaffin tissue (Fig. 10.9) is unusual amongst endocrine tissues in that its cells receive a direct innervation, this being derived from the autonomic nervous system, through sympathetic secretomotor fibres running in the splanchnic nerve. Stimulation of this nerve, therefore, evokes an increased output of secretion, just as do a variety of natural stimuli such as pain, fear, cold, muscular activity, and a fall in blood-sugar levels.

This innervation has a particular significance which derives from the fact discussed in a broader context elsewhere (p. 59), that secretion is a fundamental property of conventional nerve cells. This is because their functioning involves the release of chemical transmitter substances (neurohumours) at their axon endings, the transmitters in vertebrates

being either acetylcholine (released at cholinergic endings) or noradrenaline (at adrenergic endings). It will be recalled that the autonomic nervous system comprises two divisions, the parasympathetic and the sympathetic divisions, and that the neural pathways in both of these differ from those in the cerebrospinal nervous system in including relays between preganglionic nerve cells and postganglionic ones. The relay points are located in peripheral ganglia, and it is the postganglionic fibres that innervate the effector organs. The preganglionic endings of both the parasympathetic and the sympathetic divisions are cholinergic. So also, in general, are the postganglionic endings of the parasympathetic division, while those of the sympathetic division are adrenergic.

Nerve endings, because of this secretory activity, always contain membrane-bound synaptic vesicles, each of which represents a quantum of the appropriate neurohumour, and such vesicles, resembling those of other sympathetic fibres, are visible in the nerve endings of the adrenal medulla. The secretomotor function of the innervation is readily shown, for the appearance of these vesicles varies, under experimental stimulation, in a way that can be correlated with fluctuations in the output of catecholamines from the gland. However, the innervation of the adrenal medulla is exceptional in consisting not of postganglionic fibres, but of preganglionic ones (although the innervation in elasmobranchs has been thought to be postganglionic). Thus the chromaffin cells have the same anatomical relationship as postganglionic sympathetic nerve cells, and, of course, they resemble them biochemically in being able to synthesize catecholamines.

This close relationship is further emphasized by the common embryonic origin of the chromaffin cells and the postganglionic cells of the sympathetic ganglia from the neural crest. At an early stage of development in mammals the ganglion rudiments consist of only one type of cell: the primitive sympathetic cell. Some of the cells then differentiate into sympathoblasts, which give rise to sympathetic neurones. Others differentiate into phaeochromoblasts which move out of the ganglia (Fig. 11.1, p. 197) and give rise to chromaffin tissue, usually in close relationship with the developing adrenocortical rudiment. (We have noted elsewhere (p. 154) the wider endocrinological interest of this activity of the neural crest.)

In comparing the chromaffin cells with the postganglionic neurones we thus find community of biosynthetic activity, of embryological origin, and of anatomical relationships. It seems highly probable, therefore, that they have had a common evolutionary origin, and since, as we shall now see, their functional relationship is equally close, it becomes helpful to regard them as constituting a sympathetico-chromaffin complex.

Our conception of the functional significance of this complex is based upon an analysis which was developed particularly by W. B. Cannon. This proposes that the two catecholamine hormones, because they resemble in many of their effects the results of stimulation by the sympathetic division of the autonomic nervous system, serve to reinforce and to prolong the effects of that stimulation when the body is responding to stress. Animals have to maintain themselves in a constantly fluctuating environment, and they must, in consequence, be able to respond to fluctuations by making rapid internal adjustments.

This need would have become more acute in the vertebrates when they adopted terrestrial life, with its more rigorous and variable conditions. Doubtless this is why we find the two divisions of the autonomic nervous system developing an increasingly well defined antagonism in the higher vertebrates (cf. p. 22), and finally giving birds and mammals the capacity for remarkably precise control of their internal medium. We have found the same principle of antagonism governing the endocrine regulation of carbohydrate metabolism, although in this instance the equilibrium is maintained by the interaction of opposing hormones.

The explanation of the association of the adrenal medulla specifically with the sympathetic division of the autonomic nervous system lies in the organization of that division, which differs from the parasympathetic division in having its relay points widely separated from the effectors. The sympathetic division is thus adapted to bring about widely diffused responses, included in which are many reactions that increase the capacity of the animal to deal with the emergencies presented by such stresses as cold, pain, fear, and asphyxia. Amongst these responses are the acceleration of the heartbeat, the redistribution of blood, the dilatation of the bronchioles, and transient hyperglycaemia. Cannon showed that such stresses evoke action in the sympathetic system, and also secretory discharge from the adrenal medulla, the latter response resulting from the sympathetic innervation of the chromaffin tissue. The adrenal secretion, he supposed, would then develop and prolong the animal's reactions, for it was already apparent at that time that adrenaline was very similar to the chemical transmitter released at the sympathetic nerve endings.

His formulation antedated the demonstration of the physiological importance of noradrenaline, although he had recognized that the sympathetic transmitter (called at that time sympathin) was not identical with adrenaline. The discovery by later workers that noradrenaline is the transmitter, and that the medulla releases both this and adrenaline, complicates his argument, but it certainly does not weaken it. However, it now becomes necessary to assume that the two catecholamine hormones must be concerned with more than a simple prolongation of the effects of sympathetic stimulation, and that the differences in their properties must be of some physiological significance. It has been suggested, for example, that the release of adrenaline predominates in emotional stress, and the release of noradrenaline in circulatory stress. As an extension of this, it may

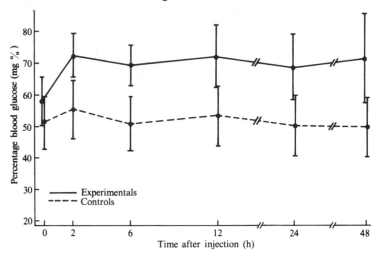

FIG. 10.10. Effect of an intramuscular injection of adrenaline (0·5 mg per kg) on blood glucose levels in dogfish. A significant hyper-glycaemia ($p < 0.02$) occurs 2–6 hours after injection of adrenaline, and blood glucose concentrations in hormone-treated animals are elevated for the duration of the experiment. —— experimentals; ——— controls. Vertical bars represent standard errors. (From Patent (1970). *Gen. comp. Endocrin.* **14.**)

be that the main response to emotional stress, pain, or hypoglycaemia is a massive release of adrenaline, while the sympathetic nervous system is the main agent in dealing with circulatory disturbances, aided by some output of noradrenaline from the chromaffin tissue. There is evidence that differential release of the two hormones does occur, and we have seen that there is a histological basis for it, but its significance needs further elucidation.

Uncertainty applies even to the interpretation of one of the best-defined effects of the catecholamine hormones: the production of a rise in metabolic rate with a consequential elevation in heat output. This calorigenic effect might be expected, in conjunction with the calorigenic action of the thyroid hormones, to play some part in the regulation of body temperature in homoiotherms. Probably it does, but its physio-logical basis remains obscure. One suggestion is that it may be a secondary effect, consequent upon the oxidation of the free fatty acids that are released into the blood from adipose tissue in response to catechol-amine stimulation.

However, these uncertainties do not weaken the concept of the sympathetic system and the chromaffin tissue as a complex which organizes the body for resisting emergencies by 'fright, flight, or a fight'. Cannon showed that the complex is not essential for life in a limited sense, for he was able to keep alive for three and half years a cat from which all parts of the sympathetic nervous system had been re-moved. Nevertheless, such animals can only survive in carefully controlled laboratory conditions. They

have a reduced capacity for work, and they lack the ability to respond to emergencies, so that the com-plex is essential for life in the more realistic sense of that word.

10.5. The catecholamine hormones in other animals

Both adrenaline and noradrenaline are present in extracts of chromaffin tissue from a wide range of vertebrates, including fish, and, as already men-tioned, they have also been identified in the ventral nerve cords of annelid worms. In addition, both are present in insects, more particularly in larvae and imagos, but they are said to be lacking in a number of other invertebrate groups. The physiological significance of this distribution is not clear, and it cannot be assumed that the catecholamines are neces-sarily acting as transmitters in all these groups.

However, adrenaline has a stimulatory influence upon the heart of vertebrates in general, and also of many invertebrates, and this property is shared by noradrenaline. In the isolated and perfused heart of *Raja batis*, for example, both substances produce a marked increase in the amplitude of the beat, and a slight increase in its frequency; identical effects are evoked by extracts of the chromaffin tissue of *Squalus acanthias*.

The hormones also have metabolic effects. Elasmo-branchs secrete both adrenaline and noradrenaline, the latter constituting 60–80 per cent of the catechol-amine content of the chromaffin tissue. Both hor-mones may increase blood-sugar levels after injection, with adrenaline as the more certain and effective of the

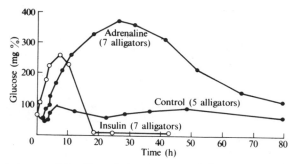

FIG. 10.11. The effect of adrenaline ($2\,\mathrm{ml\,kg^{-1}}$ of $1/1000$) and commercial insulin ($1\cdot0\,\mathrm{units/g^{-1}}$) on blood glucose in *Alligator mississippiensis*. The results are qualitatively similar to those obtained with mammals, but the response to adrenaline is considerably delayed. (From Coulson and Hernandez (1953). *Endocrin.* **53**.)

two. The response is rapid, and persists for a long time (Fig. 10.10). As regards other vertebrate groups, both hormones promote glycogenolysis in the perfused and isolated liver of the toad, while the injection of adrenaline evokes hyperglycaemia in all groups of vertebrates, but it is not clear whether such actions contribute to the handling of emergencies. Considerable delay has been noted in the blood-sugar response of the alligator to the injection of adrenaline (Fig. 10.11). This delay is also shown in the contraction of the pupil, which does not begin until after two hours and then persists for a long time, so that the animal remains nearly blind for several hours. The mode of response is evidently different from that of elasmobranchs, but comparisons are difficult, particularly since it is uncertain how far the results are truly physiological.

Of particular interest is the curious situation in the cyclostomes. The hearts of both *Lampetra* and *Myxine* contain exceptionally large amounts of adrenaline and noradrenaline, present both in the chromaffin cells in the heart wall and to some extent in the muscle cells themselves. In contrast to the typical situation in vertebrates, the isolated hearts of these two animals respond only weakly to these catecholamines, and it has been suggested that this may be because their metabolism is normally influenced by catecholamines released from their own tissues. If this is so, a further significant fact is that while the heart of the lamprey is innervated by the vagus nerve, the heart of *Myxine* has no innervation and possesses no nervous tissue in its wall. This animal is such a remarkable blend of primitive and specialized characters that it is impossible to decide the status of this particular condition. It has been suggested, supposing the condition to be primitive, that chromaffin tissue may initially have been concerned with the peripheral regulation or support of metabolism, and that its preganglionic innervation may be a secondary development. This suggestion, as already mentioned, runs counter to the view that the chromaffin cells have evolved from post-ganglionic sympathetic neurones, but it need not be dismissed out of hand. Clearly much remains to be learned about the evolution of the sympathetico-chromaffin complex in the lower vertebrates, and of the function of the catecholamines in invertebrates.

However, in vertebrates as a whole, and in the light of the present fragmentary information, there does seem to be a fundamental uniformity of response to the catecholamines. This suggests that increased output of these hormones in response to activation of the sympathetic nervous system was established early in vertebrate evolution; perhaps to facilitate rapid responses to environmental stresses which must have borne heavily upon a group that was so actively pelagic in its early pattern of life.

11

The adrenocortical tissue of the adrenal gland

11.1. Development and organization of adrenocortical tissue

We have seen that chromaffin tissue shares a common embryological origin with the sympathetic nervous system, and we have considered the significance of this. Of equal interest is the fact that the adrenocortical tissue and the gonads are closely related in their development, for they share an equally close biosynthetic relationship in being the main sources of steroid hormones in the vertebrates. The situation is well seen in the gymnophionan amphibian, *Hypogeophis*, where, as in other vertebrates, the adrenocortical cells are budded off, like the gonadal tissue, from localized thickenings of the coelomic epithelium (Fig. 11.1). They lose their connection with the epithelium, and come to lie ventro-lateral to the dorsal aorta, in the angle between it and the median cardinal vein. Tracts of cells growing out from the sympathetic ganglia then connect with these adrenocortical rudiments and give rise to the chromaffin tissue, and in this way the compound gland arises from two entirely separate sets of rudiments.

As finally established in placental mammals, the adrenal gland is surrounded by a connective-tissue capsule which extends inwards to ramify amongst the secretory cells of the cortex. It carries blood vessels with it, but, in sharp contrast with the chromaffin tissue, the adrenocortical cells receive no secretomotor nerve supply. These cells are arranged mainly in cords which normally give rise to three distinct zones (Fig. 11.2). Exceptions to this may, however, be found, and even the division between cortex and medulla is not always uniformly defined. The outermost of the zones is the zona glomerulosa, characterized by the cells forming loops or clusters, the middle one is the zona fasciculata, where there are long, straight cords, while the innermost is the zona reticularis, where the cords form a network. The histological differentiation is an expression of a functional differentiation, related to the production of the hormones that we consider later. Aldosterone is produced by the zona glomerulosa, while corticosterone and cortisol are produced by the zona fasciculata and perhaps also by the zona glomerulosa.

A feature of the adrenocortical tissue as a whole is the presence in its cells of lipid droplets, associated with cholesterol and 3β-HSDH activity. These droplets, which, as in the gonads, are indicative of the production of steroid hormones, are particularly richly developed in the outer part of the zona fasciculata, while in the zona reticularis they are scarce and, when present, rather large. Considerable amounts of ascorbic acid are also present in the cells. Its significance is obscure, but its depletion by corticotropin is the basis of one method of assay of that hormone.

11.2. Corticosteroids in mammals

One of the significant dates in the development of endocrinology was 15 March 1849, which saw the publication by Thomas Addison of a preliminary note on a chronic clinical condition which was later to be called Addison's disease. Six years afterwards he developed the subject into a monograph entitled *On the constitutional and local effects of diseases of the suprarenal capsules.* Addison's disease comprises a complex of symptoms, including general debility, muscular weakness, low blood pressure, disturbed ionic balance, and darkening of the skin. This was the condition which, it is now thought, struck down Jane Austen, and it is a sad irony that her acute observation provides, in her correspondence, the first recorded account of a disease which had not then been defined.

The ascription of this syndrome to disorder of the adrenal glands was clearly established by Addison's studies, but the importance of the distinction between medulla and cortex was not then apparent. When, therefore, Oliver and Schäfer discovered, in extracts of the gland, the active principle that was later identified as adrenaline, it was natural to suppose that this was the agent involved, particularly

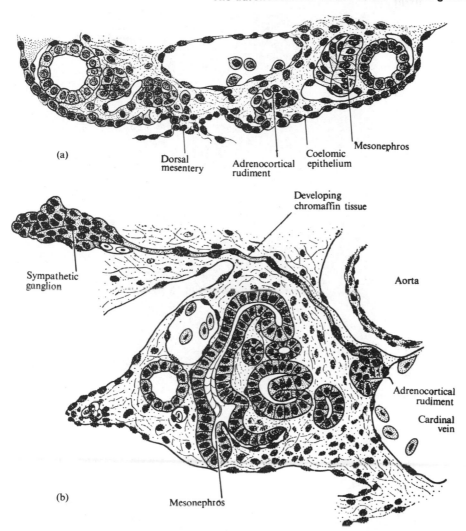

(a)

Dorsal mesentery

Adrenocortical rudiment

Coelomic epithelium

Mesonephros

Developing chromaffin tissue

Sympathetic ganglion

Aorta

Adrenocortical rudiment

Cardinal vein

(b)

Mesonephros

FIG. 11.1. Transverse sections of embryos of *Hypogeophis* (Amphibia, Gymnophiona). In the upper figure the adrenocortical rudiment is developing from the coelomic epithelium. In the lower figure the developing chromaffin tissue is extending from the sympathetic ganglion to the adrenocortical rudiment. (From Brachet (1921). *Embryologie des vertébrés*. Masson et Cie, Paris.)

since it was observed to increase muscular tone and blood pressure. Nevertheless, this supposition was incorrect, for Addison's disease is due to destruction of the adrenocortical tissue.

We have seen that cats can survive the removal of the sympathetic nervous system, and similarly animals can survive the removal of the whole of one adrenal gland and enucleation of the other. The complete removal of both glands, however, is fatal. This result, and the progressive development of Addison's disease, are due to deprivation of adrenocortical hormones, which have a far-reaching and complex influence upon the maintenance of life. The extent of this influence can be judged from the effects of total adrenalectomy in mammals. They include the following.

Digestive. Loss of appetite; delayed or incomplete absorption from the intestine; nausea and vomiting; ulceration of the alimentary tract; diarrhoea.

Circulatory. Increased concentration of the blood, and decrease in its pressure, flow, and volume; decrease in the sodium, chloride bicarbonate, and glucose of the serum, and increase in its potassium and non-protein nitrogen.

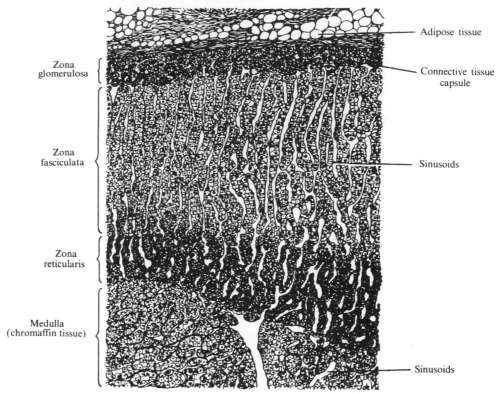

Zona glomerulosa

Zona fasciculata

Zona reticularis

Medulla (chromaffin tissue)

Adipose tissue

Connective tissue capsule

Sinusoids

Sinusoids

Fig. 11.2. Section of the adrenal gland of the monkey (*Macacus*). (From Young (1957) (2nd edn 1975). *The life of mammals*. Clarendon Press, Oxford.)

Tissues. Muscular weakness and reduction in muscle mass; decrease in sodium and increase in potassium and water in muscle; decrease in glycogen in the liver and muscles after fasting.

Kidney. Increased excretion (renal wastage) of sodium, chloride, and bicarbonate; decreased excretion of potassium and total nitrogen; inability to excrete ingested water

Growth. Hypertrophy of the thymus and lymphoid structures; cessation of body growth; loss of weight; fall in body temperature.

Resistance. Decreased resistance to all forms of stress (e.g. toxins, injury, environmental changes), leading to death in untreated animals.

The analysis of adrenocortical functions can be simplified by grouping them under two main headings. The first includes effects exerted upon the metabolism of water and electrolytes, and hence upon the serum concentrations of sodium and potassium; the second includes those exerted upon carbohydrate and protein metabolism. Effects in the former category result largely from disturbances of the

functioning of the kidney; they are shown, for example, in the increased non-protein nitrogen of the blood which follows adrenalectomy. This can be restored to normal by injection of suitable adrenocortical extracts. The renal wastage of sodium and chloride shown in the above list is another example; injection of adrenocortical extracts results in sodium retention, which is reflected in the decrease in the sodium/potassium ratio in the urine. This disturbance of ionic balance, with which is associated disturbance in water metabolism, is one of the factors contributing to the death of adrenalectomized animals. Their condition can be alleviated greatly by the administration of sodium and chloride, preferably as a mixture of sodium chloride and bicarbonate in order to allow for the fact that sodium is lost at a greater rate than chloride; this treatment will permit the survival of such animals for long periods.

The effects upon carbohydrate and protein metabolism are shown by the importance of the part played by the adrenal steroids in antagonizing the action of insulin (p. 55). They are illustrated, too, by the fall in blood sugar and in liver glycogen which are amongst the consequence of total adrenalectomy in mammals.

Loss of muscular strength is probably associated with such effects, in so far as it may reflect disturbance of glucose metabolism, and is manifested in the rapid development of fatigue after adrenalectomy. This can be measured quantitatively, either by making rats swim in water until they are exhausted, or by making the gastrocnemius muscle contract against a weight in response to faradic stimulation. In an untreated adrenalectomized animal, exhaustion of the muscle may occur in less than ten hours, while in one that is appropriately treated with adrenocortical extracts the muscle may be able to continue working for more than twenty-four hours.

We have seen that the analysis of the function of a supposed endocrine organ ideally involves a study of the effects of replacement therapy. From 1928 onwards, investigators were overcoming the normally fatal results of complete adrenalectomy by injecting the animals concerned with extracts of adrenocortical tissue, and attempts were being made to isolate and characterize an active principle. By analogy with what had been learned of other glands, it was at first supposed that this would prove to be a single hormone which was provisionally designated as cortin; but this supposition, although properly in accord with the principle of Occam's razor, was ill-founded.

By 1931 it was already apparent that the activity was concentrated in the lipid fractions of the extracts, and its further analysis was a part of the developments in steroid chemistry which we have already mentioned (p. 108). Systematic investigation of these fractions, following the isolation of oestrone in 1929, were carried out simultaneously by several groups of workers, and a large number of adrenocortical steroids conveniently called corticosteroids were soon isolated and characterized.

A turning point came in May 1949, with the announcement that one of these substances, cortisone, appeared to be of strikingly beneficial value in the treatment of rheumatoid arthritis. With the large doses that were customary during the early trials some very dramatic results were achieved, patients who had been dependent on others for years being able within forty-eight hours to dress themselves. Further study showed that prolonged treatment with this substance might be associated with undesirable side-effects, such as peptic ulceration, sodium retention (leading to oedema), and increased risk of bone fracture, but the discovery was none the less of fundamental importance. The belief that literally millions of patients might be demanding treatment with a substance at a time when the world supply of it amounted to only a few grams provided an immense

stimulus to research into methods for its bulk preparation; particularly since in the early days of insulin therapy some patients had died, owing to shortage of the hormone, after their condition had been temporarily alleviated. Thus it was found, for example, that cortisone could be prepared from progesterone, which could itself be prepared from diosgenin, a plant glycoside available in commercially workable quantities. The rapid fall in the price of cortisone was a sufficient testimony to the success of such studies.

Some fifty steroids have been isolated from adrenocortical material, but, as we have earlier emphasized, the presence of active substances in tissue extracts is no proof that they are a normal secretory product, or that they are of physiological importance. Many of these steroids are probably intermediary metabolites, or artifacts of the method of extraction, yet some of them may still be of great potential importance. For example, they include androgens, oestrogens, and progesterone, and we shall see later how defects of adrenocortical metabolism may result in the overproduction of these, with dire consequences for the sexual differentiation of the affected individual. Decisions as to which steroids are of major importance in normal endocrine regulation rest on technical developments (p. 108) which have made it practicable to identify these substances on the microscale, so that it has been possible to determine which of them are actually released into the blood stream in physiologically significant quantities.

The biologically active corticosteroids are derivatives of pregnane (Fig. 11.3), and are C_{21} steroids, carrying two carbon atoms in a side chain at carbon-17. They also have a ketonic group at carbon-3, a double valence bond at carbon-4, and another ketonic group at carbon-20. In addition, there may be a hydroxyl group at carbon-17. Using the functional distinction made earlier (p. 198), those that exert their effects mainly upon carbohydrate metabolism are called glucocorticoids, while those that act mainly upon the metabolism of water and of salt-electrolytes are called mineralocorticoids. The distinction is helpful in dealing with the mammalian hormones, but is of doubtful validity in dealing with those of the lower vertebrates.

Three corticosteroids are important as hormones in mammals. Two of these, corticosterone and cortisol (hydrocortisone), are glucocorticoids, while the third, aldosterone, is a mineralocorticoid. Cortisone, already mentioned for its clinical significance, is not a major component of the mammalian adrenocortical secretion, but is important in various lower

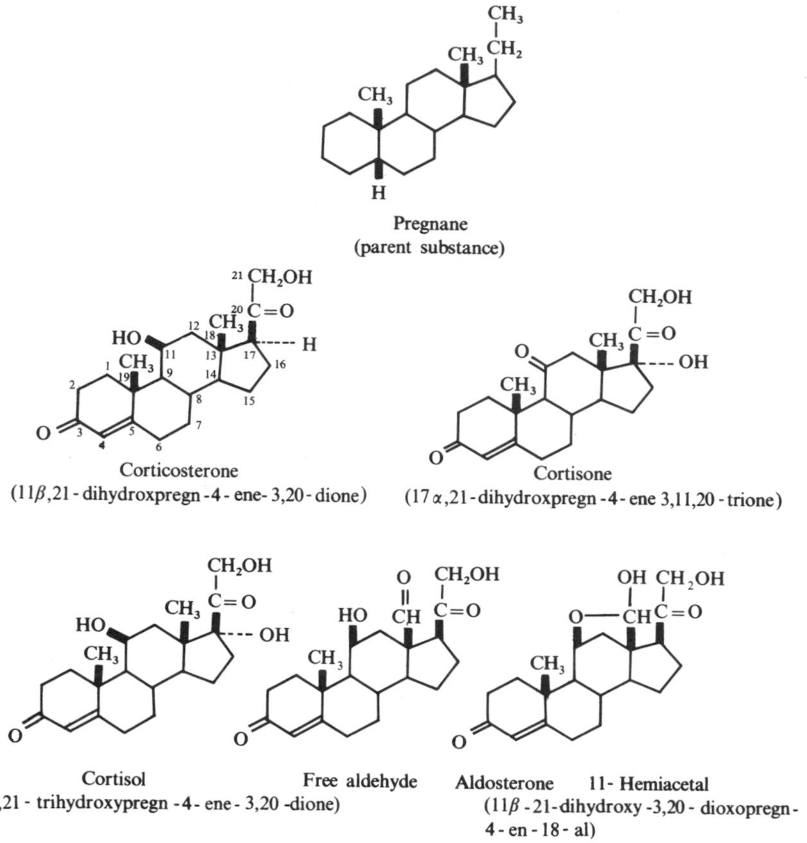

FIG. 11.3. Corticosteroids.

Pregnane
(parent substance)

Corticosterone
(11β,21 - dihydroxypregn -4- ene- 3,20- dione)

Cortisone
(17α,21 -dihydroxypregn -4- ene 3,11,20 - trione)

Cortisol
(11β,17α,21 - trihydroxypregn -4- ene- 3,20 -dione)

Free aldehyde   Aldosterone   11- Hemiacetal
(11β -21-dihydroxy -3,20- dioxopregn-
4 - en - 18 - al)

forms. Corticosterone and cortisol, both of them isolated in 1937, differ markedly in the proportions in which they are secreted in various mammalian species. Man, monkey, and sheep secrete mainly cortisol, the rat and the rabbit mainly corticosterone, while the cow, ferret, dog, and cat secrete more equal mixtures of both. The influence of the glucocorticoids on the regulation of carbohydrate metabolism has been mentioned earlier (p. 55). Lack of them results in low blood-glucose levels, and increased sensitivity to insulin. They promote gluconeogenesis in the liver, this effect being associated with decreased uptake of amino acids by the muscle cells, and an increased uptake of amino acids by the liver. The latter action leads to increased production of the enzyme systems required for the conversion of amino acids to glucose.

Aldosterone differs from these glucocorticoids in possessing an aldehyde substitution at carbon-18, which is normally masked by acetal formation with the hydroxyl group at carbon-11. Its discovery in 1952 had been long delayed because it is present in the adrenal venous effluent in only trace amounts,

representing, for example, less than 1–2·5 per cent of the total corticosteroid production in the dog. Functionally, however, it is a potent mineralocorticoid, and strikingly illustrates the principle that biological importance is not to be judged solely in terms of quantitative abundance. The action of aldosterone is mainly exerted on the distal tubule of the nephron, where it promotes increased permeability to sodium and also an increase in its active transport. There is thus increased uptake of the ion from the glomerular filtrate, while potassium and hydrogen ions pass into the tubule fluid by an exchange mechanism. Aldosterone also promotes sodium retention in the salivary glands, sweat glands, and colon, and the excretion of magnesium in the urine.

11.3. Corticosteroids in other vertebrates

Information regarding the biosynthetic capacity of adrenocortical tissue in non-mammalian vertebrates, and the nature of the circulating hormones, is very limited and fragmentary. It is derived in part from *in vivo* studies and in part from *in vitro* ones, and from only a few species. Further, much of the

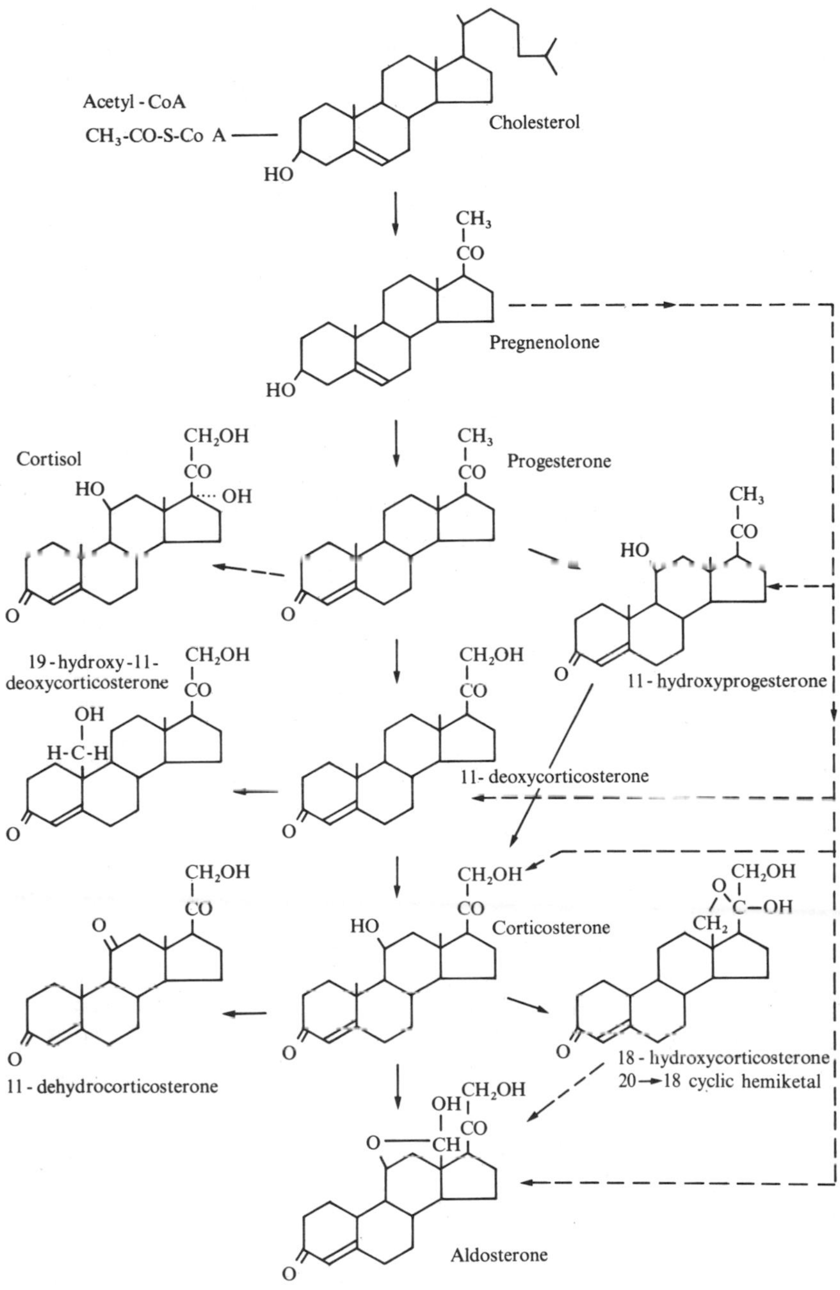

FIG. 11.4. Schematic representation of the biosynthesis of cortico-steroids by the adrenals of amphibians, reptiles, and birds, based on results obtained by *in vitro* methods, using exogenous substrates.

All the reactions shown have their parallels in mammalian adrenals. (From Sandor (1972). In *Steroids in nonmammalian vertebrates* (ed. D. R. Idler), p. 253–327. Academic Press, New York and London.)

evidence is subject to the reservations made earlier (p. 199), so that only the most tentative generalizations are possible.

Within these limits, it can be said that the same corticosteroid biosynthetic pathways are found throughout the vertebrates. They are shown in Fig. 11.4, which presents a scheme that is well established for mammals, but which will serve also for the other groups. Table 11.1 shows, and again within the limited information available,

TABLE 11.1

Distribution of corticosteroids in the main vertebrate groups.

Many of the identifications in this field of study are tentative, and the table should be regarded as approximate.

Cyclostomata	Cortisol, corticosterone
Elasmobranchii	1α-hydroxycorticosterone; cortisol; corticosterone
Teleostei	Cortisol; cortisone; 11-deoxycortisol
Amphibia Reptilia Aves	Corticosterone; 18-hydroxycorticosterone; aldosterone
Mammalia	Cortisol; cortisone; corticosterone; 18-hydroxycorticosterone; aldosterone

what are the main hormones produced in these groups. Cortisol is clearly a common product, but two other features are particularly noteworthy. One is the production in elasmobranchs of 1α-hydroxy-corticosterone; these animals are unique in having this steroid as their principle corticoid. Its production requires 1α-hydroxylase, an enzyme which was identified for the first time in these animals. Particularly striking is the contrast between elasmobranchs and holocephalans in this respect, for no 1α-hydroxy-corticosterone has been found in the ratfish (*Hydrol-agus colliei*). Its expected precursor is converted to cortisol by a 17α-hydroxylase; an enzyme which is present in elasmobranchs in only very small amounts. A second important feature is the apparent restriction of significant amounts of aldosterone to lung-fish and tetrapods. This situation, however, is not yet wholly clear. For example, the enzymes required for the synthesis of this hormone (18-corticosteroid hydroxylase and 18-ol dehydrogenase) are present in the adrenocortical tissue of the herring. (*Clupea harengus*), yet it is doubtful whether significant amounts of aldosterone are discharged into the blood of any teleost.

The universal distribution of corticosteroids in vertebrates is a sure indication of their functional importance, yet it is difficult to define what this is in the lower members of the group. Complete adrenal-ectomy is often fatal to these animals, although seasonal conditions may affect the result. The meta-bolic consequences of the operation are sometimes of the general character that would be associated in mammals with glucocorticoid deprivation, such as muscular weakness, circulatory disturbances, hypo-glycaemia, and loss of liver glycogen, but information remains very incomplete. As for injection experi-ments, much of the data are only of pharmacological value, while there is also the problem of ensuring that the experimental animals are not showing the

effects of generalized stress, which is particularly easily evoked in lampreys and fish under laboratory conditions. Diuresis and hyperglycaemia are both readily produced in lampreys by handling, and, to judge from cytological observations, are associated with increased secretory activity of both the chrom-affin and the interrenal tissues. Some evidence that the adrenocortical tissue may influence mineralo-corticoid metabolism in fish is suggested by the results of adrenalectomy in eels, which affects urine flow and the flux of sodium across the gills. In fresh-water eels the urine flow is reduced by this operation, as also is the uptake of sodium by the gills. In sea-water eels the outflow of sodium across the gills is reduced. These responses, which affect the adjust-ment of sodium outflux in fresh-water eels transferred to sea water (Fig. 11.5), can be corrected by injec-tions of cortisol, which, as shown in Table 11.1, is one of the corticosteroids of teleosts.

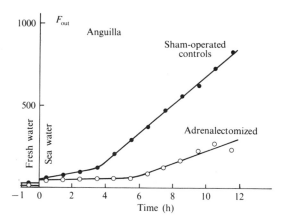

FIG. 11.5. Effect of adrenalectomy on the transfer of eels from fresh water to sea water. Ordinates: time in hours. Abscissae: Sodium outflux (F_{out}) in μequiv h^{-1} per 100 g for successive periods. (From Maetz (1961). *Gen. comp. Endocrin.*, Suppl. 2 (ed. M. R. N. Prasad).)

Little of value is known about amphibians, although mineralocorticoid symptoms are suggested by the way in which removal of the adrenocortical tissue from frogs results in a loss of sodium and accumulation of water. Immersion of such animals in isotonic saline may prolong their lives, by enabling them to maintain a more normal water and electro-lyte balance.

A feature of great potential interest in this field is the presence in certain reptiles and birds of paired nasal glands, which seem to be under adrenocortical

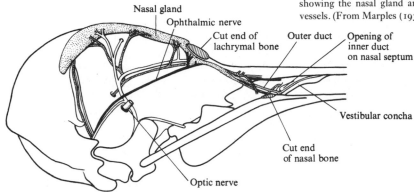

FIG. 11.6. Diagram of a dissection of the head of an oystercatcher, showing the nasal gland and its ducts and the associated blood vessels. (From Marples (1932). *Proc. zool. Soc. Lond.* pp. 829–44.)

influence. These glands (Fig. 11.6), which lie above the orbits, discharge a fluid which contains sodium chloride at a level hypertonic to that of the plasma. This is an adaptation, particularly well developed in marine birds, which counteracts the consequences of the ingestion of salt in the food and drinking water. Secretion is readily evoked in normal ducks, for example, by administering a salt load, but those which have undergone unilateral adrenalectomy give only a reduced response, while those that have been totally adrenalectomized give no response at all (Fig. 11.7). A normal response can, however, be evoked in

these operated animals by cortisol treatment. Converse experiments, in which either corticosteroids or corticotropin (p. 205) are administered to normal birds, result in an enhanced secretory discharge.

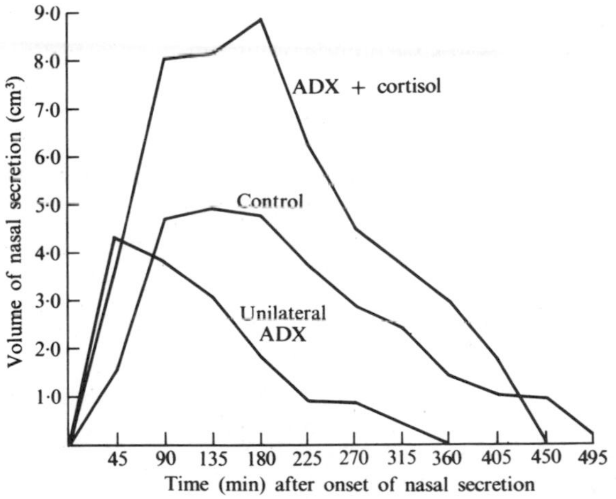

These results suggest that corticosteroids are required to ensure the response (the hormone thought to be involved is corticosterone), and the same may be true of reptiles. However, the evidence is not clearcut, and other factors are involved. For example, if glucose is given simultaneously with a salt load to normal birds, the secretory response is enhanced, while a response can also be evoked by cholinergic stimulation from the parasympathetic nervous system. The situation is typical of the difficulty of interpreting adrenocortical regulatory actions. The difficulty is compounded by the need to take account of the possible interactions of the corticosteroids with other hormones, such as the neurohypophysial hormones and prolactin, which have closely related physiological effects, and which themselves probably act directly upon the salt gland.

11.4. Stress

One line of thought which has attracted much attention over many years arises from a point that has already been made: that the adrenocortical hormones are so far-reaching in their effects that they must have provided an essential basis for the adaptive responses of vertebrates to a wide range of environmental pressures. Such adaptive responses have been generalized, under the influence of Selye, into the concept of resistance to stress, a term that may be taken to cover the situation arising when animals are exposed to stimuli that are actually or potentially harmful. Under such circumstances they manifest a complex and generalized response which is termed

FIG. 11.7. Effect of adrenalectomy and cortisol administration on the secretory activity of the nasal gland of the domestic duck, following the introduction into the stomach of 20 ml of 20% NaCl solution. *Middle curve*, normal control animals; *lower curve*, animals with one adrenal gland removed, showing reduced activity; *upper curve*, animal with both adrenal glands removed, but receiving cortisol, showing that secretory activity is fully restored by treatment with the hormone. (From (Phillips *et al.* (1961). *Endocrin.* 69.)

the Stress Syndrome or General Adaption Syndrome, and this is regarded, according to Selye's interpretation, as falling into three phases.

The first of these, the alarm reaction, is conceived as a 'generalized call to arms' of the defensive forces of the organism; it is accompanied by excitation of the sympathetico-chromaffin complex and increased adrenocortical secretion, together with enlargement of the adrenal gland and depletion of its lipid content. If the exposure to the stressful stimulus continues, and if the animal is able to survive, the second stage is established, the stage of resistance. The body now adapts to the stimulus, under the influence of the adrenocortical secretions; these may be involved, for example, in the regulation of water balance, carbohydrate metabolism, and neuromuscular irritability. After still more prolonged exposure the animal may lose this acquired adaptation and pass into the third stage, the stage of exhaustion. From this, it is thought, there might result in man certain diseases of adaptation such as gastro-intestinal ulcers, arteriosclerosis, and rheumatoid arthritis, which are thus conceived as arising at least in part from disorders of the endocrine system. Indeed, it has even been suggested that the Stress Syndrome might contribute to the heavy mortality that results from overcrowding in populations of wild mammals. Population size can obviously be regulated either through control of births or deaths, and both of these can be influenced by population density. Crowding evokes behavioural responses, which, by their effect upon the pituitary–gonad relationship, can influence fertility, antenatal death, and lactation. They can also influence mortality through increased corticoid secretion resulting from their effect upon the pituitary–adrenocortical relationship.

How far the responses to stress can be adequately interpreted in the way outlined, and how far there may be other causative agents at work in promoting diseases of adaptation, are matters needing more discussion than is possible here. It has been said that 'one important key to increased understanding of the nature of man's psyche and emotional behaviour, and the intimate details of complex enzyme systems residing in the liver, brain, heart, kidney and muscles, lies in the study of the response of tissue cells to steroid hormones'. If this is so, the application of the principle will certainly not be restricted to man. We may therefore expect that future research will disclose increasing evidence that the corticosteroids are involved not only in the day-to-day adjustments of vertebrates to their environment, but also in the periods of intense activity and physiological crisis

which are a regular feature of their life-cycles (p. 182). Pointers in this direction are reports of increased levels of corticosteroids in the blood of migratory salmon and steelhead trout, and of hyperplasia of their adrenocortical tissue.

As usual, however, results are contradictory and difficult to interpret. For example, carp which have been forced to swim in aquaria tanks have been found to have elevated plasma corticosteroid levels. Salmonids, by contrast, can show considerable enforced activity without significant rise in plasma levels. The difference in this instance might be that carp are not adapted for considerable exertion, whereas salmonids are. But it cannot be emphasized too often that all such experiments carry little value unless they also take account of the fluctuations in physiological condition and endocrine status of fish (and, indeed, of other vertebrates as well), in relation to age, season, and reproductive cycle.

We have seen earlier (p. 106) that steroid metabolism is a widespread and probably universal property of living organisms. It will now be apparent that the production of steroid hormones in the gonads and adrenocortical tissue, and the common origin of these tissues from the coelomic epithelium, are highly characteristic features of vertebrate organization, and of fundamental importance for survival. A suggestive interpretation of the evolution of these features has been proposed by Willmer. He has emphasized the possible evolutionary significance of the obvious tendency of the coelomic epithelium to give rise to cords and tubules. This tendency, well seen in the sex cords of the early stages of the gonads and in the characteristic histological pattern of the adrenocortical tissue, may, he suggests, be related phylogenetically to the production of coelomoducts. These are thought to have been concerned initially with the removal of the genital products and later to have become involved in excretion and osmoregulation, and he suggests that all three organs, kidneys, gonads, and adrenal cortex, may be derived from them. He argues that an important function of such tubules in the early stages of their evolution would have been the regulation of the composition of the fluids bathing their walls, and that this activity would have resulted in the formation of metabolites which could later have become modified into hormones. For example, the metabolites arising from the responses of the adrenocortical cells to fluctuation in the sodium/potassium ratio in the blood might have acquired the capacity to control those cells of the kidney tubules which are directly concerned with the regulation of this ratio.

11.5. Corticotropin

The adrenocortical cells, unlike the chromaffin cells of the adrenal medulla, are not innervated. Instead, the zona reticulata and zona fasciculata (but not the zona glomerulosa, as will be explained later) are controlled through a negative feedback relationship with the pars distalis of the pituitary gland, similar in principle to that involved in the regulation of the steroid-secreting tissue of the gonads. The hormone concerned is termed corticotropin or ACTH (for adrenocorticotropic hormone). Hypophysectomy in mammals results in atrophy of the adrenocortical tissue, an effect which can be counteracted by implants or injections of pars distalis extracts. There is experimental evidence for the existence of the same situation in lower vertebrates, from fish upwards, but it is not clear whether corticotropin is present in cyclostomes.

H.Ser-Tyr-Ser-Met-Glu-His-Phe-Arg-Try-Gly-Lys-

Pro-Val-Gly-Lys-Lys-Arg-Arg-Pro-Val-Lys-Val-Tyr-

Pro-Asp-Gly-Ala-Glu-Asp-Glu-Leu-Ala-Glu-Ala-Phe- $\overset{\displaystyle\ulcorner NH_2}{}$

Pro-Leu-Glu-Phe.OH

FIG. 11.8 Amino-acid sequence of pig corticotropin. (After Shepherd *et al.* (1956). *J. Am. chem. Soc.* 78.)

Corticotropin has been obtained in a pure form, and has been fully characterized as a straight-chain polypeptide composed of 39 amino-acid residues (Fig. 11.8). The corticotropins of the sheep, ox, and pig differ from each other in respect of substitutions between positions 25 and 39, while fragmentation studies have shown that this region is not essential for biological activity. This activity depends upon positions 1–24; attempts to degrade this part of the chain result in loss of activity, and it is significant that it is this region which is identical in all three species. Amino-acid substitutions are presumably unacceptable there (p. 100).

An important characteristic of the molecule is the presence of a heptapeptide sequence (positions 4–10) which is identical to that found also in α and β melanocyte-stimulating hormones (p. 213). This sequence, which has been synthesized, has been shown to have a very slight action upon melanophores, evoking some dispersion of their granules (p. 213). It has been thought that this property accounts for the darkening of the human skin noticed

in the Addisonian syndrome, for the malfunctioning of the adrenal cortex in this condition evokes, by negative feed-back, an increased output of corticotropin. The bearing of this molecular feature upon the possible evolution of the molecules concerned will be discussed later (p. 213).

The regulatory action of corticotropin is exerted primarily upon the zona reticulata and zona fasciculata, where it evokes increased growth and protein synthesis. The regulation of aldosterone secretion in the zona glomerulosa, however, involves a different mechanism, which is associated with the renin–angiotensin system, best known at present in mammals. Renin is an enzyme which is formed in the kidneys, probably in the afferent arterioles supplying the glomeruli. It is released into the blood stream, where it acts upon a substrate to form angiotensin; this product appears first as a biologically inactive decapeptide, which is then converted to an active octapeptide. Angiotensin is so called because it raises blood pressure through an action upon smooth muscle. It reduces sodium excretion in man, probably by direct action on the kidney, and it is possible that it should be regarded as a true hormone, aiding sodium retention. In addition, however, it contributes to sodium retention by increasing aldosterone secretion. The exact physiological significance of the renin–angiotensin system is still obscure. Probably, however, it is widely distributed in vertebrates, for renin occurs in fish, although its origin is uncertain.

With corticotropin, as with thyrotropin and the gonadotropins, feedback relationship with the pars distalis is maintained along two pathways. One of these is a direct pathway between the adrenal cortex and the pars distalis, provided by the blood stream. The other is an indirect pathway, involving the hypothalamus and the hypophysial portal system, as well as the systemic circulation. Injection of adrenocortical extracts may result in a reduced output of corticotropin, which can be accounted for in terms of the direct pathway. Evidence of the indirect one is that pituitary transplants situated at points remote from the hypothalamus cannot maintain an entirely normal adrenal cortex. This should clearly not be so if the only factor involved in its maintenance was the direct action of its circulating adrenocortical steroids upon the pars distalis. Particularly striking is the fact that the transfer of a pituitary transplant back to the median eminence, after it has been situated on the kidney for one month (p. 125), will result in restoration of the reduced adrenal cortex to normal size and function.

Equally impressive is the evidence obtained by assaying the concentration of circulating corticotropin. This confirms the existence in the rat of the direct feedback relationship, in that the concentration of circulating corticotropin is substantially increased after adrenalectomy. On the other hand, the application of stress (in the form of exposure to ether, with or without a standardized scald) results within two minutes in an increase in the circulating corticotropin, not only in the intact rat but even in the adrenalectomized animal, from which it follows that the discharge of corticotropin can be evoked in the complete absence of adrenocortical steroids. Possibly, then, the direct feedback relationship is a homeostatic mechanism providing delicate adjustments under normal or basal conditions, as we have suggested also for the thyroid gland (p. 174), with other factors coming into play when there is a marked departure from normal.

Evidence that the release of corticotropin is regulated by the hypothalamus, through the mediation of a specific releasing hormone, comes from experiments analogous to those discussed earlier in relation to the gonadotropins and thyrotropin. For example, electrical stimulation, by remote control, of the posterior region of the tuber cinereum or mammillary body in the rabbit, results in a reduction of lymphocytes (lymphopenia), which is also one of the results of adrenocortical response to stress. With the dog, it has been possible to measure the concentration of 17-hydroxycorticosteroids in adrenal venous blood, and to use this as another index of cortical activity. In this way, it has been shown that the output of these steroids in normal dogs which are subjected to surgical stress is over twice that in dogs which are similarly treated after lesions have been made at the anterior end of the median eminence. Lesions elsewhere do not have this affect.

It is thus concluded that lesions in the anterior median eminence impair the ability to secrete corticotropin, and this has been confirmed by direct measurements of the blood level of the hormone. This level rises in normal animals subjected to surgical stress, but does not do so in those with the lesions. Still further evidence comes from *in vitro* studies, which have shown that corticotropin release from the pituitary of the rat is increased by adding pieces of hypothalamus to the incubate. Purification studies of hypothalamic material have yielded substances with corticotropin-releasing activity, but chemical characterization has been slow to progress,

although the existence of a polypeptide hormone seems highly probable.

We have already noted the capacity of the adrenocortical tissue for producing steroids that can affect the gonads; oestrone and progesterone have been identified amongst the many compounds which have been isolated from tissue extracts, while androgens are known to be secreted in small amounts *in vivo*. It seems doubtful whether such substances have any normal physiological role to play, but their production can have grave results in man when the normal balance of activity of the tissue is disturbed, with consequential interference with corticotropin output.

It may happen that the cortical tissue of genetic females will produce an excessive amount of androgens, either as the result of the development of a tumour, or sometimes because of an inherited defect in the enzyme equipment of the tissue. The early sexual differentiation follows the pattern appropriate to the genetic sex, but signs of masculinization (virilization) appear when the androgen production becomes sufficiently great. This condition (the adrenogenital syndrome), which provides an instructive example of hormonal interaction, is characterized by increased excretion of 17-oxo-steroids. The disturbance of the normal metabolic pathways of the gland also results in a reduction of cortisol production; this leads to an excessive output of corticotropin, which then stimulates the adrenocortical tissue to an increased output of corticotropin, which then stimulates the adrenocortical tissue to an increased output of intermediary metabolites. Thus a condition of adrenal hyperplasia is established.

Tumours can be removed by surgery, while if cases of metabolic defect are detected sufficiently early they can be satisfactorily feminized by treatment with cortisone; the supposition is that this depresses corticotropin output, and thereby leads to a lowering of the secretion of the adrenocortical sex steroids, this in its turn promoting the output of pituitary gonadotropin with a consequent restoration of normal ovarian function. If, however, such cases are untreated, they may result in a genetic female coming to attain a completely masculine physique, aptitude, and drive, and actually developing a guilt complex as a result of being sexually attracted towards females. Under such circumstances it has sometimes been found advisable to recommend the acceptance of complete masculinity, the 'change of sex' involving a combination of legal action and minor surgical adjustment.

12

Colour change in vertebrates

12.1. Chromatophores

The colour changes of lower vertebrates, from cyclostomes to reptiles, depend upon cells called chromatophores, which can be defined, following Parker (1948), as pigmented cells, with dendritic processes, in which the colouring matter can be dispersed or aggregated, with consequent changes in the colour of the animals (cf. Fig. 12.2).

These cells are of various types, and have been variously classified, but they can conveniently be regarded as comprising: melanophores, with black or brown pigment (melanin); xanthophores, with yellow pigment; erythrophores, with red pigment; and iridophores, with reflecting crystals or platelets of purine, usually guanine, although adenine or other purines may be present. Of the pigmented cells, xanthophores and erythrophores are found only in poikilotherms, whereas cells with melanin are found also in birds and mammals. It is upon this last-named cell type, therefore, that research has mainly been directed, and this account will be largely based upon it.

Melanophores are derived from melanoblasts, which originate from the neural crest, in common with other cell types that we have already considered (pp. 154, 193). From the melanoblasts arise melanocytes, a term applied to cells that can synthesize melanin, which is laid down in intracellular bodies called melanosomes. These bodies, which arise within membrane-bound vesicles, are formed of fibrillar protein that is synthesized by the rough endoplasmic reticulum; melanin is then deposited upon the protein matrices.

Melanins are a group of polymeric pigments of high molecular weight, which are formed from tyrosine by its oxidation through the mediation of the copper-containing enzyme tyrosinase. The process begins with the deposition of this enzyme upon the lattice of the melanosome (which at this stage, before the appearance of the melanin, is termed a pro-melanosome). Tyrosine is converted by this oxidation to dihydroxyphenylalanine (dopa); indole-5,6-quinone is formed from this through several intermediates, and is then polymerized. The biosynthetic pathway is subject to intracellular control, which can be further modulated by environmental influences. For example, the amount of tyrosine present in the amphibian skin is not necessarily correlated with the amount of pigment that is normally found there; presumably, then, there must be some control of enzymatic activity.

Melanocytes, with their characteristic dendritic processes, are universal in the vertebrates. Melanophores are simply a particular category of melanocyte in which the melanosomes can be dispersed or aggregated by movement within the cell, the effect being respectively to darken or to blanch the animal. These cells are characteristic of the poikilothermal vertebrates. The melanocytes of mammals lack the property of melanosome movement, but nevertheless can contribute to long-term change of colour, either through changes in the number of cells present in the skin or hair, or through changes in the total amount of pigment present in the cell. This long-term change is called morphological colour change. It contrasts with physiological colour change, which results from short-term and relatively rapid changes in the dispersal or aggregation of the melanosomes, and which thus depends upon the presence of melanophores.

The melanocytes of mammals lie in the epidermis, with their processes closely applied to the cells of the Malpighian layer (keratinocytes). Through this relationship a melanocyte is associated with a group of epidermal cells, the whole forming an epidermal melanin unit, in which melanosomes can be transferred from the melanocyte into the keratinocytes, probably by phagocytosis. It is these units which provide the basis for variations in the colour of the human skin, resulting from genetically based racial differences, or from the influence of environment. This is exemplified in the effect of suntanning, which results from the capacity of ultraviolet light to in-

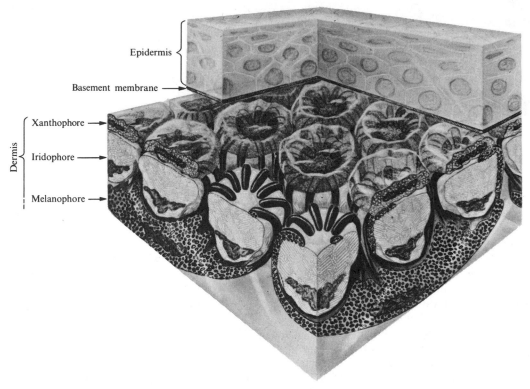

Epidermis

Basement membrane

Dermis

Xanthophore

Iridophore

Melanophore

FIG. 12.1. Schematic interpretation of the dermal chromatophore unit from several anurans. Adaptation to a dark background is represented. In this condition the bright colours imparted by the iridophores are modified by the obscuring of the light-reflecting capacity of these cells. This is effected by a migration of melanosomes into melanophore fingers between the xanthophore and the iridophore; thus the xanthophore–iridophore relationship is also interrupted or modified. (From Bagnara *et al.* (1968). *J. Cell. Biol.* **38**.)

crease both the activity and the numbers of the melanocytes.

Much attention has been given to determining the mechanism of movement of the melanosomes, as seen in physiological colour change, but there is no agreement on this matter. An early view that it depended upon sol–gel changes in the cytoplasm was related to the supposition that the melanosomes were attached to a gel framework. On this view, aggregation (it is also termed concentration) is brought about by a shrinkage of the framework, sol being squeezed out into the cell processes; dispersion is then effected by an unfolding of the gel framework, with sol flowing back into the cell body. Another suggestion is that microtubules play some part, for these have been observed in the cell processes of teleostean melanophores. However, they are thought to be absent from amphibians, so that at best this view could only be of limited application. Other suggestions are that dispersion may depend upon either the uptake of water or the entry of sodium ions, but it remains impossible to extract from any of these

views a comprehensive and satisfactory generalization. Evidently much more analysis is needed of the physiology and ultrastructure of these highly specialized cells.

12.2. Hormonal regulation of colour change in Amphibia

In examining the regulation of melanophore responses, it will be convenient to deal first with amphibians, for this group has provided much of the foundation of our present knowledge. Physiological colour change in these animals is brought about mainly by dermal melanophores; this, indeed, is true of vertebrates in general, morphological change being associated mainly with the epidermal melanophores. In anuran amphibians the response is mediated by dermal chromatophore units (Fig. 12.1). These include xanthophores, situated superficially, and forming there a yellow pigment layer. Below these are reflecting iridophores, and below these again are melanophores, with cell processes extending upwards. The skin appears dark-coloured when the melanosomes are dispersed, and pale-coloured when they are aggregated. In this latter condition, incident light is reflected back from the iridophores, and passes through the yellow pigment of the xanthophores. This absorbs the shortest wavelengths, so that the animal appears green.

The colour responses of amphibians, like those of other lower vertebrates, may be of two types: non-visual, which do not depend upon the eyes, and that are therefore shown by eyeless animals, and visual, which depend upon optic stimulation. *Xenopus*, for example, shows a non-visual response in which the melanosomes disperse in light and aggregate in darkness. The response, which is maintained after hypophysectomy, combined with destruction of the spinal cord, is supposedly due to direct action of light upon the melanophores; because of the absence of hormonal and neural regulation it is termed an unco-ordinated visual response. A variant occurs in larval *Xenopus*, in which illumination evokes dispersion in the head and aggregation in the tail. This, too, is an unco-ordinated response, for it occurs in isolated tails.

Studies of amphibian colour change have, however, been mainly concentrated upon the co-ordinated responses of adults to background and illumination. These are evoked when animals (usually *Rana* or *Xenopus*) are transferred from one to another of three different types of background: an illuminated white one, an illuminated black one, and a completely dark (i.e. non-illuminated) one. In order to reduce the subjective element involved in estimates of relative pallor and darkness, Hogben and Slome introduced a quantitative measure, which requires the distinguishing of five melanophore phases, ranging from fully aggregated to fully dispersed. An arbitrary numerical value is given to each phase, so that the mean condition of the melanophores of an individual can be expressed as a melanophore index (M.I.), lying between 1 and 5 (Fig. 12.2). This index continues to be widely used, although other procedures have also been introduced. There is, for example, a photo-electric procedure which allows the recording of the responses in pieces of excised skin. These pieces can be stretched over a ring, placed in the test fluid on the stage of a microscope, and the colour change recorded by means of a photo-electric cell inserted in place of the eyepiece.

The effects produced in anurans by the above-mentioned background changes are well defined. On a black background, with overhead illumination, the animal darkens to an index of 4·5 or even higher. On an illuminated white background it blanches to

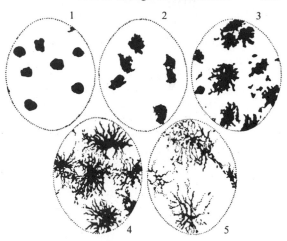

FIG. 12.2. The melanophore (melanocyte) index of Hogben and Slome (diagrammatic). (From Young (1962). *The life of vertebrates.* Clarendon Press, Oxford.)

an index of 1·5. In complete darkness the index is at an intermediate value of about 3·0. In *Xenopus*, which is completely aquatic, light is the main effective stimulus, but in more terrestrial forms other factors may also influence colour. These factors include temperature and humidity, so that *Rana temporaria*, for example, tends to be pale in a warm and dry environment, and dark in a cold and moist one.

These colour changes are slow processes, their completion involving hours or even days, rather than minutes. This at once suggests hormonal regulation, although naturally this could not be appreciated by nineteenth-century workers. They recognized that the eyes were an essential factor, and because of this, and because of the importance attached at that time to neural co-ordination, it was supposed that colour change was mediated by nervous reflexes; an interpretation analogous to that developed in connection with studies of the control of alimentary activity (p. 7). The demonstration in 1898 that injection into frogs of adrenal extracts resulted in the development of pallor suggested that glandular activity might also be involved, but this possibility did not attract serious attention until the introduction of experiments involving the hypophysectomy of tadpoles in connection with studies of metamorphosis. It quickly emerged that tadpoles lacking a pituitary gland were permanently pale, and it was this fact that led Hogben to initiate in 1922 his investigations of the pigmentary effector system.

The fundamental conclusion which resulted from this work is that darkening is brought about in amphibians by the release of a pituitary hormone. There is no histological evidence of innervation of the melanophores, and no physiological evidence of their responses being regulated by nerve fibres. Initially, the hormone, which was referred to as the B-substance, was regarded as a secretion of the 'posterior lobe', but it will be recalled that this region includes both the pars nervosa and the pars intermedia, so that both contributed to the commercial preparations that were employed in the earlier studies of colour change. It was soon shown, however, that the hormone actually originated in the pars intermedia, and for this reason it was named intermedin. The term now preferred is melanophore-stimulating hormone (MSH), or melanocyte-stimulating hormone (since, as we shall see, it has some action in mammals), because it is usual to name a hormone by reference to its point of action rather than to its point of origin. However, it should be borne in mind that the action of MSH is not restricted to melanophores and melanocytes. It concentrates the crystals in itidophores, and it may also evoke a morphological reaction in these cells by decreasing the amount of purine in them. It also disperses the pigments of xanthophores, more particularly in fish.

The cells producing the hormone have proved difficult to characterize. Secretory cells in the pars intermedia are stained by the PAS reaction, with lead haematoxylin, and with other stains as well. Sometimes these methods differentiate two cell types (in teleosts, for example), but this is not always so; many amphibians, for example, are thought to have only one. But even when two types are present, it does not follow that they are releasing two different secretions, nor is it certain which of them is secreting MSH. In short, the cytological basis of MSH production is not well understood, and there is probably more yet to be learned regarding the functions of the pars intermedia.

The action of MSH is thought to be mediated by cyclic AMP, acting here, as elsewhere, as a second messenger. MSH has not been shown actually to activate the adenylate cyclase of melanophores, but it does increase the amount of cyclic AMP in dorsal frog skin, where the melanophores and iridophores are the only known targets of the hormone. Further evidence is that cyclic AMP has a dispersing action on frog melanophores, both *in vivo* and *in vitro*, and that it promotes the formation of cell processes by melanocytes in tissue culture. The concept has a bearing upon the view (p. 208) that dispersion depends upon an obligatory Na^+ requirement, for the activity of cyclic AMP is not sodium dependent. This would not, however, exclude the possibility that sodium may still play some part in melanophore

response, perhaps in facilitating the binding of MSH to its target receptors.

The evidence for the hormonal control of amphibian colour change has been discussed so often that only the salient steps of the argument need be recapitulated here. First, hypophysectomy of both anurans and urodeles results in permanent pallor, even under conditions, such as the provision of a dark background, which favour darkening in the intact animal. Secondly, the injection of pituitary extracts into animals that are pale, either because they are on a pale background, or because they have been hypophysectomized, results in darkening; the effect then slowly wears off as the hormone is metabolized and excreted. In such experiments, the pituitary of one frog has been found to contain sufficient stored hormone to induce melanophore dispersion in at least fifty other animals. Thirdly, the presence of the hormone in the blood can be demonstrated by introducing into a pale animal some blood drawn from a dark one; this results in dispersion.

The separation of the parts of the pituitary is not always very easy, but it has been possible to darken a hypophyectomized tadpole by implanting into it a pars intermedia, while albino tadpoles of the treetoad *Hyla* have been produced by an experimental treatment which inhibits the development of the pars intermedia while allowing the rest of the pituitary to grow normally. That the hormone is acting directly upon the melanophores is shown by the fact that isolated pieces of amphibian skin in Ringer's fluid will react to the presence of pituitary extracts in the medium, and that the reactions are not affected by the presence of nerve paralysants such as atropine.

That the receptor organ for these responses is the eye can readily be shown by covering or removing them; this eliminates the responses. The animal's ability to discriminate between black and white backgrounds depends upon the retina being differentiated into two regions, the B and the W areas (Fig. 12.3). When *Xenopus* is on a black background under water, it can receive light only from above. The rays are thus restricted to a cone which illuminates only the B area, and this evokes dispersion. On a white background, with light entering from all around, the W area is also illuminated, and this evokes aggregation. No histological differentiation is apparent between these two areas, but there is some evidence that they may be sensitive to different wavelengths. In general, then, the amphibian response depends upon the albedo or ratio of the amount of direct incident light to the amount of light reflected from the background.

The release of MSH after appropriate stimulation

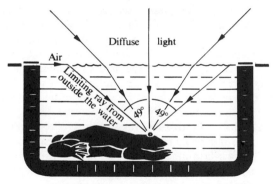

FIG. 12.3. (a) Light rays entering the eye of *Xenopus* in a black tank with overhead illumination. (From Waring (1963). *Colour change mechanisms of cold-blooded vertebrates*. Academic Press, New York.)

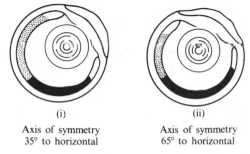

(i) Axis of symmetry 35° to horizontal

(ii) Axis of symmetry 65° to horizontal

(b) The B (black) and W (stippled) areas of the eye of *Xenopus*. The region which can be illuminated only by rays reflected from subaqueous surfaces is stippled. (From Waring, as above.)

some of these cells have aminergic, cholinergic, and peptidergic nerve terminals ending on them. On the other hand, there is evidence that releasing and inhibitory hormones may pass in mammals from the hypothalamus to the pars intermedia by the hypophysial portal system (p. 127). Of course, it need not be supposed that the mechanism of control is uniform throughout the vertebrates. Moreover, even if releasing and inhibiting hormones are involved, their output may be regulated by adrenergic or cholinergic endings in the hypothalamus.

Control of the pars intermedia by the hypothalamus becomes established during the life history of the tadpole, just as does control of the thyroid gland (p. 179). Young tadpoles which lack this hypothalamic regulation, and which (in the context of colour change) are called primary stage tadpoles, become characteristically blanched when they are maintained in darkness. (So also do many fish.) This response is attributed to the release from the pineal gland of melatonin. This substance (Fig. 12.4), which is a potent aggregating agent, is widely distributed in vertebrates, including birds and mammals as well as lower forms. It is formed from serotonin (5-hydroxytryptamine), which is first acetylated to *N*-acetylserotonin, this being then methylated to melatonin by the enzyme hydroxyindole-*O*-methyl transferase (HIOMT). Alternatively, serotonin can be metabolized by monoamine oxidase to 5-hydroxyindole acetaldehyde. These enzymes, together with their substrates, are found in the lateral eye as well as in the pineal, so that both organs contain melatonin.

This substance evokes aggregation in the dermal melanophores of primary stage larvae, and also in

of the eye is mediated by the hypothalamus, which, as we have seen (p. 86), is primarily inhibitory. Darkening thus results from the removal of this inhibitory action. However, the path of communication between the hypothalamus and the pars intermedia is by no means clear. In lower vertebrates (fish and amphibians), the pars intermedia is poorly vascularized, but it is richly innervated by nerve fibres which contain biogenic amines, and which arise from hypothalamic nuclei. In higher forms (lizards, for example, and mammals), the innervation is reduced or absent, but vascularization is well developed. It seems possible that inhibition of MSH release was initially neural, and that it remains so still in lower forms. Then, in the course of vertebrate evolution, the pathway of communication shifted towards a neurosecretory one, with blood vessels arising either in the median eminence or in the vascular plexus which separates the pars nervosa from the pars intermedia. But direct innervation of the pars intermedia cells still persists; in the cat, for example,

Serotonin (5-hydroxytryptamine)

Melatonin

FIG. 12.4. Melatonin and serotonin.

those of secondary stage ones, which are larvae in which hypothalamic control of the pars intermedia has been established, so that an MSH-mediated response is also possible. Thus both melatonin and MSH contribute to the responses of these secondary larvae. The evidence obviously suggests that the gland may function as an endocrine element of the chromatophore response in tadpoles, and this view is strengthened by the fact that blanching of these animals is abolished by removal of the pineal, but persists if the eyes are removed and the pineal left intact. No less significant is the fact that melatonin affects only the dermal melanophores of the larvae and not the epidermal ones, for it is the dermal ones that are responsible for the blanching reaction of the intact larvae. The action of melatonin is an exclusively larval one, for it does not significantly influence chromatophore responses in adults, nor do adults usually blanch in darkness. Thus there is no reason to suppose that the pineal contributes to colour change in adult amphibians, and this applies also to lampreys, elasmobranchs, and teleosts. It is important to appreciate this limitation, as will now become apparent.

Hogben, having firmly established the action of MSH, went on later to propose an extension of the argument by postulating that a second (probably pituitary) hormone was also involved. This he believed to be an aggregating hormone (W substance), supposedly secreted by the pars tuberalis or perhaps elsewhere. On this interpretation, the change from an index of 4·5 to one of 1·5, when the animal was transferred from an illuminated black background to a white one, was effected by the release of the W substance as well as by the inhibition of the release of the B substance (MSH). The argument, which rested upon an ingenious but highly theoretical interpretation of certain evidence, never carried complete conviction. The supposed aggregating hormone has never been isolated, and, for reasons explained above, it could not (as later work at first suggested) be melatonin. In any case, the experimental results can now be explained in simpler terms, which can be reconciled with the one-hormone interpretation.

To give only one example of this, extirpation of the 'anterior lobe' complex of *Xenopus* causes permanent darkening, whereas its extirpation from *Rana* has no effect. The difference was ascribed, on the two-hormone interpretation, to the pars tuberalis of *Xenopus* being removed with the 'anterior lobe', thus depriving the animal of the W substance. In *Rana*, the pars tuberalis was left *in situ* after the operation, so that the W substance continued to cause aggrega-

tion. However, an alternative explanation became apparent when the importance of the median eminence was discovered, and this explanation has been confirmed by experiment. Removal of the 'anterior lobe' in *Xenopus* damages the median eminence, and severs the nerve fibres which would normally inhibit the release of MSH from the pars intermedia; the animal thus darkens. In *Rana*, by contrast, the removal does not disturb these fibres; the animal therefore retains its control of MSH release.

The two-hormone interpretation has thus been abandoned, but it was of great value in its day, for it promoted research that has extended our understanding of the regulation of colour change. It can now be stated, in terms of the one-hormone interpretation, that maximal dispersion in amphibians on a black background is due to maximal release of MSH. Aggregation on a white background is due to inhibition of this release. The intermediate condition observed in complete darkness may be ascribed to tonic release of the hormone.

Nevertheless, despite the rejection of the two-hormone interpretation, MSH is not the only hormone influencing the chromatophores of adult amphibians. In these animals, as in other poikilotherms, the catecholamine hormones, in conjunction with the sympathetic nervous system, cause changes in pigment distribution that are shown during stress, and that are termed 'excitement darkening' and 'excitement pallor'. The effects, which depend upon the reacting cells containing either α- or β-receptors, are complex, partly because species differ in the predominance of one or other of the two types of receptor. Moreover, iridophores may also be affected, while, as indicated earlier, catecholamines may be involved in the release of MSH from the pars intermedia.

12.3. Melanophore-stimulating hormone (MSH)

The physiology of melanophore-stimulating hormone has been mainly studied in the lower vertebrates, where its role in colour change is well substantiated. Somewhat paradoxically, however, its chemistry is known almost entirely from mammals, in which group the function of the hormone, and the reason for its persistence, is little understood. It has been isolated from mammalian pituitaries (cattle, horse, pig, sheep, man) in two forms, which have been fully characterized as α-MSH and β-MSH. α-MSH, which has the greater biological activity, is a tridecapeptide, of constant composition in the mammals studied. β-MSH, of which the bovine and human hormones have been synthesized, has 18

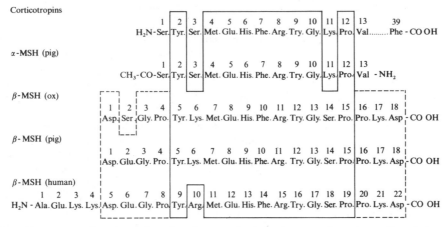

FIG. 12.5. Amino-acid sequences of corticotropin and melanocyte-stimulating hormones from mammalian pituitary glands. (After Harris (1960). *Br. med. Bull.* **16**.)

amino acids in cattle, the horse, and the pig, but 22 in man, and it also varies in amino acid composition (Fig. 12.5). All of these molecules, however, possess a common heptapeptide sequence (positions 4–10 in α-MSH) which is essential for their biological activity. Evidence for this is that a small amount of activity (estimated to be 10^5–10^6 times less than that of the natural hormone) is present in a synthetic pentapeptide corresponding to positions 6–10 of α-MSH. The addition of appropriate amino acids increases the activity, a maximum being attained with the tridecapeptide sequence of α-MSH.

What little is known of the chemistry of MSH in lower vertebrates suggests that the situation in these is similar in principle. Electrophoretic studies of bullfrog pituitary extracts indicate the presence of α-MSH, β-MSH, and a third unknown variant, but electrophoresis cannot give conclusive evidence for amino-acid sequences. Sequence studies of pituitary extracts of the dogfish, *Squalus acanthias*, however, show that two forms of α-MSH are present. Ten of their residues are identical with those of the mammalian hormone, while the similarity is increased in one-fifth of the molecules by the presence of an additional tyrosine residue at the NH$_2$-terminus. About half of the dogfish molecules have a free carboxyl group at the COOH-terminus, the remainder being amidated. The apparent absence of β-MSH suggests that this may be a later derivative of α-MSH, but this is only supposition, and no firm conclusions can be drawn from these limited data.

MSH provides a particularly instructive illustration of the evolutionary implications of amino-acid substitutions in polypeptide hormones (p. 101). This is because the active heptapeptide sequence is found

in corticotropin (Fig. 12.5), which also carries a sequence of 13 amino acids that is identical with that of the α-MSH molecule. The presence of the heptapeptide explains the small amount of MSH-like activity found in that hormone; an amount equivalent to about 1 per cent of that of the β-MSH of the pig. Presumably the activity of the sequence is largely masked by the remaining structural features of the corticotropin molecule, but it is likely that its remaining activity accounts for the darkening of the skin that we have seen to be a feature of Addison's disease, and that was recorded by Jane Austen in her own illness.

The same heptapeptide sequence is also present in lipotropin, a substance, present in the pituitary, which has a fat-mobilizing action, the physiological significance of which is obscure. Lipotropin (LPH), initially discovered by accident during the purification of corticotropin, has been isolated from the adenohypophysis in two forms. One of these, β-LPH, has 90 amino acids and a molecular weight of 9500. The other, γ-LPH, has a molecular weight of 5810, and comprises the first 58 sequences of the β-molecule. It has been suggested that β-LPH is a parent molecule of β-MSH, which, it is thought, could be split off from β-LPH by hydrolytic action in the pars intermedia. As an extension of this proposition, it is further suggested that α-MSH could be formed in a similar way from ACTH, and that this accounts for the small amounts of the latter which are identifiable in the pars intermedia.

Whether or not these ideas prove to be correct, all of these structural relationships suggest very strongly that the molecules have had a common origin within the adenohypophysis, and that they have diverged, according to the principles discussed earlier, through gene duplication and amino-acid substitution. Suggestive evidence that they belong to a single molecular family is that the pituitary of a single individual sheep may contain no less than seven of these molecules: two different corticotropins, one α-MSH, two different β-MSHs, and β-lipotropin. This implies some persistence of gene duplication and mutation. Clearly, however, this evolutionary diversification has been accompanied also by a good deal of molecular stability, and it is particularly remarkable to find the two forms of MSH in mammals, despite the absence from this group of physiological colour change. To suggest that they may be vestigial hormones, as has sometimes been done, is merely to conceal ignorance. It is altogether more likely that they persist because they have functions that are still unknown. Indeed, it is not excluded that these hormones may, in lower forms, have functions additional to the regulation of colour change. Experience with the hypothalamic polypeptides shows that the history of MSH, corticotropin and lipotropin will not be unravelled until very much more is known of the chemistry of these molecules in lower vertebrates. It is unfortunate, from this point of view, that the structure of MSH is best known in the group in which least is known of its function; what little information that is available suggests a promising field for research.

α-MSH produces darkening of the skin in man, with increase in the numbers of melanosomes, but it is uncertain whether or not this is of physiological significance. MSH also increases deposition of melanin in the hair of mice, but even more striking is an action in the weasel, *Mustela erminea*, which seems to be clearly adaptive. This animal, under the influence of photoperiod, develops brown fur in summer and white in winter, the change of pelage being under hormonal control, as is shown by the effects of hypophysectomy. This results in the growth of white fur regardless of the season. Hair growth can be evoked in this animal by plucking, and the new hair will be brown in hypophysectomized animals if they are treated during its growth with MSH or corticotropin. Moreover, hypophysectomized weasels grow brown hair, even in winter, if pituitaries are grafted into their kidney capsules; removal of the grafts will then evoke moulting, followed by the growth of white hair. The facts indicate that the development of the brown pelage is promoted by output of MSH, and that hypothalamic inhibition of the production or release of the hormone is responsible for the white pelage of winter.

12.4. Cyclostomata

Larval lampreys show a well-marked diurnal colour change, being pale by night and dark by day (Fig. 12.6). Adult brook lampreys (*Lampetra planeri*) behave similarly, but adult river lampreys (*L. fluviatilis*) show little change. This rhythm is undoubtedly influenced by external stimulation, for it can be stopped by reversing, with artificial illumination, the normal diurnal alternation of light and darkness (Fig. 12.6). The effect of continuous darkness is less clearly defined, and under this condition there may be some persistence of the diurnal rhythm. This suggests an interaction of exogenous and endogenous factors analogous to what we have found in sexual cycles.

The colour change, like that of amphibians, is due to the movement of pigment within melanophores, and is assumed, on good evidence, to be regulated by MSH. Destruction, by cauterization, of the whole pituitary, or of the pars intermedia alone, results in permanent pallor, while intraperitoneal injection of mammalian 'posterior lobe' extracts causes dispersal of pigment.

Larval lampreys are blind, with imperfectly developed lateral eyes buried beneath the skin, but the pineal eyes serve as the external receptors; if these are destroyed, the animals lose all capacity for colour change, and become permanently dark. In adults, the paired eyes are well developed, and become involved as receptors in cooperation with the pineal complex. The exact path of communication between the central nervous system and the pars intermedia is not known, but it may be that hypothalamic neurosecretion plays a part, since the neurosecretory granules of the preoptic nucleus cells, and of their axons, are depleted in continuous light and accumulate in continuous darkness (cf. Fig. 5.14(b), p. 74). There is certainly no evidence of innervation of the melanophores, so that the regulation of colour change by means of MSH must be a very primitive feature of vertebrate organization.

12.5 Elasmobranchii

Elasmobranchs show types of colour change, both non-visual and visual, which are essentially similar to those found in amphibians, although there are considerable variations in the degree of response. *Mustelis canis*, for example, changes from a grey colour on a black background to a pale colour on a white one in some two days, the reverse change taking only half an hour to two hours, while *Raja erinacea* will develop pallor on a white background in twelve hours and will darken on a black one in

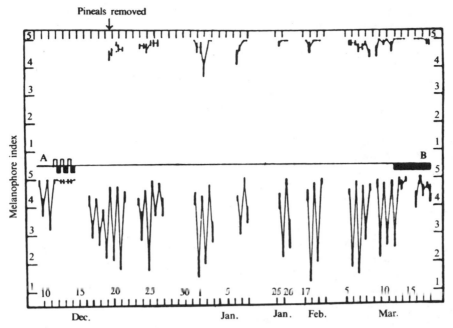

FIG. 12.6. Colour changes of larval lampreys. Animals kept out of doors except as shown along the line AB, where rectangles above the line show illumination with electric light and below the line total darkness. Normal animals show a regular daily rhythm which stops when the normal diurnal alternation of light and darkness is reversed. On 19 December the pineal eyes were removed from 5 out of the 10 individuals and these thereafter remained dark (upper chart); the other 5 continued to show the normal rhythm, until placed in total darkness. (From Young (1962). *The life of vertebrates*. Clarendon Press, Oxford.)

nine hours. On the other hand, there are many elasmobranchs which are extremely sluggish in their responses; examples of this are the common dog-fishes, *Scyllium catulus*, *Squalus acanthias*, and *Scyliorhinus canicula*, the last-named requiring from eighty to one hundred hours to change from its pale-background response to the dark one, and vice versa. The ray *Raja clavata* has been said not to show any colour change when it is transferred from a black background to a white one and, like the dogfish, is normally dark. However, when it is hypophysec-tomized it develops a pallor, which shows that its melanophores have certainly not lost their capacity for pigment movement. The assumption is that its normal colour is maintained by a tonic production of MSH by the pituitary, and that the activity of the gland is not markedly influenced by incident light.

The conclusion that the dark phase in the re-sponses of these fish is evoked by the secretion of MSH by the pars intermedia is well established, particularly with the identification of α-MSH in one species (p. 213). The physiological evidence derives from the early studies on *Mustelus canis*. These showed that removal of the pituitary gland resulted in blanching, which reached a maximum in twelve

hours and which, as with the corresponding phenom-enon in amphibians, could be temporarily overcome by the injection of mammalian 'posterior lobe' extracts. They further showed that removal of the 'neurointermediate lobe' (p. 75) also resulted in blanching, and that removal of the 'anterior lobe' did not, while injections of extracts of the former into such experimentally blanched fish produced a tem-porary darkening. It was thus concluded that the 'neurointermediate lobe' must be the source of the supposed hormone. Later, it was shown that the injection into a pale dogfish of blood from a dark one resulted in the development of a dark area at the site of the injection, whereas the injection of such blood into a dark fish, or of blood from a pale fish into either a dark or pale one, had no such effect. There was thus some evidence for the presence of the hormone in the blood stream.

As regards the possibility of an innervation of the melanophores in this group, there is no completely convincing evidence for this, although Parker argued that nerve fibres bring about concentration of the pigment in certain species. His interpretation hinged upon the significance to be attached to caudal bands similar to those that have been obtained in teleosts.

The arguments against it are substantially the same as those outlined below, with the additional consideration that such bands have only been observed in *Mustelus canis* and *Squalus acanthias* and that they have not been found in at least six other species of rays and dogfish in which investigators have looked for them. If we add to this the fact, often overlooked, that no grey rami arise from the sympathetic ganglia in elasmobranchs and that there is, in consequence, no outflow of sympathetic fibres from the sympathetic chain to the skin, it becomes difficult to justify a belief in autonomic innervation of the melanophores in this group.

12.6. Teleostei

The colour changes of teleosts are more complex than those of the groups so far discussed. The equipment of chromatophores includes all the types previously mentioned, while the background responses may be varied and remarkably rapid. They may be effected in a matter of seconds or at most minutes, while some species of flat-fish can contrive a creditable imitation of the pattern of their background. These characteristics suggest innervation of the chromatophores, and this suggestion is amply substantiated. The skin of teleosts differs from that of elasmobranchs in being innervated by the sympathetic component of the autonomic system, the fibres concerned running in recurrent grey rami (Fig. 12.7), which, as we have seen, are absent from elasmobranchs. Moreover, it has been known since 1893, from histological evidence, that the melanophores of teleosts are innervated, but even earlier than that, in 1872–6, Pouchet had shown that the colour responses of flat-fish were controlled by the sympathetic nervous system; characteristic patterns of localized darkening were produced by nerve section or by destruction of the sympathetic chain (Fig. 12.8).

Subsequently, this aspect was investigated by von Frisch, who established the course of the sympathetic fibres in *Phoxinus* by studying the effect of nerve section on the background responses of the fish, and on the reaction of its melanophores to electrical stimulation of the nervous system. He was able to show, as have many subsequent workers, that concentration of pigment takes place when the nerve fibres supplying a particular group of melanophores are stimulated. The response is a localized one, and does not spread to adjacent areas that have been denervated. It must therefore result from the direct action of the nerve fibres upon their effector cells, and cannot be due to a blood-borne hormone.

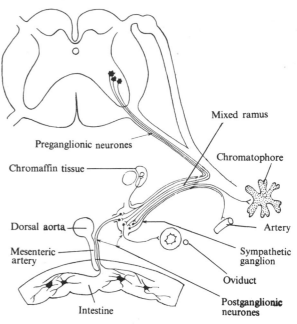

FIG. 12.7. Diagram of some sympathetic pathways in a teleost fish. (From Nicol (1952). *Biol. Rev.* **27**.)

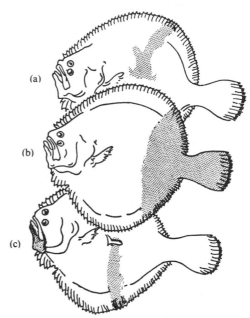

FIG. 12.8. Evidence from the work of Pouchet that nerve impulses cause concentration in the chromatophores of the turbot, *Scopthalamus* (*Rhombus*) *maximus*. The darkening results from (a) cutting spinal nerve branches, (b) cutting spinal nerve branches and the inferior maxillary branch of the trigeminus, and (c) destroying the sympathetic chain in the posterior haemal canal. (From Nicol (1960). *The biology of marine animals.* Pitman, London.)

Nevertheless, hormonal regulation of colour change also occurs in teleosts, and we shall see that the relative importance of neural and hormonal co-ordination varies from species to species.

Hormonal regulation, assumed to be mediated by MSH, is well documented for the eel, *Anguilla anguilla*. The background responses of this animal are much as in amphibians and elasmobranchs, the responses being very slow to develop. The achievement of maximum pallor after removal from a black background to a white one takes as much as 20 days at 6–8 °C, the corresponding time for *Xenopus* at the same temperature being 12 days. This is not due to insensitivity of the chromatophores, for in perfusion experiments, using pituitary extracts in saline, these cells may give a maximal response in 10 minutes. The time taken *in vivo* is presumably required for the building up of a suitable concentration of MSH in the blood stream. The chromatophores of the eel are innervated, and electrical stimulation of suitable preparations shows that aggregating fibres are present. However, it must be concluded, from the time relations of the background responses of intact animals, that innervation of the chromatophores plays no part in normal colour responses.

Phoxinus phoxinus, the European minnow, presents a complete contrast to the eel, for the nervous system is here the predominant, and perhaps the only, regulator of colour change. Von Frisch, in the work already mentioned, was able to trace the preganglionic melanophore fibres from the medulla down the spinal cord, which they leave at about the level of the fifteenth vertebra to enter the sympathetic chain (Fig. 12.9). This chain extends into the head, and the melanophores of that region are innervated by sympathetic fibres running in the trigeminal nerve. The effect of this arrangement is that section of only a few spinal nerve roots, at the particular level at which the melanophore fibres leave the spinal cord (between A and B in Fig. 12.9), will influence the colour of the whole body surface. Denervation of the melanophores in *Phoxinus*

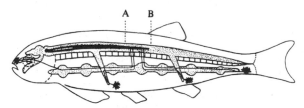

FIG. 12.9. Paths of aggregating nerve fibres in the minnow *(Phoxinus)*, after von Frisch. (From Healey (1954). *J. exp. Biol.* **31**.)

results in dispersion of their pigment. By analogy with the other vertebrates so far considered, it might be thought that this was due to the action of MSH, but there is no satisfactory evidence that this is so. Injections into *Phoxinus* of extracts of the pituitary of the same species causes pallor, while extracts of other teleosts have variable effects. Some produce darkening, some produce pallor, and some produce no response at all. In short, there is little evidence of a dispersing hormone being involved in the normal responses of this species, and it seems likely that dispersion is simply a result of release of the chromatophores from neural control.

Fundulus, the North American killifish, will serve as a third example, and a somewhat puzzling one. Dispersion takes place on a black background, and is certainly a result of stimulation of the eye, but the nature of the co-ordinating mechanism is obscure. That MSH plays a part is suggested by the fact that hypophysectomized animals cannot achieve as dark a condition as can intact ones, yet, despite this, the effect of pituitary injections is difficult to interpret. Contrary to what might be expected, pituitary preparations have no dispersing effect when they are injected into intact pale animals on a white background, although they do produce some dispersion in areas that have been denervated.

A possible explanation of this may lie in the fact that in *Fundulus*, as in *Phoxinus*, aggregation is produced by direct innervation of the chromatophores, the response being a rapid one which is prevented by denervation. Various lines of evidence confirm the adrenergic nature of the fibres. Synaptic vesicles of about 500Å in diameter are present in the nerve endings, and formalin–induced fluorescence can be demonstrated in fibres ending around the melanophores. Perhaps, then, the aggregating influence of these fibres can override the dispersing effect of the hormone, and thus minimise the effect of pituitary injections.

A further problem presented by *Fundulus* arises from the suggestion, formulated by Parker, that the melanophores also receive dispersing fibres which antagonize the concentrating ones. This proposition largely arose from experiments in which transverse cuts were made across pale fins. These caused the appearance of dark bands lying peripheral to the cuts, and persisting for some time. Parker's explanation of the dark bands, which are due to pigment dispersion on the distal side of the cut, was that they were produced by the firing of nerve impulses propagated along dispersing fibres, and initiated by the injury at the cut ends of these fibres. This argument is difficult to sustain within normal physiological tenets. There is no evidence that cut fibres actually continue to fire in this way. Moreover, it is not easy to understand why cutting should predominantly stimulate the dispersing fibres, while electrical stimulation predominantly stimulates the aggregating ones. For these reasons, this interpretation has never received full acceptance; yet the formation of the bands is not in dispute, and it remains to be explained.

vesicles of a cholinergic type, about 1000 Å in diameter and with electron-dense contents, occur in nerve endings in the skin, and it has been suggested that a melanosome-dispersing transmitter substance may leak from the cut ends of some of the fibres. Thus there is still some support for the existence of dispersing fibres in this animal, and it can be coupled with a further suggestion, which is that dispersion, set up in this way, might be sustained by Brownian movement of the melanosomes after the chemical transmitter has been exhausted. However, these dark bands still present an essentially unresolved problem. This is even more true of the bands which can be produced in certain species of elasmobranch (p. 215). No satisfactory explanation exists for these; the difficulties are exactly the same as those outlined, and the best that can be suggested is that they could perhaps be due to vasomotor disturbance.

12.7. Reptilia

The only group of reptiles showing marked colour changes is the Lacertilia (lizards), although some snakes and the alligator are said to have a slight capacity for this. Within the Lacertilia, as far as can be judged from the very limited evidence, there is great variation in the mode of regulation of the response, which is what might be expected of so ancient and specialized a group. The spectacular responses of *Chamaeleo* are certainly regulated by the sympathetic nervous system. The distribution of the nerve fibres is somewhat like that in *Phoxinus* (p. 217), so that the effect of cutting the nerve cord depends upon the level at which this is done (Figs 12.10 and 12.11). There is no evidence for hormonal regulation in chamaeleons, although this does not necessarily mean that it is absent. It is certainly present, however, in two other genera which have been studied in some detail: the horned lizards, *Phrynosoma blainvilli* and *P. cornutum*, and a Florida lizard, *Anolis carolinensis*.

Colour change in *Phrynosoma*, which bears dark bands, involves paling and darkening of the background colour of the skin. Eyeless animals tend to

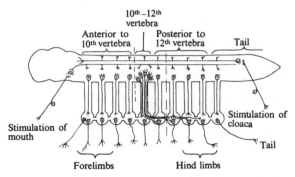

Fig. 12.10. Diagrammatic representation of the nerve paths involved in the control of the pigmentary effector system of the chameleon. (From Hogben and Mirvish (1928). *J. exp. Biol.* **5**.)

darken in bright light and to blanch in darkness; reactions which are probably due in part to independent response of the melanophores, since they occur in animals that have been hypophysectomized, and that also have the pineal eye covered and the skin denervated. In addition to this non-visual response, the intact animal shows a typical background response, blanching in light surroundings and darkening in dark ones. This reaction is dependent upon MSH, essentially as in the groups already considered.

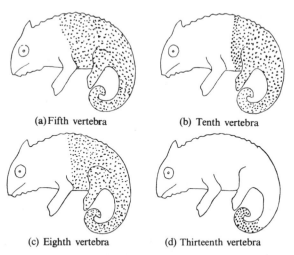

(a) Fifth vertebra

(b) Tenth vertebra

(c) Eighth vertebra

(d) Thirteenth vertebra

Fig. 12.11. Demonstration of the direct innervation of the pigmentary effector system of the chameleon through the central nervous and sympathetic systems. Section of the nerve cord anterior to the 11th vertebra restricts the pallor following faradic stimulation of the mouth to the region in front of the cut (a), (b), and (c). Section of the cord at the thirteenth vertebra results in generalized pallor as a result of impulses being distributed to posterior parts of the body through preganglionic fibres leaving the cord at about the level of the tenth to twelfth vertebrae (d) (cf. Fig. 14.10). (From Hogben and Mirvish (1928). *J. exp. Biol.* **5**.)

Hypophysectomy is followed by pallor, which can be maintained for at least five weeks, while temporary darkening can be induced in hypophysectomized animals by injection of pituitary preparations. The presence of the hormone in the blood is demonstrated when blood from a dark animal is injected subcutaneously into a pale one; this induces a dark spot, whereas a similar injection into a dark animal is without effect.

It follows, therefore, that darkening in *Phrynosoma* is evoked by an increased level of circulating MSH, and pallor by a decline in this level. However, the situation is complicated by Parker's assertion that aggregation is further promoted by direct innervation of the melanophores. Unfortunately, the evidence for these aggregating fibres, in contrast to the evidence from certain teleosts, remains incomplete and unconvincing, for it rests in large measure upon the results of experiments involving faradic stimulation of the nervous system. These experiments are difficult to interpret, since their results could often be due to vasomotor disturbances.

Colour change in *Phrynosoma* is expressed not only as a background response, but also as a diurnal rhythm; individuals are dark in the early morning, pale at midday, dark in the evening, and pale again during the night. It is not clear whether this is a response to light, or to temperature, or to both, but whatever the cause, the changes could well make a contribution to thermoregulation. Lizards have a well-developed pattern of behaviour which enables them, by taking advantage of the physical conditions of the environment, to maintain a remarkably constant temperature during their hours of activity. The colour changes of *Phrynosoma* would favour absorption of radiant heat during early morning and late evening, when the body can benefit from warming, and reflection of it during the middle of the day, when there could be a danger of overheating.

Anolis carolinensis has a much more elaborate play of colour than *Phrynosoma*, ranging from brown to green through shades of light brown and yellow. Brown is the dark phase, with maximum dispersion in the melanophores, and green the pale phase, with maximum aggregation. The green colour, much as in *Rana* (p. 209), is a result of the reflection of light from iridophores and its passage through the overlying xanthophores.

There is the usual background response, but its form depends upon the intensity of illumination. Animals are brown in strong sunlight, for example, but green under weaker laboratory lighting, and they are also green in complete darkness. These changes are assumed to be mediated by MSH. Hypophysectomy results in permanent green colour, pituitary injections produce temporary darkening, and MSH preparations darken isolated pieces of skin *in vitro*. Blinded animals show a non-visual response, being brown in strong light and green in weak light, or in darkness, irrespective of the background. This response, too, is hormonally co-ordinated, for it is eliminated by hypophysectomy, which makes the colour of all animals bright green. The only plausible explanation of this non-visual response (although it has never been confirmed) is that stimulation of dermal photoreceptors brings about reflex stimulation of the release of MSH from the pituitary.

The melanophores are not innervated in *Anolis*, and there is no evidence for direct involvement of nervous regulation in the background responses. Cutting of the spinal cord and sympathetic chains has no effect upon these responses; even when the posterior part of the cord is destroyed by pithing, the animal can still respond as a whole to light and dark backgrounds. Nevertheless, electrical stimulation of the cloaca, muscles, or spinal cord evokes a generalized pallor. This, however, is shown also by denervated regions of the body as well as by intact animals, which conforms with the view that the response is not due to direct innervation of the melanophores. Nor is there any evidence that the pineal complex is involved in this response. The explanation of it is that the aggregation is evoked by catecholamines, released from the adrenal gland. Normally, this release takes place in conditions of stress, but plays no part in the normal background response. A further complication is that the catecholamines may also produce a localized dispersion, so that parts of the body become mottled, notably in the post-orbital region. Experiments with blocking agents show that dispersion depends upon β-receptors in the chromatophores, and aggregation on α-receptors. Mottling could therefore be due to some cells having only the β-receptors, but it may also be that the circulating level of catecholamines influences the response, which certainly depends in addition upon the degree of dispersion or concentration initially present in the skin.

13

Hormones in invertebrates I

13.1. Invertebrates and vertebrates

Invertebrates and vertebrates (or, more strictly, chordates), are often discussed as though they occupied totally unrelated segments of the animal kingdom, with the one offering little towards the understanding of the other. However, this approach (which may be a matter of convenience in the writing of text-books) is based on too narrow a vision, and obscures the point made earlier: that unrelated groups, by the exploitation of common principles and materials, may independently evolve analogous systems that are remarkably similar in form and function (p. 4). We shall find this to be well shown by the endocrine systems of invertebrates as compared with those of vertebrates, particularly in relation to the use made of neurosecretion. Because of this, there has been continuous cross-fertilization of comparative endocrinological studies, regardless of the systematic position of the animals under investigation. Care, however, is needed in interpreting the results in terms of evolutionary history. It cannot be assumed that similar arthropodan systems are necessarily homologous because they are found within the same phylum, or that they have been derived from those of annelid worms. It is doubtful whether there is a direct relationship between the phylum Annelida and the phylum Arthropoda. Moreover, it is difficult to avoid the conclusion that arthropods may very well have had a diphyletic origin, and that parallel evolution (perhaps homoplastic, p. 5) has contributed to their specializations.

Even without this latter complication, it is clear that the crustaceans and insects can at best be only very remotely related, for these two groups must have become separated at a very early stage, possibly in the pre-Cambrian. Crustaceans are already highly organized as an independent group in the Cambrian (some 500 million years ago), and in their subsequent history, with their failure to make effective use of the possibilities of terrestrial life, they have pursued a course very different from that of insects. It follows that in this field of comparative endocrinology comparisons must not be pressed further than can be justified by the classical principles of comparative zoology, although, for reasons explained earlier, the analysis may sometimes be a subtle one, and classical principles not always a sufficient basis for it.

13.2. Invertebrates and neurosecretion

Neurosecretion plays such an important part in the lives of vertebrates that one would expect it to contribute to physiological regulation in other groups as well, and this proves to be so.

As we shall see, the arthropods are by far the most fully documented, but convincing, if circumstantial, evidence comes from *Hydra*, in which animal, as in so many others, a mechanism exists for dissociating growth from reproduction. It has long been known, from classical studies of development and regeneration, that the apical region of the body is of special importance in the promotion of growth. Associated with this is the presence, immediately below the hypostome, of a growth zone from which cells are continuously forced towards the tentacles and towards the base of the body. Cytological studies, grounded on current understanding of neurosecretion, have now enlarged our understanding of this process.

The growth phase of *Hydra*, which is characterized by the transformation of interstitial cells into cnidoblasts, is accompanied by asexual reproduction (budding). During this phase, the nerve cells in the hypostomal region (Figs 13.1 and 13.2), and at the bases of the tentacles, contain stainable droplets which are found only in very small amounts in other regions of the body. They appear, however, in the nerve fibres of the hypostomal region of a bud just before it forms its own tentacles and growth region. Further evidence comes from studies of regeneration. For example, removal of the hypostome and tentacles results in this apical fragment regenerating a trunk

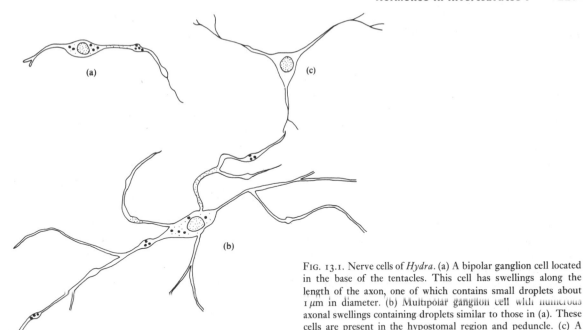

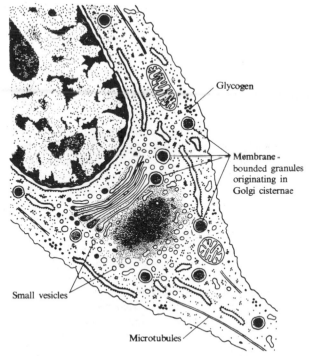

Fig. 13.1. Nerve cells of *Hydra*. (a) A bipolar ganglion cell located in the base of the tentacles. This cell has swellings along the length of the axon, one of which contains small droplets about 1 μm in diameter. (b) Multipolar ganglion cell with numerous axonal swellings containing droplets similar to those in (a). These cells are present in the hypostomal region and peduncle. (c) A tripolar ganglion cell without droplets, common in tentacles and peduncle. (From Burnett and Diehl (1964). *J. exp. Zool.* **157**.)

Glycogen

Membrane-
bounded granules
originating in
Golgi cisternae

Small vesicles

Microtubules

Fig. 13.2. Ultrastructure of neurosecretory cells of *Hydra*. Membrane-bounded granules of moderate density seem to originate within Golgi cisternae. (After Lentz (1968), from Scharrer and Weitzman, in *Aspects of neuroendocrinology* (eds W. Bargmann and B. Scharrer). Springer–Verlag, Berlin.)

region and thus forming a complete body. During the first four hours of regeneration, the droplets in the hypostomal region increase, and are then passed into the surrounding tissue.

All of this suggests that these nerve cells are neurosecretory cells, secreting a neurosecretory growth-promoting factor. The facts do not, of course, prove this to be so, but electron microscopy (Fig. 13.2) supports this view, and further support comes from the sexual phase. This is marked by the transformation of interstitial cells into germ cells, and by the cessation of budding. At the same time, the supposedly neurosecretory droplets of the hypostomal region cease to be visible, and the nerve fibres of that region seem to disappear. In some way, then, sexual reproduction in *Hydra* is correlated with a decline in the supposed neurosecretory activity of the hypostomal region. It is not known what factors normally bring about this decline, although sexuality can be induced by various laboratory procedures. We shall see, however, that the situation as a whole is remarkably similar in principle to the regulation of growth and reproduction in polychaete worms.

Evidence of neurohormonal regulation comes from many other invertebrate groups; probably no group that has been at all closely studied has failed to yield some such evidence. Here we can mention only a few examples. Regeneration of the eyes in the planarian

Polycelis nigra will not take place in the absence of the brain, which contains cells that appear to be neurosecretory. Homogenates of it, added to the ambient water, induce regeneration of the eyes in decerebrate animals. This is suggestive of neuro-secretory regulation, but the evidence in this instance is slim, for other substances as well can induce regeneration in these animals.

Maturation and shedding of gametes from sexually ripe starfish is regulated by two hormone-like substances. One is a polypeptide of some 23 amino acids, with a molecular weight of 2200, present in aqueous extracts of the radial nerve fibres. This substance acts by evoking in the ovary the local synthesis or release of a meiosis-inducing substance which has been isolated from *Asterias amurensis* and character-ized as a purine, *l*-methyladenine. It evokes morpho-logical changes in the entire ovary, including the ovarian wall and the follicle cells, as well as in the oocytes.

Molluscs are less well understood from this point of view than might be hoped, having regard to their advanced level of physiological organization. This is partly because of the experimental difficulties involved in operating upon their nerve ganglia, and partly because results obtained are not always easy to interpret. For example, presumptive neurosecretory cells are found in the cerebral ganglia (Fig. 13.3) of various gastropods. These show a cycle of activity in the fresh-water snail, *Lymnaea stagnalis*, which appears to be correlated with germ-cell production, yet removal of them has no clear-cut effect upon the development of the ovotestis. This negative finding

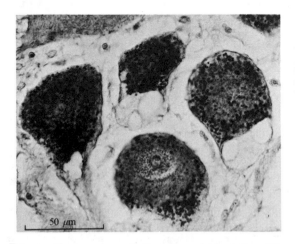

FIG. 13.3. Neurosecretory cells from the cerebral ganglion of the opisthobranch snail, *Aplysia limacina*. Bouin's fluid, chrome-alum–haematoxylin and phloxin. (From Scharrer and Scharrer (1954). *Rec. Prog. Hormone Res.* **10**.)

may seem disappointing, but it is nevertheless a very useful one, for it shows how dangerous it is to assume endocrine activity from cytological observations that are unsupported by experiment. Equally, however, this finding may be replaced by a positive one in due course.

More satisfactory evidence comes from studies of water balance in *Lymnaea stagnalis*. Its neuro-secretory system is complex, with at least nine types of presumed neurosecretory cell, but two particular categories are here involved. One com-prises dark green cells in both of the pleural ganglia, while the other comprises yellow cells in both of the parietal ganglia and in the single visceral ganglion. *L. stagnalis* has a high internal osmotic pressure, so that it is subjected to an influx of water and an outflux of ions. Maintenance of a steady state thus depends on an active uptake of ions and the production of a copious hypotonic urine.

Placing the animals in de-ionized water activates water elimination, and concomitant activation is also demonstrable in these neurosecretory cells, shown in a decrease in the number of neurosecretory granules in their axon endings. That this relationship is causally determined is strongly indicated by the fact that removal of the pleural ganglia leads to swelling of the animals in de-ionized water, while injection of homogenates of these ganglia reduces body weight. This evidence, in conjunction with other observations, has been held to indicate that the dark green cells secrete a diuretic hormone, and that the yellow cells are implicated in the activation of ion uptake.

The most convincing evidence for neuroendocrine regulation in invertebrates, outside the arthropods, comes from annelids. Cells with stainable inclusions are widespread in the cerebral ganglion of these animals (Fig. 13.4), and also in the ventral nerve cord. Not all are neurosecretory, but some certainly are, and these probably include cells of more than one type. They are associated with tracts of neuro-secretory fibres, visible, for example, in the ventral nerve cord of the leech (Figs 13.5 and 13.6). In this animal, section of the cord results in the accumulation of presumed neurosecretory material at the posterior side of the cut. This implies that there is a move-ment of this substance forwards from its cells of origin towards the brain; an effect similar in principle to that which has been demonstrated in the neuro-secretory systems of arthropods and vertebrates, although in these groups the movement is normally in the opposite direction.

A situation more directly comparable with that of

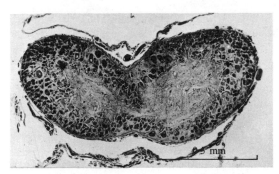

FIG. 13.4. Section through the cerebral ganglion of the earthworm, *Lumbricus terrestris*. The numerous neurosecretory cells are conspicuous by their darker coloration. Zenker-formol, chrome-alum–haematoxylin and phloxin. (From Scharrer and Scharrer (1954). *Rec. Prog. Hormone Res.* **10**.)

arthropods and vertebrates is well documented in polychaete worms. In *Nephtys* (Fig. 13.7), a tract of nerve fibres runs within the cerebral ganglion to the pericapsular membrane surrounding the ganglion. Here the fibres give rise to swollen nerve endings on the brain capsule, very close to a coelomic sinus and blood vessels which overlie the capsule. Granules similar to elementary neurosecretory granules are visible by electron microscopy, together with others resembling synaptic vesicles, and there is evidence of their discharge. Thus the whole of this cerebro-

vascular complex satisfies the requirements of a neurohaemal organ. An essentially similar condition is found in *Nereis*, except that here there are several neurosecretory tracts instead of one.

However, there is a further complication in both *Nereis* and *Nephtys*, which concerns the coelomic epithelium covering the ventral surface of the posterior part of the ganglion. This epithelium is formed of glandular cells, constituting what has been termed the infracerebral gland. Some neurosecretory fibres end near this gland, while others penetrate it and directly innervate some of its cells. These observations suggest a real possibility that cerebral neurosecretory fibres may be regulating an epithelial gland, and not only in these genera—an infracerebral gland has also been reported in phyllodocid and polynoid worms. Some similarity to the arthropod secretory systems, not to mention the pituitary organization of vertebrates, is sufficiently obvious; however, the interpretation of the cerebral organization of polychaetes awaits much further study. Nevertheless, we shall see that there is convincing experimental evidence that the brain is an important centre of endocrine regulation in these animals. Initially, the cerebral ganglion was thought of simply as a source of neurosecretion which was discharged into the circulation through the neurohaemal organ, but the

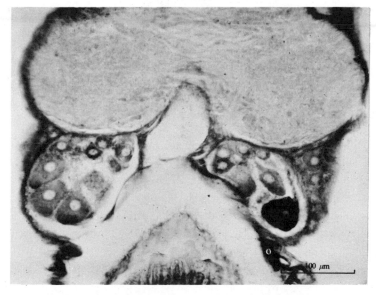

FIG. 13.5. Frontal section through the cerebral ganglion of the leech, *Theromyzon rude*. The dorsal commissure is at the top, partly surrounding the subcommissural blood vessel, at the sides of which are seen two of the 36 compartments of cells which make up the cerebral and sub-oesophageal ganglia. The neurosecretory cell at the extreme right has contents which are intensely stained with aldehyde–fuchsin and which extend into the axon. (From Hagadorn (1958). *J. Morph.* **102**.)

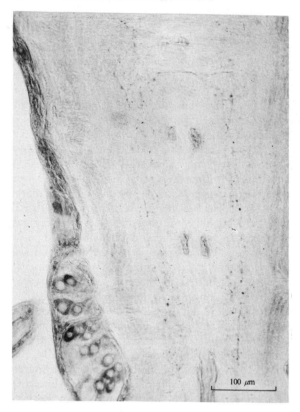

100 μm

FIG. 13.6. Frontal section through the cerebral ganglion of the same species as in Fig. 15.5. Axons containing neurosecretory material, which stains with aldehyde–fuchsin, form two well-defined tracts of fibres, one on each side of the mid-line. (From Hagadorn (1958). *J. Morph.* **102**.)

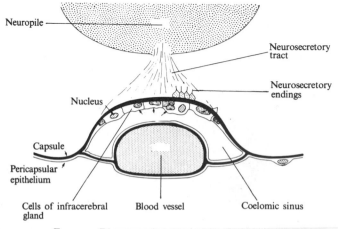

FIG. 13.7. Diagrammatic representation of the elements comprising the infracerebral gland of *Nephtys*. (From Golding (1970). *Gen. comp. Endocrin.* **14**.)

discovery of the infracerebral gland makes it necessary to envisage that it, too, may also play a part. This possibility remains to be clarified, but it does not affect the general principles of endocrine regulation which are now to be outlined.

13.3. Growth and reproduction in polychaete worms

Growth and reproduction constitute two distinct phases of life which are separated in some species of polychaetes, just as they are in *Hydra* and in many other animals. The endocrine basis of this separation has been particularly closely studied in nereid worms. Young (i.e. sexually immature) nereids have a marked power of regeneration, which is associated with their normal capacity for growth. Amputation of a group of posterior segments is followed by muscular contraction, to protect the surface of the wound. New ectoderm and mesoderm then form from a blastema of undifferentiated cells, while new endoderm arises from the existing alimentary tract. Wound-healing, which may last for one week, is followed by the regeneration of new segments, which match in number those that have been lost. As may be seen from Fig. 13.8, the regenerative process lasts for some weeks. Its adaptive significance in creeping and burrowing animals is obvious, and it is not surprising to find that it is regulated by an endocrine mechanism which is simple in principle but elegantly and efficiently organized.

Removal of the brain removes the power of posterior regeneration, except that the pygidium and anal cirri can be formed, owing to the local inductive action of the ventral nerve cord, which is always needed for regeneration. Implantation of the brain of an immature worm into the coelom of a young decerebrate one restores the power of regeneration, regardless of whether the donor worm was intact or was itself regenerating. For reasons that we shall see, however, the brain of a mature worm cannot do this. Only one ganglion is needed to demonstrate this effect, for one ganglion contains all the capacity that is needed to promote full regeneration. One half of a ganglion produces less effect than a whole one, while two separate halves can be equivalent to a whole one.

Apparently, then, the brain of an immature worm is capable of secreting a growth hormone, for, since it can produce its growth-promoting action whether it is in its normal position in an intact worm, or whether it is an implant in the coelom, its action is clearly humoral. The same conclusion follows from the fact that a frozen ganglion cannot evoke regeneration. A single dose of the hormone is not,

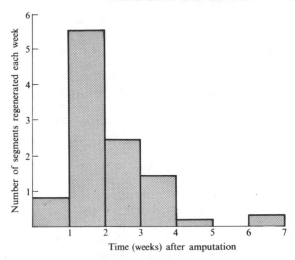
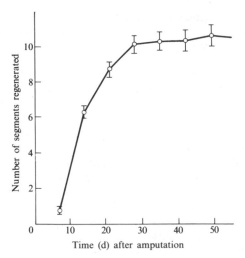

FIG. 13.8. The rate of segment proliferation during regeneration in specimens of *Nereis diversicolor* with *in situ* ganglia. (From Golding (1967). *Gen. comp. Endocrin.* 8.)

therefore, enough; continuous production from a living tissue is required. This continuous secretion can be maintained for a very long time, certainly longer than is needed for normal regeneration. This can be demonstrated by implanting brains into parapodia. Repeated transplantation of the same ganglion from one recipient to another shows that it retains its growth-promoting effect for at least seven months. Further evidence that it is actively secreting throughout regeneration, and is not merely triggering a process which can then continue in its absence, is derived by removing the ganglion from its normal position after regeneration has been in progress for a few days (Fig. 13.9). The result is a slowing down of the regenerative growth.

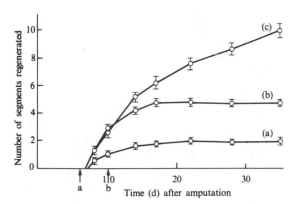

FIG. 13.9. The effect on regeneration of decerebration carried out on *Nereis diversicolor* at different times after segment loss. (From Golding (1967). *Gen. comp. Endocrin.* 8.)

We have mentioned that the number of segments regenerated matches the number removed. How is this ensured? In theory, it might be that there is some type of feed-back from the regenerating tissue to the brain; or the hormone might be more concentrated in the shorter trunk that is left after removal of more segments. However, these possibilities have not been supported by the results of experiments. The most likely explanation seems to be that the brain secretes the growth hormone at a steady rate, and that the number of segments regenerated is determined by the competence of the blastema, which is itself influenced by the level of the body at which it is formed.

Nereids become sexually mature at limited breeding seasons, an arrangement that facilitates successful fertilization of the eggs. The onset of reproduction is marked by the maturation of the sperm, and, in the female, by a phase of rapid growth of the oocytes, associated with vitellogenesis. In some species, there is a metamorphosis into the heteronereid phase; this is an adaptation for sexual swarming, which involves metabolic and structural changes affecting, amongst other parts, the eyes, parapodia, chaetae, and musculature.

Removal of the brain from an immature worm evokes precocious sexual maturation. This can be prevented by implanting a brain from an immature worm, but the brain from a mature one will not have this effect. Clearly, some form of inhibition is operating in immature worms. One explanation could be that the brain secretes an inhibitory hormone which is withdrawn at sexual maturity. It will be noted, however, that this withdrawal coincides with the loss of the power of regeneration. It is possible, therefore, that only one hormone is involved, the growth hormone of immature worms serving also to inhibit sexual maturation in them. Whatever the correct alternative, the endocrine mechanism for separating growth and sexual reproduction seems in principle a simple one.

Yet it is not quite so simple as the facts so far stated may indicate. The precocious sexual maturation induced by removal of the brain from young worms does not lead to normal reproduction, unless the worms are already close to sexual maturity. If they are not, then vitellogenesis is abnormal and fertilization impossible. Ingenious experiments, involving implantation of brains into different-sized pieces of recipient, have shown the explanation of this. A high concentration of hormone inhibits all oocyte development, an intermediate concentration promotes growth and vitellogenesis, while too low a concentration, attained too quickly, leads to abnormal response of the oocytes. Normal development of the oocytes depends upon a progressive decrease in the amount of circulating hormone, and hence upon a delicately organized relationship between the hormone and its target tissue. This suggests a remarkably close parallel with the mode of action of thyroxine during the life of the larval amphibian.

In other respects, too, the simple regulatory mechanisms of nereids suggest comparisons with the more advanced ones of higher forms, but it would be an over-simplification to suppose, because of this, that the polychaete systems necessarily exemplify the foundations upon which further evolution has been based. Even with the polychaetes themselves, there is much variation, and it cannot be assumed that nereid worms, just because they provide favourable experimental material, provide also the best starting point for evolutionary speculation.

For example, sexual maturation is hormonally inhibited in the Syllidae much as in the Nereidae, yet in syllids the hormone concerned is secreted by the pharynx instead of by the brain. Then again, sexual maturation in the lugworm *Arenicola* is controlled by the brain, but in this instance the regulation is mediated not by an inhibiting hormone but by a stimulatory one which is secreted after vitellogenesis is completed. If the brain is removed, the maturation divisions of the eggs are arrested in the prophase of the first division. Moreover, the eggs are not accepted by the funnels of the nephromixia, through which the ripe eggs are discharged. Presumably,

then, the maturation hormone has some effect upon these organs, although *Arenicola* does not undergo the far-reaching somatic changes that accompany reproduction in nereids.

One further variant is found in *Cirratulus cirratus*, which differs from the other species mentioned in breeding throughout the year, instead of having a restricted spawning season. Here an important factor in the regulation of reproductive activity is a negative feedback relationship between the coelomic oocytes of gravid females and the ovaries of the segments which contain them. The presence of these ripe oocytes inhibits the proliferation of young oocytes. When the ripe oocytes have been released, either by natural spawning, or by artificial stripping through longitudinal incisions, the ovaries start to proliferate a new generation of oocytes into the coelom (Fig. 13.10). In contrast to the situation in *Nereis*, the

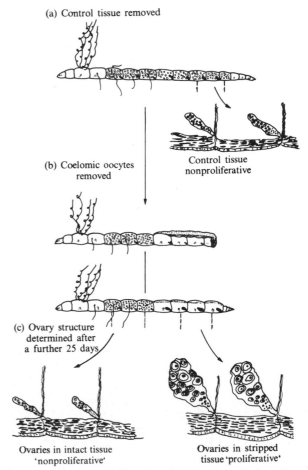

(a) Control tissue removed

Control tissue nonproliferative

(b) Coelomic oocytes removed

(c) Ovary structure determined after a further 25 days

Ovaries in intact tissue 'nonproliferative'

Ovaries in stripped tissue 'proliferative'

Fig. 13.10. Diagrammatic illustration of the partial stripping of coelomic oocytes from gravid *Cirratulus cirratus* females. (From Olive (1973). *Gen. comp. Endocrin.* **20**.)

brain does not influence the growth rate of the oocytes, but it partially inhibits spawning, and is necessary for the proliferation response of the ovary to spawning or stripping.

The principles illustrated in polychaete worms are found operating also in oligochaetes and hirudineans, but again with diversity of detail. Neurosecretory cells occur in the cerebral ganglia of the earthworm *Lumbricus terrestris*, and, as earlier mentioned, in the brain and ventral nerve cord of leeches. Removal of the brain from earthworms inhibits regeneration of the hind end, but in some species the hormone involved is needed for only the first one or two days after the amputation. Moreover, the suboesophageal ganglion may also be involved, for regeneration in *Allolobophora icterica* is only prevented if this ganglion as well as the brain is removed. Reproduction in earthworms also depends upon a cerebral neurosecretion, which evokes maturation of the germ cells and the development of the clitellum. This may also be true of leeches.

These regulatory systems provide the basis for the synchronization of the spawning of polychaetes at a more or less sharply defined breeding season, and the correlation of this with the lunar cycle. In the Mediterranean *Platynereis dumerilii*, for example, there is maximal swarming at the surface of the sea, from March to October, at around the time of new moon. This is because the secretion of the inhibitory (or growth) hormone ceases at the time of the prolonged illumination provided by the full moon. The animals then come into full reproductive condition at about two weeks later, which is the time needed to complete sexual maturation. Thus the cerebral neurosecretory cells are influenced by photoperiod, and this is true even of blinded animals, so that perhaps light directly affects the brain, although, of course, dermal photoreceptors may be involved. In some way unknown the effect of the light can be imprinted upon the animals, for they will spawn at new moon in a given month even though the immediately past full moon may have been obscured by cloud. Indeed, under laboratory conditions, the worms will spawn synchronously after three months of continuous illumination, the time of spawning being determined by the photoperiod which ended before the continuous illumination began. The photoperiod is thus being used by polychaetes to provide predictive information, as we have already seen in birds (p. 135).

13.4. Colour change in crustaceans

Our present understanding of crustacean hormones can fairly be said to originate from studies of the

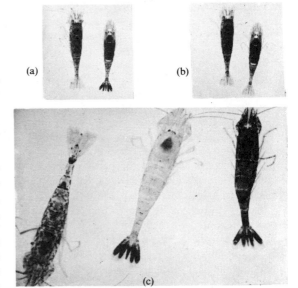

FIG. 13.11. Influence of the eyestalk, and the circum-oesophageal and tritocerebral commissures, on the colour of the shrimp, *Crangon*. (a) Eyestalkless animals; *left*, after injection of sea water; *right*, after injection of an extract of *Crangon* circum-oesophageal commissure, which has darkened the tail. (b) The same two animals as in (a); *left*, after injection of sea water; *right*, after injection of an extract of *Crangon* eyestalk, which has blanched the tail. (From Brown and Ederstrom (1940). *J. exp. Zool.* **85**.) (c) Eyestalkless animals; *left*, after injection of sea water; *centre*, after injection of one-sixth of the sea-water-soluble contents of one *Crangon* tritocerebral commissure; *right*, after injection of one-sixth of the alcohol-insoluble contents of one *Crangon* tritocerebral commissure. All three animals were matched and resembled the left one before the injections, which were made about nine minutes before the photograph was taken. The results indicate that the sea-water extract contains a body-lightening and a tail-darkening principle, the latter alone being present in the alcohol-insoluble fraction. (From Brown and Klotz (1947). *Proc. Soc. exp. Biol. Med.* **64**.)

control of colour change (Fig. 13.11), a field that invites direct comparison with the problems that we were considering in Chapter 12.

Several groups of Crustacea, and particularly the Decapoda, possess chromatophores which are similar to those of vertebrates, being highly branched cells in which pigment granules can be either dispersed or concentrated (aggregated). In general they lie under the hypodermis or in the deeper part of the body, but details of their arrangement and colour vary greatly from species to species. The pigments are of several kinds, including red, yellow, brown, and white, and these can respond independently of each other; probably this is because each is in a separate cell, two or more of which may, however, unite to form a syncitial complex. Whether these cells are in any way homologous with those of the vertebrates is not clear; conceivably they might all have been derived from some primitive pigmentary effector, for colour change is reported to occur sporadically in other groups of invertebrates, including polychaetes, leeches, and echinoderms, but it is certain that this property has been the centre of much independent and unrelated evolution.

The insect *Carausius* (*Dixippus*) *morosus* (p. 257), for example, is able to change its colour without possessing true chromatophores, but best known from this point of view are the peculiar chromatophores of the cephalopod molluscs, each of which is a single cell to which smooth muscle fibres are attached. The action of the latter brings about changes of colour by causing the cell to range in its form from a contracted spherical body to an expanded and very thin disc, but they do not create an endocrinological problem, for these fibres have a direct innervation.

The experimental study of crustacean colour change derives from Pouchet, whose work on the teleosts we have already considered. He made the fundamental discovery that the adaptive responses of shrimps to the colour of their background could be eliminated by the removal of the animals' eyestalks. He had also shown that blinded teleosts failed to show these background responses, and from the results of experimental sectioning of nerves, had rightly concluded that the chromatophores of these animals were innervated (p. 216). He went on to infer that a similar mode of control existed in crustaceans. This was a reasonable interpretation at a time when the principles of endocrinology had still to be established, but it can be seen in retrospect as an example of assuming too readily the existence of similar organization in unrelated groups. In fact, the chromatophores of crustaceans are not innervated, and Pouchet, not surprisingly, failed to demonstrate any effects of nerve section of the sort that were evident in teleosts. Crustacean chromatophores are regulated exclusively by hormones, which are variously referred to as chromactivating hormones, chromophorotropins, or pigmentary effector hormones. As we shall see, the evidence that the chromactivating properties of crustacean tissue extracts are indeed hormones is not yet as complete as that for the hormones of vertebrates, because of the technical difficulties involved in isolating and characterizing them. Nevertheless, it has become sufficiently complete to justify acceptance of their endocrine status.

Our current understanding of these matters dates from the work of Perkins and Koller who, in 1928, published the results of independent studies carried out respectively on the shrimps *Palaemonetes* and *Crangon* (cf. Fig. 13.11). Both of these animals have a range of pigments, the independent responses of which enable them to adapt to a diversity of background colours; *Palaemonetes* to white, grey, black, yellow, red, green, and blue, and *Crangon* to white, grey, black, yellow, orange, and red. The reactions, which may differ in different parts of the body (Fig. 13.11) often depend as in vertebrates upon the albedo, or ratio of direct incident light to the amount of light reflected from the background.

Amongst the facts established by Perkins and Koller were that section of the ventral nerve cord had no effect upon the background responses, but that if the dorsal blood vessel was cut or interrupted, the chromatophores lying posterior to the point of interruption passed into the dispersed state and remained so. If the cut was restricted to a lateral branch of the dorsal vessel, then the chromatophores supplied by that branch became permanently dispersed, while the remainder continued to show normal colour changes. There was no sign of any nerve fibres accompanying the vessels, so that these observations were presumptive evidence of hormonal control. A further indication of this was the fact that if blood from a dark *Crangon* was injected into a pale one, the latter would darken even though it was on a light background. This went some way to meeting the classical requirement that the hormone should be shown to be present in the circulation. As for the source of the hormone, it was found, following up Pouchet's observation, that the chromatophores would pass into the dispersed state in animals that had been blinded by removal of the eyestalks, but that they could be made to concentrate by injecting an extract prepared from crushed eyestalks taken from pale animals. This indicated that the eyestalks were the source of a concentrating hormone.

Background responses are not the only types of colour change in crustaceans. Some of these animals show rhythmical colour change, a well-known example being the fiddler-crab, *Uca*. This animal shows little capacity for background adaptation, but shows a diurnal rhythm resulting in it being pale at night and dark by day (Fig. 13.12). This rhythm, which is independent of the nature of the background, or of the intensity of the illumination, can be maintained under uniform conditions in the laboratory, and will persist for up to 26 days in constant darkness. Evidently, then, the regulation of the rhythm involves an endogenous component of

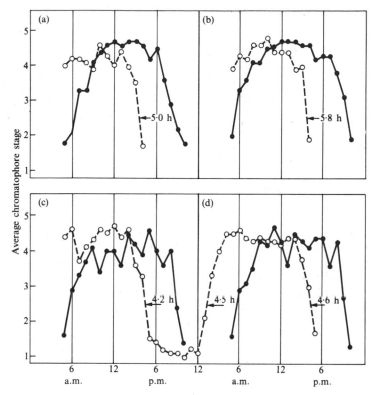

FIG. 13.12. The diurnal colour rhythm in control specimens of *Uca* (solid line) and those with the rhythm shifted backwards (broken line) by three periods of midnight to 6 a.m. illumination; (a) and (b) from one experiment, and (c) and (d) from another. Taking a melanophore index of 2·5 as a reference point, the rhythm is shifted back about 5·4 hours in the first experiment and about 4·4 hours in the second. (From Brown *et al.* (1953). *J. exp. Zool.* **123**.)

some precision, and here the endocrine system is certainly involved.

Eyestalkless animals soon became permanently pale, although the rhythm can be maintained for the first three days after the operation. Presumably the eyestalks secrete a black-pigment-dispersing hormone, but, since the rhythm can be expressed for at least a short time in the absence of the eyestalks, it can hardly depend upon rhythmical release of the hormone. This conclusion is reinforced by the fact that implanting sinus glands (p. 230) into eyestalkless animals restores the diurnal rhythm. One cannot suppose that the isolated gland contains within itself the provision for rhythmic discharge of the dispersing hormone. It is therefore supposed that a black-pigment-concentrating hormone is also involved, and that the rhythmic discharge of this, perhaps from the postcommissure organs, establishes the diurnal colour change by antagonizing the dispersing hormone. The restoration of the rhythm after implantation is ascribed, on this hypothesis, to a continuous output of concentrating hormone from the implanted gland interacting with a rhythmically fluctuating output of a dispersing hormone from elsewhere. The effect of the concentrating hormone can thus be maximally expressed when the level of the dispersing hormone falls around the middle of the day. We shall see that this principle of hormone antagonism has other applications in crustacean chromatophore regulation.

The complications inherent in crustacean endocrinology are well exemplified by the existence in *Uca* of a 12·4 hour rhythm of colour change, which is superimposed upon the diurnal cycle. This rhythm, which corresponds in its periodicity with the phases of the tides, is correlated with the times of high and low tide in the habitat, dispersion of black pigment occurring shortly before low tide. Double peaks of dispersion are therefore seen if low tide occurs in the early morning, because the two cycles are out of phase. With low tide at midday, however, they are in phase with each other, and then there is a single peak (Fig. 13.12).

Such rhythmical properties are a deep-seated and

widespread physiological phenomenon in animals and plants, but no biologist should be satisfied with a statement of their existence unless their adaptive significance can be understood. Unfortunately, this aspect of the rhythmical colour changes of *Uca* is far from clear. The significance of the diurnal rhythm is obscure, for the animal is said to be as active by day as by night. It has, however, been suggested that this rhythm may contribute in some way to the maintenance of the tidal rhythm of colour change. An adaptive significance for the latter is a little easier to formulate for the animal shows a tidal rhythm of feeding activity; the 12·4 hour rhythm may, therefore, be functionally associated with this in some way.

With this recognition of the importance of the eyestalk, a search was initiated for the secretory tissue concerned. Within a few years Hanström had drawn attention to two possible structures. One of these was at first called the blood gland, but was later given the name by which it is now known, the sinus gland, because it lies in the wall of a blood sinus. In its simplest form, as seen in the Mysidacea, this structure is a disc-shaped thickening of the neurilemma of the eyestalk ganglia, but it becomes elaborated in other groups by folding and by separation from the neurilemma, although it retains its close association with the sinus. This position, as

we shall see, has an important bearing on its functioning.

Extraction experiments showed that this sinus gland was a potent source of chromactivating material, but it proved unexpectedly difficult to interpret its histological structure. It contained numerous stainable droplets, and there were indications also of what looked like delicate canals, yet it proved impossible to establish the presence of secretory cells. It was, in fact, difficult to justify calling it a gland, although its physiological importance was not in doubt, and it was clearly innervated by the central nervous system. A further complication was Hanström's identification of a second structure which seemed to have secretory characteristics, and which he designated the X-organ (see later, p. 231).

The resolution of these difficulties provided a powerful demonstration of the value of comparative studies, for it was directly linked with the analysis of the neuroendocrine activity of the hypothalamus and of the nature of the relationship of this with the neurohypophysis. It immediately became evident that this was the key to the interpretation of the secretory activities of the eyestalk, and this led to the recognition that it is the nervous system of the Crustacea which is their most important endocrine tissue. Within the eyestalk it is now possible to recognize many groups of neurosecretory cells (Fig.

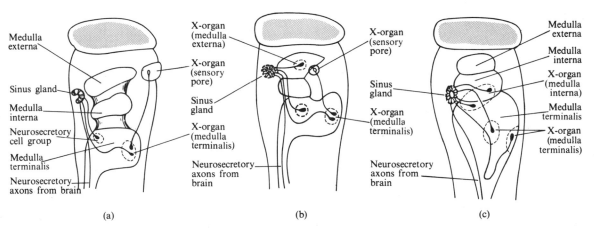

FIG. 13.13. Arrangements of neurosecretory cell groups within the eyestalks of different crustaceans. Dark areas represent neurosecretory cells, light ovals their axon terminals. (a) *Lysmata seticaudata*. The X-organ consists of neurosecretory cells in the medulla terminalis, with the sinus gland as its major neurohaemal organ. The sinus gland also receives axons from neurosecretory cells in the brain. But some neurosecretory cells in the medulla terminalis send axons to the sensory pore X-organ which, despite its name, is another neurohaemal organ. (b) *Palaemon serratus*. There are two areas of neurosecretory cells, called ganglionic X-organs, one in the medulla terminalis and one in the medulla externa, both of which send axons to the sinus glands where they are joined by neurosecretory axons from the brain. The sensory pore is absent in this species, but the sensory pore X-organ remains, supplied by neurosecretory axons from the medulla terminalis. (c) *Gecarcinus lateralis*. In this species there are several ganglionic X-organs in the medulla terminalis and the medulla interna with axons terminating in the sinus gland together with those from the brain. (After Gorbman and Bern, from Highnam and Hill (1969). *The comparative endocrinology of the invertebrates*. Edward Arnold, London.)

13.13), but their anatomical interrelationships are complex, and vary from species to species. We shall not attempt to describe these variations in detail, but shall examine the situation in one or two selected examples.

13.5. The X-organs and the sinus gland

The nervous tissue of the eyestalk is concentrated into three lobes. The most proximal is a brain centre, the medulla terminalis (Fig. 13.15), which is connected with the rest of the protocerebrum by the peduncle of the optic lobe. The other two are primary optic centres, the medulla interna and the medulla externa, the latter being directly connected with the most distal optic centre, the lamina ganglionaris. An important source of neurosecretory material is to be found in one or more groups of cells which lie in the medulla terminalis, for stainable droplets have been identified in these cells, and also in the axons which arise from them (Fig. 13.14). Unfortunately, the term X-organ has been applied to these cell groups in the mistaken belief that they are the homologue of the X-organ described earlier by Hanström and other workers

of the 1930s. In fact, however, the two are quite distinct, so that the medullary cell group is now called the ganglionic X-organ. Where they are more than one, they are named according to the particular medulla with which they are associated.

Many nerve fibres from the ganglionic X-organ run to the sinus gland, a structure which is largely and perhaps exclusively a storage and release centre for neurohormonal products arising elsewhere, mainly in the ganglionic X-organ. The two structures thus form a functional unit which can be called the ganglionic X-organ/sinus gland complex, the sinus gland being the neurohaemal organ of the unit. This, of course, is the explanation of its association with a blood sinus, and of its puzzling histological structure; like the neural lobe of vertebrates, it consists largely of the terminations of neurosecretory axons. We shall see that it is not the only neurohaemal organ in crustaceans. There is some reason for thinking that such centres may have arisen simply as local thickenings of the neurilemma, as is still seen today in the mysids, the development of more elaborate forms serving to facilitate the release of their contained secretions into the circulation.

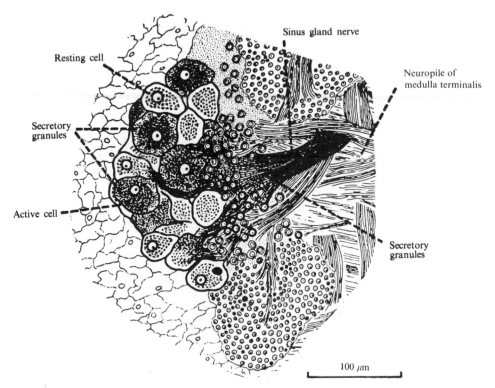

FIG. 13.14. A section which indicates the passage of secretory granules from giant neurosecretory cells of the medulla terminalis of the crab *Sesarma* into the sinus gland. (From Enami (1951). *Biol. Bull.* **101**.)

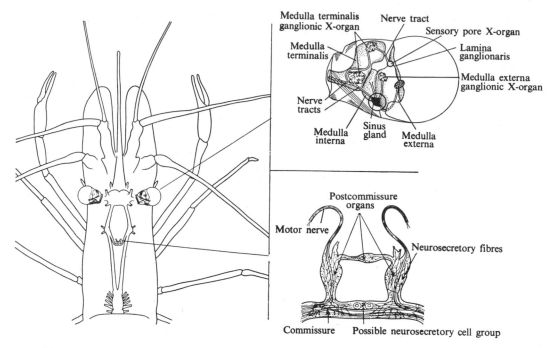

FIG. 13.15. Diagrams illustrating the approximate positions of the sinus gland, X-organs, and postcommissure organ of *Palaemon* (*Leander*) *serratus*. In this species the sensory pore has been lost, but the sensory-pore X-organ retained. (From Knowles *et al.* (1955). *J. mar. biol. Assoc. U.K.* **34**, and Carlisle and Knowles (1959). *Endocrine control in crustaceans.* Cambridge University Press, London.)

The presence of neurosecretory material gives to the sinus gland in the living animal a characteristic opalescence which greatly facilitates its recognition and experimental removal. In the fixed gland, this material shows a diversity of staining reactions, responding positively both to acidic and to basic dyes. This presumably reflects a corresponding diversity of secretions, although the possibility that some transformation or processing of these secretions takes place within the sinus gland cannot be excluded. The question whether cells are present in it is still a matter of dispute, but even if they are, it is doubtful whether they make any contribution in the form of an actual synthesis of secretion. The term gland is therefore a misnomer. What is certain, however, is that the products released from it must be of a varied nature and this, as we shall see, is in line with the results of physiological studies.

In the blue crab, *Callinectes sapidus*, for example, no less than six distinct types of neurosecretory fibres can be distinguished on the basis of their staining reactions, some staining red with azocarmine, others yellow with orange G, blue with aniline blue, or red with aldehyde fuchsin, a situation reminiscent of the complexity of the staining reactions of the pars distalis. We need to know much more about the

significance of these reactions, but they provide some evidence that each fibre may carry one particular type of secretion, for the colours can be traced back to individual cells. It has thus been possible to unravel something of the pattern of distribution of nerve connections; this has shown not only that the sinus gland receives neurosecretory fibres from the ganglionic X-organ (Fig. 13.15), but that other structures are also involved.

We have seen that the ganglionic X-organ is not the same as the X-organ of Hanström. The latter (Fig. 13.15) is typically associated with a sensory papilla or with a sensory pore derived from this by reduction, and for this reason it is called the sensory papilla X-organ or sensory pore X-organ. Its histological organization is more complex than that of the other structures so far mentioned. It is composed in part of the club-shaped endings of neurosecretory fibres, but sensory cells are also present, together with epithelial secretory cells and neurosecretory cell bodies, at least in some species. Thus in the natantian *Lysmata*, the sensory papilla X-organ is widely separated from the medulla terminalis ganglionic X-organ and receives neurosecretory fibres from it (cf. Fig. 13.15), so that it evidently acts in part as a neurohaemal release organ. In addition, however, axons of its sensory cells unite to form a nerve which runs to the medulla terminalis, so that at this stage of its evolution it is clearly an organ of mixed function.

The degree of separation of the two types of X-organ varies a good deal in the decapods, ranging from the condition just described to that found in the Brachyura, where the two form a single complex lying mainly within the medulla terminalis. This latter arrangement is associated with the loss of the sensory papilla and, if it can be regarded as expressing an evolutionary trend, implies an increasing concentration upon the neurosecretory functions of an originally heterogeneous organ. As yet, however, we lack an assured basis for the determination of the evolutionary history of the endocrine complex of the eyestalk.

13.6. Chromactivating hormones and the central nervous system

Our emphasis so far has been upon the neurosecretory tissue of the eyestalk, but secretions influencing the chromatophores are not restricted to that region. They are found also in the tritocerebral (post-oesophageal) commissure, which connects the circum-oesophageal commissures immediately behind the oesophagus. Two fine nerves (Figs 13.15 and 13.16) leave the tritocerebral commissure, and in *Penaeus braziliensis*, *Squilla mantis,* and *Palaemon* (*Leander*) *serratus* these each bear a flattened lamella which differs in its exact position in the several species but is formed in all three by an extension of the epineurium. Nerve fibres and chromophil droplets are found in these lamellae, which thus closely resemble the sinus gland in their organization. This resemblance is heightened by the fact that extracts of them are especially potent sources of chromactivating material, and it is clear that these structures, which have been called the postcommissure organs, are neurohaemal release organs. The fibres that enter them probably arise in the brain, and transport material formed in neurosecretory cells in the tritocerebrum. The function of neurosecretory-like cells in the commissure remains uncertain.

This exemplifies a characteristic feature of the endocrine system of Crustacea: a widespread distribution of neurosecretory cells in the nervous system. Our present information suggests that the cells dominate the organization of crustaceans to an extent far exceeding anything that we find in vertebrates, and we can feel certain that other examples await detailed analysis. Cells of supposed neurosecretory

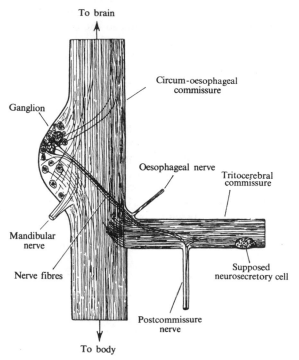

FIG. 13.16. Left connective ganglion and left half of the tritocerebral commissure of *Palaemon* (*Leander*) *serratus*. The fibres and cell bodies shown were seen in preparations stained by methylene blue. (From Knowles (1953). *Proc. R. Soc. Lond.* B141.)

character have been found in other sites, as, for example, in the commissural and thoracic ganglia of crabs. The variety of their staining reactions suggests that, if they are indeed neurosecretory cells, they constitute a variety of cell types which may eventually be found to be concerned with a wide range of regulatory functions, fully comparable with the range of activities which are now thought to be under hormonal control in these animals.

Our discussion of similar problems in vertebrate endocrinology has already shown, however, that the analysis of endocrine systems is fraught with difficulties unless supposed hormonal functions can be securely related to highly purified secretions. One need only recall in this connection how the actions of growth hormone were at one time attributed to individual but hypothetical secretions. Clearly a similar approach must be adopted towards crustacean problems, and, as already mentioned, sufficient progress has been made along these lines to give some support to the general assumption that these chromactivating substances are indeed hormones.

Early studies, based on the fractionation of extracts by differential solubility, showed that eyestalk extracts of *Crangon* could be fractionated into two principles; one of these blanched the body and tail, while the other blanched the body alone. Further, extracts of the tritocerebral commissure also contained two fractions, one of which blanched the body alone, while the other darkened both the body and tail. This suggested that movement of the black pigment in this animal might be regulated by three or even four different substances.

Electrophoresis has proved equally suggestive. For example, it has permitted separating from the sinus gland and postcommissure organs of *Palaemon* (*Leander*) *serratus* a substance with a concentrating action on the large and small red chromatophores, and from the postcommissure organs a substance which concentrates the large chromatophores but disperses the red ones of the body and tail.

Another illustration of the results of electrophoresis is seen in Fig. 13.17. This shows that eye-

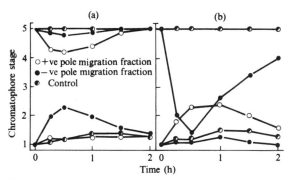

FIG. 13.17. Responses of dark red chromatophores of dwarf crayfish on white and on black backgrounds to extracts of (a) eyestalks and (b) supra-oesophageal ganglia with the circumoesophageal connectives attached. Filter paper electrophoresis was carried out on the extracts before injection. (From Fingerman and Aoto (1958). *J. exp. Zool.* **138**.)

stalks of the dwarf crayfish, *Cambarellus*, contain a fraction which disperses dark-red pigment and which migrates towards the negative pole, while the combined supra-oesophageal ganglia and circum-oesophageal commissures contain a fraction which has a similar effect but which migrates towards the positive pole. The inference is that there are here two substances which are chemically different yet similar in their physiological action. An analogous contrast is seen between the concentrating fractions of the two extracts.

Experiments of this type are open to a number of obvious objections. Chromactivating substances are unstable, so that the products of chemical separation may be artifacts. The results of injection experiments

may be confused by the sensitivity of chromatophores to the surrounding medium, while the injected material may release active principles from the recipient's neurosecretory system, rather than act directly upon its chromatophores. And there are questions that need to be answered, particularly regarding the chromactivating properties of the central nervous system. Why, if this activity is physiologically important, does it not replace the action of the sinus-gland products when the sinus gland and postcommissure organs of *Palaemon* how, given the impossibility of removing parts of the central nervous system and carrying out the classical procedures of replacement therapy, can it be shown that chromactivating substances present in the nervous system do indeed play a physiological role in colour change?

Experiments have given some help in resolving these problems. One example involved keeping *Palaemonetes vulgaris* on either white or black backgrounds for varying periods up to 14 days. Extracts of the circum-oesophageal and tritocerebral commissures prepared from animals kept for 14 days on a white background contained much more red-pigment-dispersing activity, and much less concentrating activity, than did extracts prepared from animals that had been kept on a black background for the same time. After only two hours on these backgrounds, however, the activities of the two extracts were much closer. The conclusion suggested is that continued production over 14 days of a red-pigment-concentrating principle results in a reduction in the amount present in the nervous system, and that this is evidence that it is used in normal colour responses. As regards the functional necessity for the provision of multiple neurosecretory sources for chromactivating substances, it can be argued that each neurosecretory centre may have its own characteristic sensory input, so that one centre will not necessarily be an exact functional replicate of another.

Ultimately the resolution of these uncertainties must rest upon improved methods of purification of the hormones, with chemical characterization as the ultimate goal. Here the use of gel filtration and ion exchangers has proved of particular value in purification studies, because hormonal action is localized in specific peptide peaks, revealed in the usual way by optical-density measurements. For example, a white-pigment-concentrating substance has been isolated from a shrimp, *Crangon crangon*, and from a prawn, *Pandalus jordani*, by gel filtration on columns of Sephadex G-25, and partially purified. It is found to be rapidly inactivated by trypsin and by pronase, which indicates (as has been widely assumed for these chromactivating substances) that it is a polypeptide. Moreover, comparisons of the material obtained from the two genera suggests no chemical or biological differences between the two, other than could be accounted for by the presence of contaminants; it is supposed, on this and other grounds, that these chromactivating hormones are not species-specific.

The purification of the red-pigment-concentrating hormone of *Pandalus borealis* has been carried further than this, using 20 μg of a preparation obtained from 100 g of lyophilized eyestalks. This hormone, too, is a polypeptide, and is found to contain eight amino acids (aspartic acid, glutamic acid, glycine, leucine, phenylalanine, proline, serine, and tryptophan).

Another important principle, inferred from earlier work already mentioned, and strengthened by these newer purification studies, is that the chromactivating hormones interact by antagonism. For example, aqueous extracts of the eyestalk of the crab *Rhithropanopeus harrisi* concentrates the black pigments of *Crangon*. Gel filtration of the extract, however, permits the isolation of several hormones; a black-pigment-dispersing hormone occurs in zone IB (Fig. 13.18; Table 13.1), a white-pigment-concentrating one in peak IV, and a red-pigment-concentrating one in peak VI. Why, then, does the crude aqueous extract show no dispersing effect? The answer is that the concentrating activity of the crude extract is due to the red-pigment-concentrating hormone, which concentrates other pigments as well as the red one. Black-pigment-dispersing action is absent from the crude extract, because this hormone

TABLE 13.1

Distribution of chromatophorotropic hormones from the eyestalk of the crab Rhithropanopeus harrisi *after gel filtration on Sephadex G-25, tested on pigment cells of the shrimp* Crangon crangon.† (From Skorkowski (1972). *Gen. comp. Endocrin.* **18**, 329–34.)

Fraction	Tube Number	Black-pigment-dispersing hormone activity score‡	White-pigment-concentrating hormone activity score‡	Red-pigment-concentrating hormone activity score§
IA	35–44	3·3	0·0	0·0
IB	45–55	27·0	0·0	0·0
II	56–62	0·0	0·0	0·0
III	63–71	0·0	1·7	0·0
IV	72–80	0·0	25·0	3·7
V	81–95	0·0	0·0	0·0
VI	96–109	0·0	0·0	24·6
VII	110–119	0·0	0·0	15·8
VIII	120–124	0·0	0·0	2·7
IX	125–144	0·0	0·0	0·0
X	155–170	0·0	0·0	0·0

† Activity scores by method in which 10 μl of each fraction equivalent to one eyestalk was injected into each animal.
‡ Tested on pleopods.
§ Tested on the dorsal side of the body.

is antagonized by the red-pigment-dispersing one. These antagonistic relationships make it easier to understand why aqueous extracts of decapod eye stalks have long been known to concentrate pigments in eyeless shrimps, and yet disperse black pigment in crabs. But no doubt other factors, too, are involved, including specializations of target cells, and differences in endocrine balance, to name only the most obvious.

One may reasonably conclude that the chromatophores of crustaceans are regulated by a multiple hormone system; a conclusion which, by one of life's little ironies, has become strengthened during the period in which the bi-hormonal theory of vertebrate chromatophore regulation was being weakened. But the field remains one of the utmost complexity, in which prudent investigators move cautiously, one step at a time, and avoiding the temptation to regard every active material that comes their way as being necessarily a distinct hormone.

13.7 Retinal pigment migration

It is because of historical accident and experimental convenience that the study of colour change has played such a conspicuous part in the development of crustacean endocrinology, but many other functions are also under endocrine regulation. Closely

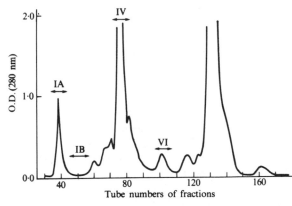

FIG. 13.18. Separation by gel filtration of the aqueous extract of the eyestalk from the crab *Rhithropanopeus harrisi*. Hormonal activities were found in zone 1B and peaks IV and VI. cf. Table 13.1 (From Skorkowski (1972). *Gen. comp. Endocrin.* 18.)

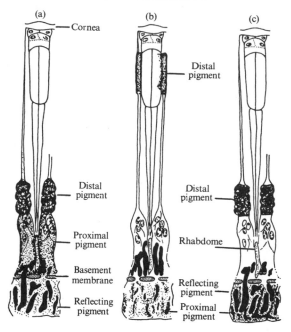

FIG. 13.19. Ommatidia from the eyes of *Palaemonetes vulgaris*. (a) Light-adapted; (b) dark-adapted; (c) light-adapted position of distal pigment in an eye of an animal which, after adaptation to darkness, was injected with eyestalk extract prepared from light-adapted animals. (From Kleinholz (1936). *Biol. Bull.* **70**.)

related to colour control is the adaptive migration of the pigment of the compound eye, which takes place in response to the intensity of light which falls upon the organ. Each eye consists of a large number of units called ommatidia (Fig. 13.19), with which are associated characteristic groupings of pigment cells. The crystalline cone is surrounded by distal pigment cells, the inner portions of which (e.g. in *Palaemon* (*Leander*) *serratus*) contain dark pigment and are distally continuous with the cornea and proximally with the retinular cells. The latter give rise at their bases to nerve fibres, but their cell bodies contain further pigment known as the proximal pigment. Finally, a group of tapetal cells at the base of the ommatidium contains a white reflecting pigment.

There is some variation in the pattern both of the pigment cells and of their responses, but in general the proximal pigment moves upwards in illuminated conditions and downwards in darkness; these two reactions, known respectively as light adaptation and dark adaptation, have the effect respectively of either screening the photoreceptor cells or exposing them to maximum illumination. There is no convincing evidence that these movements are under hormonal

control, and they may well be direct responses to illumination, but a hormone certainly regulates the responses of the distal pigment cells, in which light adaptation involves a proximal movement and dark adaptation a distal one.

It was first shown in 1936 that injection of *Palaemonetes* with eyestalk extracts would bring about light adaptation of the distal pigment in dark-adapted animals, and it was subsequently demonstrated that *Palaemon* (*Leander*) would remain permanently dark-adapted after removal of the sinus glands, even though the eyes themselves were left quite undamaged. These findings, closely analogous to those obtained in studies of background responses already discussed, indicate that light adaptation must be regulated by a hormone. Fractionation of aqueous extracts of sinus glands has separated the hormone concerned (distal-retinal-pigment hormone) from the erythrophore-concentrating hormone mentioned earlier, but it has yet to be established whether it is completely distinct from other chromactivating hormones.

13.8. Hormones and the crustacean moulting cycle

It has long been known that the eyestalks have some influence on the moulting of crustaceans, and it has been natural in recent years to look for evidence of hormonal regulation analogous to that demonstrated in insects. In dealing with this process it is convenient for descriptive purposes to divide the moulting cycle into four stages. These comprise (*i*) proecdysis (premoult), in which preparations for moulting take place, including the removal of calcium from the exoskeleton, cessation of feeding, and the beginning of secretion in the epidermis as this separates from the exoskeleton; (*ii*) ecdysis (moult), the short stage during which the exoskeleton is shed; (*iii*) metecdysis (post-moult), a gradual return to normal during which the skeleton hardens; and (*iv*) intermoult, the normal condition. The intermoult may consist either of a long period called anecdysis in those animals that have a seasonal moult, or of a short period called diecdysis in those that have a succession of moults throughout the year. In either case it is the period of maximal growth, in the sense of protein synthesis and the formation of new tissue, for the apparent growth that marks the moult stage is a swelling that results from the absorption of water (or of air in terrestrial forms).

Hormonal control of the moulting cycle is demonstrated by the observation that removal of the eyestalks from decapods during the intermoult stage initiates proecdysis, and that this effect can be counteracted by the implantation of sinus glands into such animals. The eyestalks, and more particularly the sinus glands, are thus shown to be the source of a moult-inhibiting hormone. The effect of this hormone, however, is strictly confined to delaying the inception of proecdysis; if the eyestalks are removed during proecdysis, there is no accelerating effect upon the remainder of the moult.

The experiments upon which these conclusions were initially based antedated the unravelling of the true nature of the sinus gland, and some confusion was at first caused when it was found that removal of this gland by itself had no effect at all, whereas removal of the complete eyestalk in the same species clearly accelerated the onset of proecdysis. The explanation of this apparent paradox lies in the

results from a withdrawal of this hormone, but nothing is known of the factors, exogenous or endogenous, which determine this change of activity.

The moult-inhibiting hormone does not act directly upon the tissues, but exerts its effect through an organ called the Y-organ. This structure, which is innervated from the sub-oesophageal ganglion, lies in either the antennary or second maxillary segment, depending upon the situation of the excretory organ of the species concerned, and it varies somewhat in its form. Its physiological significance is clear-cut, for its complete removal during the intermoult or early proecdysis will prevent moulting, and will also prevent either the removal of the eyestalks, or the injection of eyestalk extracts, from having any effect at all upon the moulting cycle. Thus the Y-organ

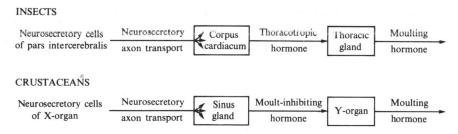

Fig. 13.20. Diagram of the control of moulting in crustaceans and insects.

organization of the neurosecretory system of the eyestalk which we have just outlined. The accelerating effect can be obtained if, instead of removing the sinus glands by themselves, these organs are removed together with the neurosecretory cells in the ganglionic X-organs which supply them. The importance of this functional relationship, already seen in our analysis of the physiology of colour change, is further emphasized by the demonstration that the precocious moulting which results from eyestalk removal can be eliminated completely by implanting both the sinus gland and the ganglionic X-organ with their nervous connections intact. If, however, they are implanted separately, or with their connections cut, the elimination is only partial. These experiments show that a moult-inhibiting hormone is secreted in the ganglionic X-organ and is transmitted through neurosecretory fibres to the sinus gland for storage and release. The hormone may be thought of as responsible for the control of the duration of the intermoult, at least in those species in which the stage is prolonged as a result of moulting being seasonally restricted. The end of the intermoult presumably

must be the source of the actual moulting hormone, the moult-inhibiting hormone of the eyestalk being a tropic hormone acting upon the Y-organ. It follows that proecdysis is initiated by the Y-organ releasing a hormone in response to a reduction in output of the moult-inhibiting hormone of the ganglionic X-organ/sinus gland complex. Removal of the Y-organ at a later stage of proecdysis has no effect upon the impending moult, but it blocks the next one.

We shall see later that this situation presents a remarkable parallel with the regulation of moulting in insects, and is a good illustration of the unity as well as of the diversity that emerges from comparative studies. The Y-organ is analogous to the thoracic (prothoracic) gland of insects, in that both produce a moulting hormone; the two organs may even be homologous, but of that we cannot be sure. However, the activity of the Y-organ is *inhibited* by its regulatory neurosecretory hormone, whereas, as we shall learn, the activity of the insectan thoracic gland is *stimulated* by the corresponding neurosecretory hormone (Fig. 13.20).

Since moulting is merely a special incident in the

growth processes of Crustacea, imposed upon them by the nature of the exoskeleton, we might expect that the hormones regulating it would, like the growth hormone of vertebrates, be closely linked with a variety of metabolic processes, but it is difficult to judge how far this is actually so. The sinus gland is certainly involved in regulating some metabolic processes, but it is not clear how many hormones are concerned, or whether any are identical with the moult-inhibiting hormone itself.

We have noted the importance of water uptake at the moult. This is probably regulated by a water-balance hormone which inhibits water uptake, for eye-stalkless *Carcinus* increase in volume at ecdysis by about 180 per cent, whereas intact animals increase by only about 80 per cent. This increase in the operated animals, which is due to abnormally large water uptake, can be counteracted by injecting extracts of the sinus gland, while injections of these glands into intact crabs result in a lowering of the increase below the normal value. This water-balance hormone is probably distinct from the moulting hormone. For example, sinus gland extracts can only delay proecdysis when they are prepared from crabs that are in the intermoult stage; water uptake, however, is reduced by extracts prepared at any stage of the moult cycle. This raises the question, not yet answered, whether the water-balance hormone comes from the same neurosecretory centre as does the moulting hormone, or from a separate one.

Two other metabolic processes for which hormonal regulation has been plausible suggested are the regulation of the blood-sugar level, and the production of digestive enzymes. Blood-sugar levels in *Callinectes sapidus* are increased after the injection of sinus gland extracts, supposedly by a hyper-glycaemic hormone. This perhaps mediates the hyperglycaemia that results from stressing intact animals, for hyperglycaemia does not appear in stressed animals from which the eyestalks have been removed. As regards the regulation of enzyme production, removal of the eyestalks from the cray-fish *Procambarus clarki* results in decreased synthesis of amylase in the digestive gland (the so-called hepatopancreas). But the effect is probably more far-reaching than this, for the removal is followed by a general decrease in the RNA content of the cells of the gland, with restoration to a normal level if eye-stalk extracts are injected.

These findings are only partial evidence for the existence of distinct hormones regulating metabolic functions, but they reinforce the impression given by studies of the chromactivating properties of sinus gland extracts. The X-organ/sinus gland complex impinges on many functions, and it follows that the deceptively simple act of injecting an eyestalk extract into a crustacean must create a profound physiological disturbance. The full extent of this will not be exposed until the active principles have been isolated and their separate properties investigated. Chrom-activation studies have already provided good pointers to the way ahead.

13.9. The pericardial organs

The pericardial organs (Fig. 13.21), discovered by Alexandrowicz in 1952–3, are groups of nerve fibres lying in the pericardial cavity, and containing membrane-bound granules of a diameter of about 120 Å. They are supposedly neurosecretory. Extracts of the organs increase the amplitude and frequency of the beat of the isolated heart. It is thus supposed that in some way they supplement the neurogenic regulation of the heartbeat, which is mediated by accelerator and inhibitor fibres connecting the intact heart with the cardiac ganglion. Perhaps the neural regulation is concerned with short-lived responses, and the pericardial organ with responses of longer duration. It was at first supposed that the active product of the pericardial organs was either serotonin or a closely related compound, since this affects the heartbeat. It is now known, however, that the active substance (there may, indeed, be two) is a peptide, like so many other neurosecretory products of animals. That serotonin is not involved follows, in any case, from the fact that its action upon the heart can be experimentally blocked, yet that organ will still respond to extracts of the pericardial organs, or to the peptide preparation.

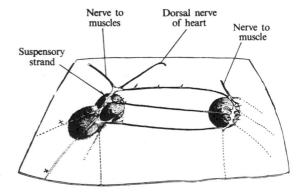

FIG. 13.21. Pericardial organs of the right side of *Maia squinado*, with part of the lateral pericardium wall showing the three openings of the branchio-cardiac veins. The nerves running from the central nervous system into the pericardial organs are drawn in dotted lines. (From Alexandrowicz (1953). *J. mar. biol. Assoc. U.K.* **31**.)

13.10. Sex hormones in crustaceans and parasitic castration

Reproduction in the malacostracan Crustacea depends upon hormones originating in several different organs. One of these is the androgenic gland (Fig. 13.22), discovered in 1954. Its functioning has been particularly studied in the amphipod *Orchestia gammarellus*, but it exists in the males of all orders

masculinized, with male copulatory appendages, and sperm appear in the ovary; such individuals may become the fathers of daughters. In the genetic female the androgenic gland does not develop at all; in this sex the gonad develops into a functional ovary without the action of any hormone.

Nevertheless, the ovary is under hormonal regulation, for the development of eggs outside the normal breeding season is prevented by an ovary-inhibiting

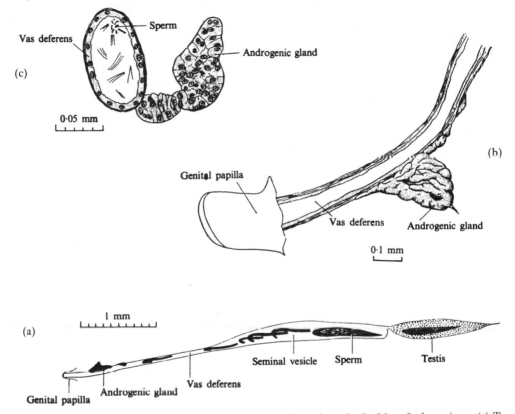

FIG. 13.22. (a) Position of the androgenic gland of *Orchestia gammarellus*. (b) Androgenic gland in a fresh specimen. (c) Transverse section of gland and vas deferens. (From Charniaux-Cotton (1957). *Ann. Sci. Nat. Zool.* **19**.)

of the Malacostraca except the Isopoda in which, however, the testes seem to act as a substitute for it. This gland, which is distinct from the gonad and is attached to the vas deferens (the duct that leads from the testis to the genital papilla), is essential for the development of the testes and of the male external sexual characters. If it is removed, the animal reverts to an indeterminate (i.e. non-sexual) stage at the next moult; an ovary transplanted into such an animal may be able to mature and thus evoke the appearance of brooding characters (see below) at a later moult. If the androgenic gland is transplanted into a female, on the other hand, the animal becomes

hormone secreted in the ganglionic X-organ/sinus gland complex. The evidence for this includes the fact that removal of the eye stalk leads in many decapods to precocious ovarian development and oviposition, which can be at least partially prevented by the implanting of sinus glands. Moreover, the normal ovarian development which ushers in the breeding season can be prevented by the injection of eyestalks, or of the separate parts of the complex. The precise effects of eyestalk removal depends upon the age of the operated animals. Removal from sexually immature *Palaemon* accelerates the moult (as explained earlier), but does not affect the development of the oocytes. This suggests that the ovary-inhibiting hormone is distinct from the moulting hormone, but, regardless of whether it is or not, we see once again the dissociation of growth from reproduction, as we have in vertebrates, *Hydra*, and annelid worms.

The ovary also exerts its own positive effect upon sexual differentiation, for it evokes the appearance of two distinct types of secondary sexual character, perhaps by the secretion of two distinct hormones. The action of the ovary is well seen in *Orchestia*. The mature female possesses a permanent brood pouch, formed by plates called oostegites, which bear long ovigerous hairs. These hairs, however, unlike the oostegites themselves, are not permanent; they appear only at the moults preceding egg laying, and

The demonstration of the hormonal regulation of sexual characters in crustaceans, and the identification of the secretory organs concerned, have clarified one of the classical problems of crustacean physiology: the phenomenon of parasitic castration (Fig. 13.23). This was first reported in 1881 but it received its name from Giard, who published a series of papers on the subject between 1886 and 1888. It is best known in crustaceans and insects, and, as found in the former group, results from parasitization either by rhizocephalan Cirripedia or by epicaridian Isopoda. Both groups of parasites are very highly specialized. The former develop through larval and endoparasitic stages into sac-like structures which are attached to the exterior of their crustacean host and which feed upon the latter by mean of a branching root-like

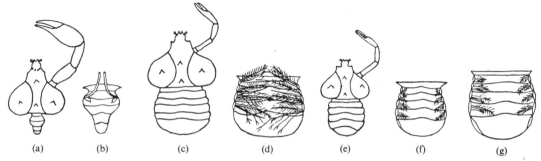

FIG. 13.23. Parasitic castration of the crab *Inachus*. (a) normal male; (b) male abdomen in ventral view; (c) normal female; (d) female abdomen in ventral view; (e) sacculinized male with 'female' characters (small chela and broad abdomen); (f) abdomen of sacculinized male in ventral view showing 'female' character (pleopod); (g) abdomen of sacculinized female. (After Smith, from Hanström (1939). *Hormones in invertebrates*. Clarendon Press, Oxford.)

are thus absent from non-reproducing females. In consequence, ovariectomy of a female bearing ovigerous hairs results in their disappearance at a subsequent moult. Implantation of ovarian tissue into an ovariectomized female, however, evokes yolk deposition, and this is followed by the reappearance of the hairs. Implantation of an ovary into a male after its androgenic glands have been removed results in the appearance of oostegites at a subsequent moult. This effect is produced regardless of the sexual condition of the donor, which implies that the hormone concerned is secreted continuously. The ovigerous hairs, however, develop only at particular stages of the sexual cycle, suggesting intermittent production of a second ovarian hormone, distinct from that regulating the development of oostegites. Nevertheless, the possibility of the effects of the ovarian secretion being modulated by target specialization does not seem to be wholly eliminated in these experiments.

system ramifying inside its body. As for the Epicaridea, one family, the Bopyridae, live either in the gill chamber or attached to the abdomen of a decapod host, while another family, the Entoniscidae, live in the haemocoele of crabs; unlike the Rhizocephala, they obtain their nutriment by the direct sucking of the blood of the host.

The literature relating to parasitic castration is extensive and complex, and the responses of the host are so variable that it would be impossible to attempt a survey of them here. The essential facts are, however, that the presence of the parasite causes changes in the external sexual characters (Fig. 13.23), and that these may be associated with a greater or lesser degree of destruction of the gonads. In general, the external changes have been said to involve a feminization of the male, which may develop, for example, the broader abdomen of the female and certain abdominal appendages normally absent in males, while the copulatory appendages characteristic of the latter are reduced. The effects upon the female are very much less and there is certainly no masculinization, although there may be some hyperfeminization shown in the precocious establishment of the female form of abdomen in an immature animal.

Earlier attempts to interpret this phenomenon in terms of hormonal control were largely based upon hypothetical analogies with vertebrates, and, in particular, upon the supposed production of sex hormones by the crustacean gonads. It was suggested that the external changes in the host were due to endocrine disturbance resulting from the destruction of the gonads, but this view was difficult to sustain, since critical examination showed no close correlation between the degree of external change and the degree of degeneration of the gonads, nor were the time relationships at all well correlated. This encouraged the development of other suggestions, such as the well-known one that the supposed feminization of *Inachus* by *Sacculina* resulted from the latter creating in its host a modification in its fat metabolism similar to that resulting in the female from the demands created by yolk deposition. Against this, however, was the fact that feminization of structure may begin in the normal life-cycle before the onset of vitellogenesis.

It is now possible to see that these difficulties of interpretation arose from the circumstance that here, as in much other invertebrate endocrinological research, physiological investigations preceded the morphological identification of the glands concerned; a course of events which has usually been reversed in the development of vertebrate endocrinology. It is now evident that the hormonal regulation of sex in crustaceans does, indeed, bear some resemblance to that of vertebrates, but yet differs from it in one crucial respect: the origin of the male hormone in an organ that is separate from the testis. 'Nature', to quote words used by Ronald Ross in quite another context, 'was more resourceful and astute than all of us'.

The effects of the parasite upon the sexual characterization of the male can now be readily explained as a result of the parasite's removal of the androgenic hormone from the blood, and, eventually, of the destruction of the androgenic gland itself, with the result that the host reverts to the non-sexual condition. The belief that the parasitized male is actually feminized is in part a misconception arising from the fact that the external form of the female departs less from the non-sexual condition than does that of the male. The situation is also influenced, however, by the fact that in the absence of the androgenic gland the gonad of a female develops into an ovary, because there is no androgenic gland present. It is thus possible for an ovary to develop in a parasitized male, and to evoke the appearance of brooding characters through the hormone or hormones which it can then secrete. To this extent parasitism may indirectly bring about sex reversal in the host. No doubt other factors may also be involved in the changes effected by parasitic castration, for the parasite may well exert the powerful metabolic and toxic influences that have often been postulated, and it is known, too, that the roots of a rhizocephalan can damage the neurosecretory cells of the thoracic ganglion of the host. There is thus much scope for profound disturbances of the complex hormonal balance of these highly organized animals.

It is interesting, in the light of our earlier discussion of evolutionary relationships (p. 220), to note that the control of sexual organization in Crustacea has much more in common with the pattern found in vertebrates than that found in insects. This applies, as we shall see, to the fundamental importance of sex hormones in the crustaceans and vertebrates, while another, although more superficial, resemblance between the two groups lies in the production by the ovaries of hormones that are concerned with making preparation for the care of the young. The unique feature in the Crustacea, however, and one which convincingly illustrates the danger of looking for too close a degree of resemblance between the plans of organization of unrelated groups, is the androgenic gland, for the production of a sex hormone, capable of determining the primary as well as the accessory characters, by a gland that is entirely separate from the gonad has no parallel within the vertebrates. Indeed, such a situation does not appear to have been described in any other group of the animal kingdom.

14

Hormones in invertebrates II

14.1. Insect life histories

The study of the endocrinology of insects, in contrast to that of Crustacea, has centred particularly around the analysis of moulting and growth, but there are also striking parallels to be noted, both in the results themselves and in the ways in which they have been achieved. Here again we encounter the difficulty that the physiological observations have sometimes been in advance of the anatomical ones, so that the full significance of the endocrine pattern has been unfolded only slowly, but the results are peculiarly satisfying, both in the elegance of the experimental treatment of the problems and in the applicability of their interpretation to species of widely different habits.

The growth of insects, like that of crustaceans, and for the same reason, is marked by a series of moults or ecdyses, at each of which the old cuticle is detached, the epidermal cells divide, and a new cuticle is laid down. Since this process is so sharply defined in time, and since it determines the size, proportions, and general appearance of the animal, it has been a major focus of endocrinological analysis. We have seen ample evidence in other groups that this kind of response, involving as it does the whole of the body, lends itself particularly well to hormonal control, so that the first questions to be answered are whether such control is operative here and, if so, where the hormones are secreted, what is their nature, and what determines the periodicity of their actions.

In seeking the answers to these questions we shall be referring particularly to two species which have proved exceptionally well suited for experimental treatment, the reduviid bug, *Rhodnius prolixus*, and the giant American silkworm moth, *Hyalophora* (*Platysamia*) *cecropia*. The former has a typical hemimetabolous life history, with five larval (nymphal) instars preceding the adult stage, while the latter is holometabolous, with five larval instars passing into the adult stage through a pupal instar. It has often been held that such life histories are composed of a sequence of stages of progressive differentiation, with the implication that the future adult begins its life in an imperfect form. However, a more acceptable interpretation is that the insect life history carries to an extreme the tendency, which is already pronounced in many lower invertebrates, for the larva and adult to undergo independent and increasingly divergent evolution in adaptation to two different modes of life. The caterpillar of *Hyalophora*, for example, is devoted to growth, and with such intense concentration that during early summer it increases its weight 5000 times; at pupation its accumulated assets are then invested, as Williams puts it, in the construction of an essentially new type of organism, a flying-machine devoted to reproduction.

The life history, on this interpretation, is regarded as an example of polymorphism, the individual having the capacity for existing in one or other of two alternative forms, with the intervening pupal stage providing the opportunity for the drastic reorganization which is involved in the metamorphosis of the holometabolous type of insect. The larva thus contains, in a latent and unexpressed form, the capacity for adult differentiation, and the reverse could also be true, except in so far as metamorphosis may involve irreversible changes which eliminate from the adult tissues the capacity for larval differentiation.

This point is illustrated by the effect of wounds upon the epidermal colour pattern in *Rhodnius*. The larva has black spots on the lateral hind margin of the segments while the adult bug has these on the lateral anterior margin. If a burn is applied between two spots in the larva, the wound is repaired by the migration of cells from the adjacent black areas, and these carry with them the potentiality for producing black pigment in the larva. So, at the next moult these black areas are found to have fused (Fig. 14.1). However, the burn has destroyed those cells which possess the particular capacity for producing black

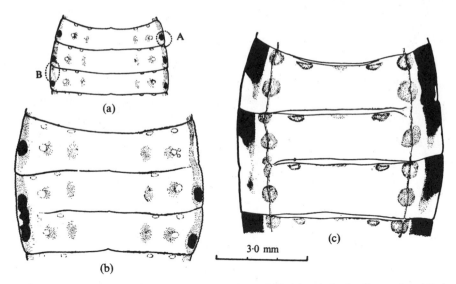

FIG. 14.1. (a) Third, fourth, and fifth tergites of a normal third instar larva of *Rhodnius*; the broken lines at A and B show the regions burned. (b) Corresponding segments in the resulting fifth instar. (c) Corresponding segments in the resulting adult. (From Wigglesworth (1940). *J. exp. Biol.* **17.**)

spots in the adult, and the migrating cells cannot replace this capacity since they do not possess it; hence, after metamorphosis the corresponding black areas will be absent. Clearly, then, each cell must be thought of as possessing two sets of potentialities, one appropriate to the larva and one appropriate to the adult, and another of our problems is therefore to establish the nature of the switch mechanism determining which particular form shall be realized at any one moult. By analogy with Crustacea, we may expect this, too, to be hormonal, for we have seen how in that group the course of a moult may be modified by, for example, the presence of an ovarian hormone capable of evoking the formation of brooding characters.

14.2. Ecdysone and the thoracic gland

The first demonstration of a probable hormonal control of an insect life-cycle dates from 1917–22, when Kopeč showed that if larvae of the moth *Porthetria* (*Lymantria*) *dispar* were tied with a thread before a certain critical stage during their last larval instar, only the portion of the body anterior to the ligature would pupate; the remainder maintained its larval form. Since the cutting of the nerve cord had no such effect, there was good reason for suspecting that a hormone was concerned, and there was reason also for suspecting an involvement of the brain, for he was able to show that removal of this before the critical stage would prevent pupation, while if the brain were reimplanted pupation would

proceed. Here at once we see how the remarkable resistance of insects to drastic manipulation makes it possible to meet some of the classical requirements of vertebrate endocrinology, such as removal and replacement of a suspected gland, by an entirely novel type of experimental procedure.

Much further evidence for the hormonal control of growth and moulting accumulated during the 1930s, more particularly under the stimulus of Wigglesworth's investigations of *Rhodnius*, to which we shall refer below, but the source of the hormone remained in doubt until the demonstration by Fukuda in 1940 of the significance of the thoracic (prothoracic) gland. This, in Lepidoptera, is a paired and much-branched organ which extends from the head into the prothorax along trunks of the tracheal system. Glands which are thought to correspond with it (Fig. 14.2) are present in most groups of insects, although their actual homology with the lepidopteran one is usually a matter of assumption. In *Rhodnius*, however, the homology can be justified on embryological grounds, for both in this animal and in Lepidoptera the gland arises in the same way from the ectoderm of the second maxilla.

The importance of Fukuda's work lay in the demonstration that if the larva of the silkworm was ligatured transversely at a level behind this gland, only the anterior portion would pupate, but that the posterior half would also do so if a thoracic gland were implanted into it. Similar results, obtained either by ligature or by transection, have since been

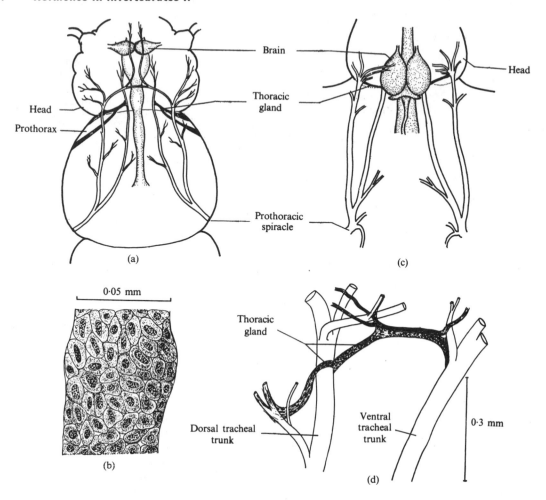

FIG. 14.2. Thoracic glands of coleopteran larvae. (a) *Nebria brevicollis*, in natural position (semi-diagrammatic); (b) *N. brevicollis*, histological appearance; (c) *Elater rufipennis*, gland in relation to dorsal and ventral tracheal trunks. (From Srivastava (1959). *Q. Jl microsp. Sci.* **100**.)

obtained for other species, including *Rhodnius* and *Hyalophora*. Isolated posterior regions of pupal stages of the latter may survive for over a year without undergoing any further development; the implantation into them of living thoracic glands will, however, promptly cause them to resume their development.

It is now accepted, as a result of this and other work, that a moulting hormone, ecdysone, is secreted by the thoracic gland or its homologue. Useful material for its further study is provided by puparium formation (pupariation) in Diptera, the stage at which the cuticle of the larva hardens by tanning of its proteins immediately before the establishment of the pupal stage (pupation). After transverse ligation of mature larvae of the blowfly, *Calliphora*, only the anterior portion forms a puparium, provided that the operation is carried out more than sixteen hours before that event (Fig. 14.3). Puparium formation can, however, be evoked in the posterior end of such a specimen by injecting into it some blood from an anterior end. This is because the reaction depends upon ecdysone, which is secreted in the anterior region. After the critical period, at about sixteen hours before puparium formation, this hormone becomes distributed throughout the body so that the whole of this is able to react, even though part may be separated by ligature from the initial source of the hormone. This source is the ring gland of Weismann, a compound organ which consists of the corpus allatum (see below) dorsally, the corpus cardiacum (see below) and hypocerebral ganglion ventrally, and

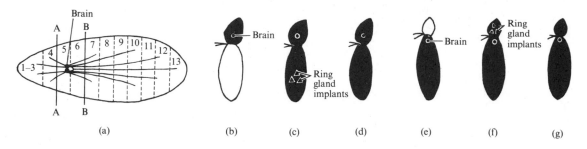

FIG. 14.3. The puparium reaction in muscid larvae. (a) Diagram of a larva. Ligatures may be placed in front of the brain and ring gland (at line A——A) or behind them (B——B). (b)–(g) the regions showing the puparium reaction are indicated in black. (b) Ligatured behind the brain before the critical period; ecdysone is confined to the anterior region. (c) As (b) but with ring glands implanted into the body posterior to the ligature; ecdysone from these evokes a reaction, provided that the larval donors have passed the critical period. (d) Ligatured behind the brain after the critical period; ecdysone has become distributed throughout the body. (e) Ligatured in front of the brain before the critical period; ecdysone is confined to the posterior region. (f) As (e) but with ring glands implanted into the body anterior to the ligature; ecdysone from these evokes a reaction provided that the larval donors have passed the critical period. (g) Ligatured in front of the brain after the critical period; ecdysone has become distributed throughout the body. (From Turner (1948). *General endocrinology*. Saunders, Philadelphia.)

the homologue of the thoracic gland (here called the peritracheal gland) on either side. The functional relationships are exactly as in *Rhodnius* and *Hyalophora*; removal of the peritracheal gland will prevent puparium formation, and this can then be induced by the implantation of peritracheal gland material from third-stage larvae, provided that these have passed beyond the critical stage. Such implants will also induce the reaction in parts of the body which have been separated by ligature from the source of ecdysone (Fig. 14.3).

The classical requirement of the demonstration of the presence of ecdysone in the blood has been met to a large extent by parabiosis experiments (cf Fig. 14.11) in which, for example, a *Rhodnius* larva decapitated before the critical period, and therefore unable to moult, is joined by capillary tube to a larva decapitated after the critical period. Both will now moult, the inference being that the former is stimulated to do so because it now shares a common circulation with the latter and receives the hormone from it in the blood stream. Actually, such insects readily become united by regenerating epidermis, so that the possibility of some stimulating agent being distributed through the tissue is not entirely eliminated in these particular experiments. However, the results of other ones have completed the proof. For example, the female pupae of certain hybrid moths which do not normally moult into adults can be induced to do so by introducing into them some blood from moulting male pupae.

The *Calliphora* puparium reaction provides the basis for a convenient bioassay procedure for the hormone. The principle of the method is to ligate

the larvae transversely in the anterior third of the body and thus to restrict puparium formation to the region anterior to the ligature, the posterior region being isolated by the ligature from the peritracheal gland. The anterior part of the puparium is then cut off and the test solution injected into the posterior region; the percentage response of the latter, as indicated by puparium formation, is a sensitive measure of the hormone content of the test solution. Commonly, the response can be evoked by 0·01 μg ecdysone, a quantity termed one *Calliphora* unit.

Ecdysone has been isolated in crystalline form, and the preparation of 250 mg from 4000 kg wet weight of *Bombyx* pupae has permitted chemical characterization and synthesis. It is a steroid, present in *Bombyx* (and in some other insects as well) in two forms, α-ecdysone and β-ecdysone (Fig. 14.4). It is thought that the hormone is secreted as α-ecdysone and then rapidly transformed into β-ecdysone outside the gland. Ecdysone has the same carbon skeleton as cholesterol (cf. Fig. 7.1, p. 106), and radioactive studies show that insects synthesize it from that substance. However, they are unable to synthesize cholesterol itself, and have therefore to obtain it from their plant or animal food. Large quantities of biologically active ecdysones have, indeed, been obtained from plants; this has led to the highly speculative suggestion that insects may initially have obtained this potentially hormonal material from plants, and that later they evolved the capacity for synthesizing it for themselves.

The name of the hormone expresses the fact that it evokes ecdysis. As part of this action, it induces the synthesis of dihydroxyphenylalanine (dopa) decar-

α-ecdysone

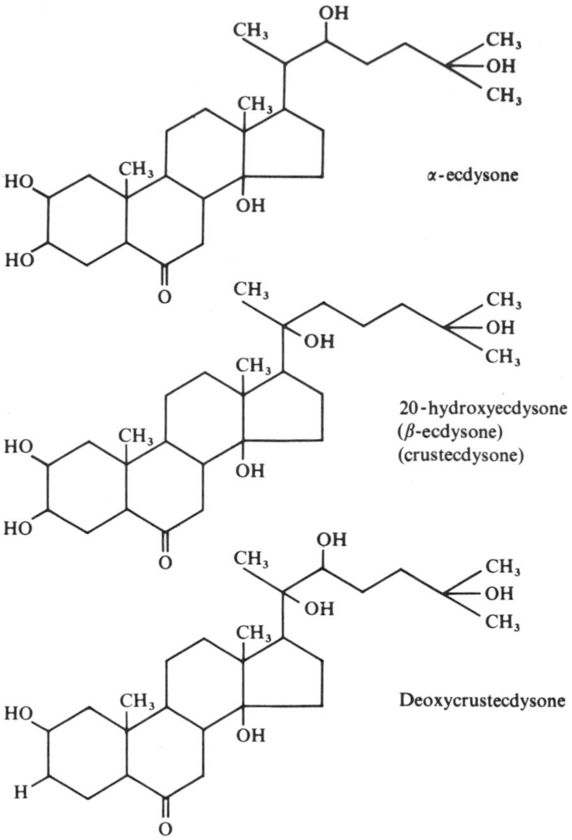

20-hydroxyecdysone
(β-ecdysone)
(crustecdysone)

Deoxycrustecdysone

FIG. 14.4. Ecdysones.

boxylase, thereby permitting tanning of the cuticle. It also regulates mitotic activity and growth processes in certain tissues, including the epidermis. Thus, if the ring gland is removed from the larva of *Calliphora*, the imaginal buds cease to grow although the animal continues to feed. Other evidence comes from *Rhodnius*, in which the ventral abdominal muscles are fully developed only when the old cuticle is actually being shed; directly afterwards, they undergo autolysis, so that only the muscle sheath and nuclei remain. Within six hours of injecting the hormone, these nuclei and their nucleoli enlarge, and increasing amounts of nucleic acid become visible (Fig. 14.5). These effects have led to ecdysone being referred to as the growth and moulting hormone, but this term needs to be used with caution, for insect growth, as reflected in increase in weight, is a continuous process. Presumably the growth of individual tissues depends upon their genetic programming, with modulation, where appropriate, by hormonal regulation.

The injection of ecdysone into *Chironomus* larvae is followed within 15–30 minutes by the appearance of swellings, or 'puffs', on the giant chromosomes of the salivary glands and other tissues. These puffs (Fig. 14.6), which are essentially enlargements of specific bands on the chromosomes, indicate RNA synthesis, each being the site of elaboration of a specific messenger RNA. Moreover, individual tissues have their own characteristic puffs, and certain of these are related to certain stages of

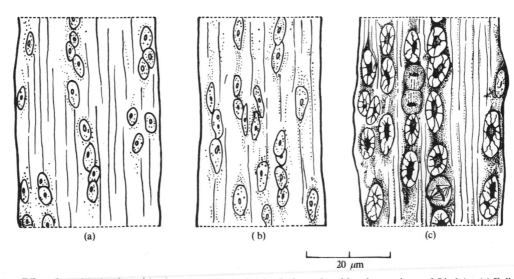

(a)   (b)   (c)

20 μm

FIG. 14.5. Effect of 'nutrition' and moulting hormone on ventral abdominal muscles of fourth-stage larva of *Rhodnius*. (a) Fully starved condition. (b) Exposed to 'nutrition' alone for 4 days. (c) Exposed to 'nutrition' plus moulting hormone for 4 days. (From Wigglesworth (1963). *J. exp. Biol.* **40**.)

FIG. 14.6. A stage specific puff in part of a giant chromosome of *Chironomus tentans*. The same bands can be identified in both the mid-larval (*left*) and late larval (*right*) stages. One of the bands is puffed in the late larval but not in the mid-larval stage. (From Highnam and Hill (1969). *The comparative endocrinology of the invertebrates.* Edward Arnold, London.)

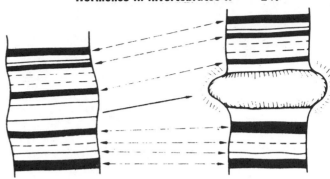

development (Fig. 14.8). Clearly, the puffs are expressions of the activity of specific genes, and it has therefore been held that their formation after ecdysone treatment indicates that the hormone regulates development by direct action on the genes. It will be recalled that a somewhat similar conclusion is suggested by biochemical studies of the action of thyroxine. However, puffing can also be evoked by ionic changes, and it has therefore been suggested that what ecdysone actually does is to modify the ionic milieu within the nucleus. We are confronted here, in these problems of the mode of action of hormones, by one of the key questions presented by the analysis of endocrine systems, and almost everything still remains to be learned about it. In any case, ecdysone does not exert an overriding control of development. We shall see that the action of another hormone (juvenile hormone) must also be taken into account, and that this, too, is involved in chromosome puffing.

The availability of the pure hormone has made it possible to show that ecdysone, like many other hormones, is not species specific. It induces moulting in *Rhodnius*, pupation in Lepidoptera, and puparium formation in Diptera; moreover, its action is not restricted to any one stage of development, for it stimulates the emergence of the imago which follows diapause in Lepidoptera and Hymenoptera (see later). Of particular interest is the question of its possible identity or relationship with the corresponding hormone of Crustacea, for there are clearly some remarkable resemblances in respect of the control of moulting in the two groups. Having regard to all these facts, it is not surprising to find it suggested that the Y-organ and the thoracic glands may be homologous. In any case, however, the evidence for this is incomplete, and the possibility needs to be weighed critically in the light of our earlier discussion of homology and phylogenetic relationships.

The Y-organ is controlled by a cerebral neurosecretion, and so also is the thoracic gland of insects (see later), although there is a difference here in that this control is inhibitory in Crustacea and excitatory in insects. The moulting hormones also function in similar ways, for the secretion of the Y-organ is required for the initiation of proecdysis, but not for its continuation, and this appears to apply also to ecdysone. Further, the Y-organ of *Maia* degenerates after the last moult, while in insects it is common for the thoracic gland to disappear at that stage.

These similarities are strengthened by chemical evidence. Ecdysone accelerates moulting in some crustaceans, while extracts of the whole body of *Crangon* contain a fraction that produces a positive puparium response. Included in this fraction is a substance called crustecdysone, which has been characterized as β-ecdysone. Another ecdysone, deoxycrustecdysone, is also found in crustacean extracts, and others may well be present. Of course, these may be steroid precursors or metabolites, and their hormonal status, if any, remains to be clarified; there is still much to be learned regarding insectan steroid biochemistry. One illustration of the possibilities is the presence of deoxycorticosterone in certain water-beetles; it has been suggested that this might act as a defence mechanism, by disturbing steroid balance in vertebrate predators, but it is hard to see how this would operate in practice.

14.3. Neurosecretion and the thoracotropic hormone

We must now consider what determines the periodicity of the insect moult. We have seen in Kopeč's work a suggestion that the brain might be involved in the moulting process, and so indeed it proves to be. Our understanding of its importance in this regard derives from Wigglesworth's studies of *Rhodnius*, which showed that the periodicity of its moult was causally related to its feeding habits.

The larva takes a large meal of blood on one occasion only during each instar, and it is this event

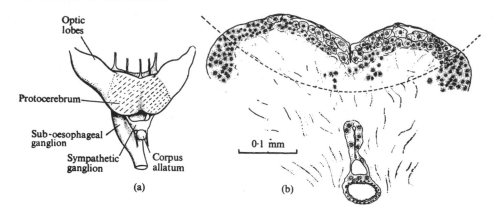

FIG. 14.7. (a) Brain of fifth-stage nymph of *Rhodnius*. (b) Vertical section through the posterior part of the protocerebrum; in the central region above are the large neurosecretory cells, while ordinary ganglion cells lie laterally. The shaded area in (a), and the broken line in (b), indicate the approximate limits of the region which, when excised and implanted into fourth-stage nymphs decapitated at 24 hours after feeding, will cause these to moult. (From Wigglesworth (1940). *J. exp. Biol.* **17**.)

which determines the onset of the moult, although a critical period of up to a week or so has to elapse before this determination becomes effective. Thus, if the animal is decapitated during the first day or two after the meal, it will never moult, although it may live for as much as a year, without growing at all during that time. A decapitated larva will, however, moult normally if the removal of its head is delayed until after the lapse of the critical period. A large meal is an essential factor in this response, for an equivalent amount of blood divided into several small meals will not result in the inception of moulting. It can thus be inferred that the stimulus arising from a large meal (actually, the stretching of the gut wall) evokes the secretion of a hormone in the head, but that the effect of this does not become fully developed during the first day or two. After the critical period, however, moulting can proceed normally without any further supply of the hormone being needed, so that decapitation will no longer have any inhibitory effect.

The next step in the analysis required the identification of the source of the hormone, and this was again made by Hanström, who drew attention, in 1938, to the presence of large secretory cells, filled with stainable droplets, in the median region (pars intercerebralis) of the protocerebrum. It was then shown that if this region (Fig. 14.7) was removed from a larva at about the critical period, and implanted into one that had been decapitated immediately after feeding, the latter was caused to moult. Since no other part of the brain had this effect, it was clear that these cells were the source of the hormone. For a time it seemed possible that this brain hormone might be the moulting hormone itself, but Fukuda's work almost immediately showed that this could not be so. What the brain hormone does is to activate the secretion of ecdysone by the thoracic gland; it is therefore named the thoracotropic hormone.

Later, when the significance of neurosecretion in the organization of the endocrine systems of vertebrates and crustaceans had been established, it became apparent that the secretory activity of the pars intercerebralis of insects provided yet another example of this; the cells concerned are, in fact, neurosecretory ones. They are usually present as two medial and two lateral groups. For example, in *Hyalophora* there are twenty-six in all; eight in each of the two medial groups, and five in each lateral one. The axons of the medial ones decussate in the middle line, and then form a pair of nerves, while those of the lateral ones form another pair without decussation. These nerves all join and run to an organ called the corpus cardiacum, which is a complex structure composed partly of secretory cells (many of which may be neurosecretory ones) and partly of neurosecretory nerve endings. At least part of it, however, is a neurohaemal organ, serving for the storage and release of secretion that has been formed in the pars intercerebralis, and perhaps also for the further processing of this secretion.

The relationship between the corpus cardiacum and the pars intercerebralis is clearly similar to that existing between the neural lobe and the hypothalamus in vertebrates, and between the sinus gland and ganglionic X-organ in crustaceans, and the nature of the complex has been demonstrated in very similar ways. For example, the characteristic granules of the cells can also be seen in their axons in the

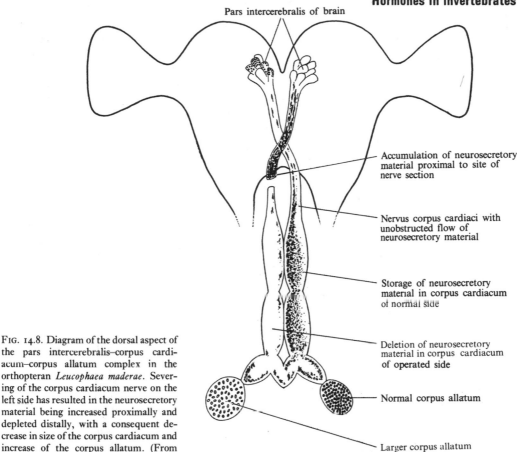

Pars intercerebralis of brain

Accumulation of neurosecretory material proximal to site of nerve section

Nervus corpus cardiaci with unobstructed flow of neurosecretory material

Storage of neurosecretory material in corpus cardiacum of normal side

Deletion of neurosecretory material in corpus cardiacum of operated side

Normal corpus allatum

Larger corpus allatum of operated side

FIG. 14.8. Diagram of the dorsal aspect of the pars intercerebralis–corpus cardiacum–corpus allatum complex in the orthopteran *Leucophaea maderae*. Severing of the corpus cardiacum nerve on the left side has resulted in the neurosecretory material being increased proximally and depleted distally, with a consequent decrease in size of the corpus cardiacum and increase of the corpus allatum. (From Scharrer (1952). *Biol. Bull.* **102**.)

medial corpus cardiacum nerves and in the corpus cardiacum itself. If one of these nerves is cut in *Leucophaea*, the secretory material accumulates proximally to the cut and disappears distally (Fig. 14.8); an experiment and a result precisely comparable with the demonstration of the transport of hypothalamic neurosecretion in the vertebrates by sectioning of the pituitary stalk. Further, ligaturing one of these nerves in the blowfly, *Calliphora erythrocephala*, results in an accumulation of secretory material in the axons above the ligature. It seems likely, therefore, that the secretion is normally released through the corpus cardiacum. Since, however, the relevant part of the protocerebrum can certainly evoke the moulting response in *Rhodnius* when it is transplanted by itself, the possibility of direct release of the secretion from the brain into the blood is not excluded.

As regards the factors promoting this release, we have seen that the initial stimulus in *Rhodnius* is the stretching of the wall of the gut by the ingested blood of a large meal. In consequence the effect of the meal can be entirely eliminated, with the prevention of any hormonal discharge from the brain, by cutting the nervous connections between the latter and the abdomen. This influence of the alimentary canal has been further confirmed by recording the passage of nerve impulses through the corpora cardiaca nerves from the brain. In an unfed larva the impulses are rare, but they are discharged at a rate of about three per second after feeding, and discharge can also be evoked in an unfed animal by stretching the abdomen. Not all the fibres in these nerves are neurosecretory, so that it cannot be assumed that it is this type which are conducting the impulses. It seems likely, however, that they may be doing so, for we know that ordinary nerve cells combine the capacity for conduction with that of secretion (p. 59), and it is not obvious what advantage would be gained if neurosecretory cells had developed the latter at the cost of completely losing control over the release of their own product. Nevertheless we cannot be sure that this is so, and we must leave open, as we did in discussing vertebrate neurosecretion, the possibility that the release of neurosecretion from nerve endings may be evoked by impulses passing in ordinary fibres lying adjacent to them.

There is also doubt as to the exact course of events which follows this discharge in the corpus cardiacum. Hormone release begins in *Rhodnius* within a few minutes of ingestion, yet it must continue for several days (to the critical period) if moulting is to result. This suggests that some interaction has to develop, perhaps between the thoracotropic hormone and the thoracic gland, or perhaps within the corpus cardiacum. An important aspect of the situation, which strengthens the comparison already made with the vertebrate endocrine system, is that ecdysone interacts by negative feed-back with the pars intercerebralis, its release leading to inhibition of the output of cerebral neurosecretion.

The chemical nature of the thoracotropic hormone is uncertain, but it seems likely to be a polypeptide. The hormone of *Periplaneta* is said to have a molecular weight of 20 000 to 40 000, but chemical evidence in this field is difficult to evaluate because of the likelihood that the preparations contain other proteins as well.

What is certain is that the thoracotropic hormone is not the only hormone originating in the brain, for the medial neurosecretory cells of blowflies (*Sarcophaga*, *Phormia*, and *Calliphora*) secrete a hormone called bursicon, which regulates tanning of the cuticle and influences other aspects of cuticular development as well, including the formation of the endocuticle. This hormone has been identified also in newly emerged adults of other insects, including locusts (*Schistocerca*, *Locusta*) and cockroaches (*Periplaneta*). Ecdysone, it will be recalled, is also involved in tanning. The contribution of bursicon, it has been suggested, may perhaps be the removal of permeability barriers, with the consequent facilitation of the tyrosine metabolism that is an essential part of the tanning process.

Bursicon is a peptide, with a molecular weight of about 40 000, which perhaps makes it a little more likely that the thoracotropic hormone is also a peptide. However, it is certainly distinct from the latter, for, although bursicon activity is found in the brain and corpus cardiacum, the hormone is mainly released into the blood from the ventral nerve cord (the fused thoraco-abdominal ganglia in blowflies, or the last abdominal ganglion in locusts and cockroaches).

14.4. Hormones and insectan diapause

An illustration of the way in which the general principles outlined above can be applied to the inter-

pretation of a specialized situation is provided by diapause in *Hyalophora*. Diapause is a condition of arrested development which depends upon physiological specialization and is quite distinct from the temporary inhibition or quiescence which may be produced by the action of adverse factors in the environment and which ceases as soon as these factors disappear. The distinction between this and diapause is of the same order as that between the simple winter sleep of certain mammals such as the brown bear and the specialized physiological adaptation called hibernation. Both hibernation and diapause are essentially ecological adaptations which enable the species to resist some unfavourable aspect of their environment, and which demand, among other things, the previous laying down of food reserves.

The experimental analysis of diapause has attracted the attention of many investigators, so much so that a reviewer of the subject writing in 1932 was able to cite 347 titles in his bibliography. Yet at that time no clear understanding of the physiology of the process had emerged, although there was some evidence that pupal development in Lepidoptera depended upon an active centre in the thorax (Fig.

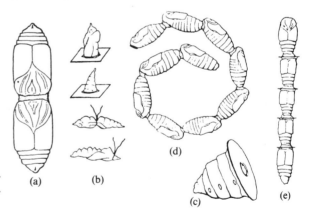

Fig. 14.9. Examples of methods used in the investigation of growth and moulting in insects. (a) One of the experiments of Crampton (1899) to show simultaneous development of *Hyalophora* pupae joined with paraffin. (b) Experiments of Hachlow (1931); pupae of *Aporia* and *Vanessa* are ligatured, or divided and sealed by paraffin to glass slides, and pupal development is shown to be initiated by a centre in the thorax (thoracic gland). (c)–(e) Experiments of Williams (1952) on *Hyalophora* pupae. (c) Isolated abdomen caused to develop by implantation of thoracic glands and chilled brain. (d) Chain of ten brainless diapausing pupae induced to develop by implantation of a chilled brain into the leading pupa. (e) Four abdomens of diapausing pupae are joined to a chilled pupa with brain and prothoracic gland; only the anterior-most abdomens develop, as only they receive adequate concentrations of ecdysone. (From Wigglesworth (1954). *Physiology of insect metamorphosis.* Cambridge University Press, London.)

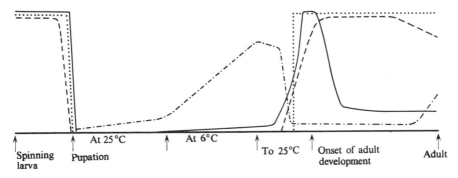

FIG. 14.10. Sequence of events associated with pupation in *Hyalophora*. —— release of prothoracotropic hormone; ...... electrical activity of brain; ——— cholinesterase in brain; —·—· acetylcholine-like substance in brain. (From van der Kloot (1955). *Biol. Bull.* **109**.)

14.9(b)). This lack must be ascribed in part to the absence of any sound foundation of endocrinological principles, and to the unsuitability of much of the experimental material. It is in this latter respect that *Hyalophora* has proved so useful, for with an adult weighing up to 8 g it is amongst the largest of American insects, while it has a particularly characteristic and well-defined form of obligatory diapause into which the pupae enter at the beginning of the instar. They remain in it during the winter and if they are kept at ordinary room temperature while they are in this condition they will never metamorphose. This diapause can only be brought to an end by chilling them for one to two months at a temperature of 3–5 °C.

Analysis of this phenomenon has been based partly upon the use of isolated abdomens sealed by wax to cover-slips; these lack the thoracic gland and are consequently unable to moult. If, however, the glands from post-diapausing (i.e. activated) pupae are implanted into such abdomens these will metamorphose, and may even lay some eggs. That the brain stimulates the thoracic glands by releasing the thoracotropic hormone has been shown by grafting pupae together with wax (Fig. 14.9(a)). If a diapausing pupa from which the brain has been removed is grafted to a chilled (activated) and intact pupa it will moult synchronously with the latter as a result of receiving some of its thoracotropic hormone. The grafting together of pupae of different species shows that this hormone is neither species nor genus specific. Its capacity for diffusion and stimulation is particularly well shown in experiments in which chains of brainless pupae have been constructed (Fig. 14.9(d)); if a single chilled (activated) brain is implanted into the most anterior member of the chain its influence will gradually spread so that they will all metamorphose as a result of the successive activation

of their thoracic glands. If, however, one is detached before this activation process has reached it, then it will be unable to metamorphose. Finally, this interaction of brain and thoracic glands is convincingly shown by experiments in which a previously chilled brain is implanted into the posterior end of a diapausing pupa together with two pairs of diapausing glands; the latter are activated by the brain hormone and will then evoke metamorphosis in the abdomen (Fig. 14.9(c)).

These facts suggest that this form of diapause must be initiated in the normal life-cycle by the withdrawal of the thoracotropic hormone, and electrophysiological studies provide some indication of the physiological adaptations which this involves (Fig. 14.10). The insertion of microelectrodes into the brain shows that after the end of diapause a spontaneous activity can readily be detected, as it can be in the brains of caterpillars. On the other hand, the brain of a pupa during diapause is electrically silent. All trace of activity disappears suddenly just before pupation, to reappear immediately prior to the resumption of development at the end of diapause, at about the time when the secretion of the brain hormone is thought to begin once again.

This is paralleled exactly by changes in the cholinesterase content, for this enzyme is present in considerable quantities in the brain of the larva, is absent during diapause, and reappears towards the end. During this same period the amount of acetylcholine-like substance in the brain slowly increases until, with the appearance once again of cholinesterase, the content falls and electrical activity can again be detected. Thus the pupal diapause of *Hyalophora* involves what amounts to a complete 'shutting-down' of the brain; a condition which is the more remarkable in that it affects no other part of the central nervous system, for the ganglia of the ventral nerve cord retain their spontaneous activity and their normal content of cholinesterase. We see in this an interesting consequence of the maintenance by the segments of the arthropod body of a considerable degree of independence; a situation which contrasts markedly with the tendency towards unification which overrides much of the initial metamerism of the vertebrates.

As regards the mode of action of ecdysone, already mentioned above (p. 247), there is some suggestion that in *Hyalophora* it may influence the cytochrome system, for this is active in the larva but inactive during diapause, as is shown, for example, by the insensitivity of the diapausing pupa to cyanide. This is associated with an absence of cytochrome c, and the synthesis of this is one of the characteristic features of the end of the diapause. However, even if this is a direct consequence of the action of ecdysone it could not be of universal significance, for diapause in insects is not always associated with reduced activity in the cytochrome system. Here, as with comparable problems in vertebrate endocrinology, we must await the results of a great deal of further investigation.

Diapause may also occur in adult insects, being usually expressed in a lack of development of the oocytes. An example is seen in the silkmoth, *Bombyx mori*. Here diapause is facultative, being determined by the conditions in which the previous generation of eggs developed, instead of being invariable, as in *Hyalophora*. Adult moths derived from eggs that developed at 15 °C lay non-diapause eggs. Those derived from eggs that developed at 25 °C lay diapause eggs, the production of those also being favoured by long photoperiod during egg development.

This situation differs from the pupal diapause just described in that it depends not upon the absence of developmental hormones but on the presence of an inhibitory one. The brain of diapause producers stimulates the release of an inhibitory hormone from neurosecretory cells in the sub-oesophageal ganglion, the influence of the brain being transmitted through the circum-oesophageal commissure, although whether by neurosecretory transmission is not clear. The adaptive significance of this facultative diapause is obvious. Non-diapause eggs are laid in the favourable conditions of summer, as a result of the development of the previous generation of eggs during the colder weather and shorter photoperiods of spring. Eggs laid in the favourable conditions of summer, however, yield adults that lay diapause eggs, which thus avoid the unfavourable conditions of winter. How the relationship between the two generations of eggs is brought about is not clear; presumably some chemical change, induced in the developing egg, persists into the cerebral tissue of the pupa (in which oocyte development begins) and of the adult.

14.5. Metamorphosis and juvenile hormone

So far we have discussed the regulation of moulting without reference to the closely associated problem of metamorphosis, and it is this which we must examine next. In *Rhodnius*, the metamorphic moult occurs at the end of the fifth larval instar and results in the appearance of the full assemblage of adult characters. It is actually an over-simplification to regard this last moult as completely different from the preceding ones, for in fact at each of the larval moults there is a slight change towards the adult characterization; nevertheless it is true that by far the greater part of this change occurs at the last one. We have suggested earlier that this situation is best interpreted as an example of polymorphism, and we have seen that the crucial problem here is to determine the nature of the switch mechanism which evokes the emergence of the adult form.

The structures concerned are the corpora allata; glands which develop from the ectoderm, and come to be closely associated with the corpora cardiaca (Fig. 14.8, p. 249). They are, in fact, innervated from the corpus cardiacum nerves and seem to receive neurosecretory products from them. The function of the corpora allata is the production of a hormone, known as the juvenile hormone, which, in association with ecdysone, promotes the development of the larval characters. It is present in *Rhodnius* during the moults of the first four larval instars; as a result, gene activity follows the programme appropriate to the production of predominantly juvenile (larval) characters. The metamorphosis which results from the moult of the fifth instar is determined by the absence of juvenile hormone at that stage. In consequence, gene activity leads to the full development of adult characters. The function of ecdysone throughout the larval moults is to activate the epidermal and other target cells. The level of juvenile hormone provides the switch mechanism which determines whether larval or adult characters shall develop. Not surprisingly, both hormones influence (whether directly or indirectly) the puffing of polytene chromosomes.

Amongst the results of experiments which support this concept is the demonstration that a fifth-stage larva of *Rhodnius*, decapitated *before* the critical stage and united in parabiosis with a fourth-stage larva that has been decapitated *after* the critical stage, will

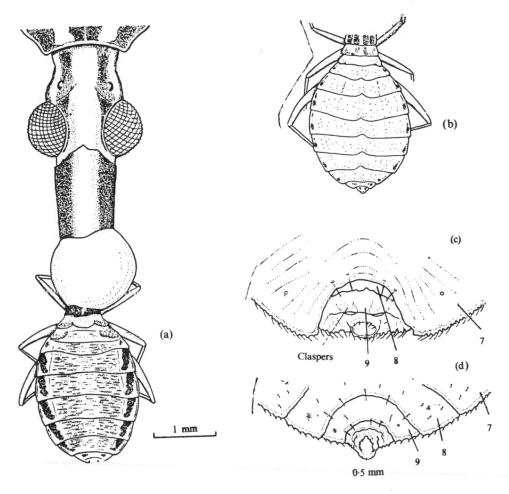

FIG. 14.11. (a) Precocious 'adult' *Rhodnius* produced from first-stage larva by joining it parabiotically to the head of a moulting fifth-stage larva. (b) Normal second-stage larva for comparison. (c) Terminal segments of the precocious 'adult' male. (d) Terminal segments of a normal second-stage larva. Figures indicate homologous sterna. (From Wigglesworth (1940). *J. exp. Biol.* **17**.)

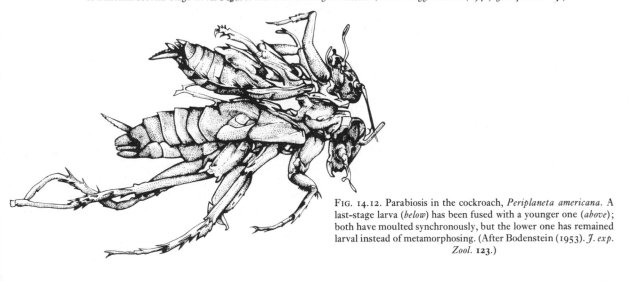

FIG. 14.12. Parabiosis in the cockroach, *Periplaneta americana*. A last-stage larva (*below*) has been fused with a younger one (*above*); both have moulted synchronously, but the lower one has remained larval instead of metamorphosing. (After Bodenstein (1953). *J. exp. Zool.* **123**.)

moult but will not metamorphose. This is because it is under the combined influence of the juvenile hormone and ecdysone from the fourth-stage larva. A similar result has been obtained with the cockroach (Fig. 14.12). Conversely, a first-stage larva, decapitated before the critical stage and then united parabiotically with a moulting fifth-stage larva, will not only moult but will undergo metamorphosis to form a small but reasonably well-formed adult (Fig. 14.11). This is because it has lacked the influence of the juvenile hormone which would normally have ensured the development of larval features.

That the corpora allata are actually the source of juvenile hormone has been shown by transplantation experiments. The transference of the glands from any of the first to fourth instars into a fifth-stage larva, at one day after it has fed, inhibits metamorphosis to a varying degree; sometimes the animal moults into a 'sixth-stage larva', but often a mixture of larval and adult characters develops, depending upon the degree of balance established in the circulating hormonal system. Corpora allata from fifth-stage larvae do not have this effect, as they are no longer producing their hormone.

This mechanism for regulating the onset of metamorphosis exists in most other groups of insects, holometabolous as well as hemimetabolous, although with variations in detail which we cannot now discuss. In *Hyalophora*, for example, the moult to the pupal stage is determined by a reduction of the secretion of juvenile hormone below the level characteristic of the earlier moults, while the final metamorphic moult of the pupa is determined by the complete absence of the hormone. Arising out of this, it has been shown that the latter is not genus- or order-specific. For example, the corpora allata of *Periplaneta* and the ring gland of the larva of *Calliphora* will promote some degree of larval characterization in *Rhodnius*.

Some reversal of metamorphosis can be induced in an adult *Rhodnius* if it is united parabiotically with fifth-stage larvae after these have passed the critical stage, and if it is supplied at the same time with an adequate number of corpora allata from fourth-stage larvae (Fig. 14.13). Such an animal will moult, and the new cuticle then formed may show a certain degree of larval characterization in, for example, the distribution of pigmentation pattern. This result not only demonstrates the positive influence of the juvenile hormone derived from the corpora allata but also illustrates the persistence throughout life of both larval and adult potentialities.

By a fortunate chance the adult male *Hyalophora*

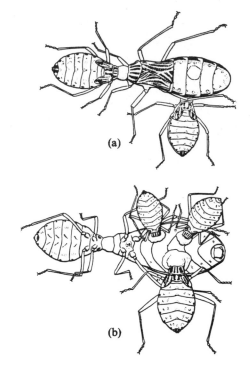

FIG. 14.13. (a) Adult *Rhodnius*, with wings cut short and corpora allata of fourth-stage larvae implanted in abdomen and joined to two fifth-stage larvae. (b) Adult *Rhodnius*, decapitated and joined to two fifth-stage larvae and two fourth-stage larvae. Adults can be caused to moult by either of these procedures and their cuticle may become partially larval in character. (From Wigglesworth (1940). *J. exp. Biol.* **17**.)

builds up a relatively enormous store of the juvenile hormone in the tissues of its abdomen. Many other Lepidoptera do this also, but to nothing like the same extent. With material from this source it has been possible to isolate the hormone, and to characterize it as methyl 10,11-epoxy-7-ethyl-3,11-dimethyl-2,6-tridecadienoate (Fig. 14.14). As with other hormones, a sensitive qualitative test is a prerequisite, and for this purpose use is made of the fact that regenerating epidermis is particularly responsive to the hormone. A small piece of the integument of the last larval stage of a hemimetabolous insect, or of the pupa of a holometabolous one, is removed. The test substance is then inserted into the animal, and the wound plugged. The presence of the hormone in the introduced material will be revealed at metamorphosis, for the adult will show a small patch of pupal cuticle at the point of injury.

With this method, in addition to ordinary injection procedures, juvenile hormone activity has been found in extracts of arthropods and of many other inverte-brates, including Hydroza, Polychaeta, Oligochaeta, a holothurian, and the hemichordate *Saccoglossus*. It is also present in extracts of the adrenocortical tissue of cattle. Usually, the active materials are mimics of the hormone; the terpene farnesol is one example of these (Fig. 14.14).

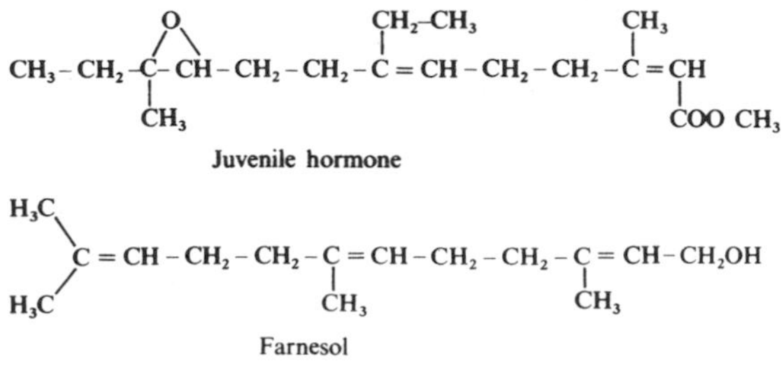

Juvenile hormone

Farnesol

FIG. 14.14. Juvenile hormone and farnesol.

Normal insect development depends upon juvenile hormone being present at definite periods in precisely adjusted amounts. This situation is closely analogous to the regulation of amphibian development by thyroid hormones, and, just as in that case, disturbance of the relationship between the hormone and its targets leads to abnormal development. This has suggested the possibility of using analogues or mimics of juvenile hormone as insecticides, on the principle that the uptake of these compounds in random concentrations would disturb or arrest the progress of the life history. The advantage over mass-distributed insecticides such as DDT is that insects would be most unlikely to develop immunity to products so similar to their normal secretions (although there is some evidence that this is not impossible), while it should be possible to select compounds which would be especially effective against particular species. It has, indeed, been possible to reduce populations of insects of stored products by application of a juvenile hormone analogue. Another approach depends upon the ability of males to tolerate higher concentrations than are needed to interfere with the development of the eggs. A preparation can thus be applied to the males in relatively high concentration, relying upon it being subsequently distributed to the females in quantities sufficient to arrest the development of their offspring. This is a field of research in which insect endocrinology has great potentialities for promoting human welfare.

14.6. Hormones in adult insects

With the completion of the metamorphic moult, there comes a change in the endocrine balance of the animal, for the thoracic gland and its homologues now disappear; as a result of this, no more moults can occur, the only known exception to this situation being in the Thysanura, which continue to moult throughout life and in which the relevant glands (ventral glands) are consequently retained. The corpora allata, however, do resume activity, and in some insects their presence in the adult is necessary for the maintenance of normal ovarian function. This is the more notable because of the fact that in insects the sex-determining chromosome mechanism retains its primacy throughout development and can determine the sexual organization of all regions of the body without being overridden by the unifying action of endocrine secretions; in this absence of a well-defined system of sex hormones, the insects, as we have already emphasized, differ fundamentally from both crustaceans and vertebrates.

In *Rhodnius*, resumption of activity in the corpora allata takes place very soon after the adult has fed. If feeding is prevented, or if the corpora allata are removed by decapitating the animal, the oocytes begin to degenerate immediately prior to the stage at which yolk disposition should be taking place, while in the male the accessory glands do not secrete properly. The normal development of the eggs can be restored, in a female that has been so treated, by joining it parabiotically with a normal adult, either male or female, which contains intact corpora allata. Moreover, corpora allata from a larva will also produce this alleviation, which suggests that the ovary-regulating hormone of the adult is the same as the juvenile hormone. This conclusion is strengthened by the observation that the gland of the adult will inhibit metamorphosis if it is transplanted into a fifth-stage larva.

In some other insects the situation is less clear. Normal egg development can take place in stick-insects in the absence of the corpora allata, but these insects are unusual in that they are thought to be neotenous, so that their reproduction may be taking place in an essentially juvenile phase. The eggs can also develop in the absence of the corpora allata in, for example, some lepidopterans, but this may mean that in these forms another secretory centre is concerned, perhaps the brain. Cerebral neurosecretion, while having no effect on egg development in *Rhodnius* and in many lepidopterans, is needed, in conjunction with the corpora allata, to ensure oocyte development in the cockroach, locusts, and the blowfly. The interpretation of this is difficult, however, because of interaction between the brain and the corpora allata. For example, the presence of the latter enhances cerebral neurosecretory activity in blow-flies.

Finally, there is some evidence that in insects, as in crustaceans and vertebrates, the hormonal control of growth and moulting is closely linked with metabolic effects. The evidence again centres around the corpora allata, which have been said to influence such processes as digestive activity, protein anabolism, oxygen consumption, and the maintenance of normal tissue growth in *Rhodnius*. They are also thought to control the synthesis in the fat body of proteins which are taken up into the yolk of the developing oocytes.

of fluid with its meal of blood, and this fluid has to be removed through the Malpighian tubules. *In vitro* studies of these tubules show that they pass more urine more quickly when they are placed in haemolymph from a recently fed bug than when the haemolymph is from a starved one. This is due to a diuretic hormone, which is a neurosecretory product, the most likely source of which is the fused thoracic and first abdominal ganglia, where there are large neurosecretory cells (Fig. 14.15; Table 14.1). Probably the release mechanism depends upon the distension of the gut by the meal, which we have seen to be responsible for the activation of the cerebral neurosecretory cells that secrete thoracotropic hormone. Evidence for this is that release of the

TABLE 14.1

The occurrence of diuretic activity in the various parts of the central nervous system of Rhodnius *(From Maddrell (1963). J. exp. Biol.* **40**, *247–56.)*

	Brain	Sub-oesophageal ganglion	Prothoracic ganglion	Mesothoracic ganglionic mass
The concentration of each part necessary to cause a resting set of Malpighian tubules in $6 \mu l$ of haemolymph to produce a further $0.5 \mu l$ of secretion (ganglia/$100 \mu l$ of haemolymph—average of 10 trials) (A).	0·7	5·0	10·0	0·07
The dry weight of each part ($\mu g \pm 1.0 \mu g$) (B).	11	3	4	13
Relative concentration of diuretic activity in each part ($1/(A \times B)$ expressed as a ratio).	5·2	2·7	1	44

In contrast to the situation in crustaceans, there is no evidence of secretion of sex hormones by the ovary. The development of the accessory glands depends upon the corpora allata, which are thus responsible for correlating the development of these organs with that of the ovary. Even so, it is only vitellogenesis which is effected; the initial stages of oogenesis are not under hormonal control at all. So also in the male, where the corpora allata control the development of accessory organs, as in the female; while the accelerated development of the testes at metamorphosis is also presumably regulated by the hormones that are involved in moulting. Thus, as already pointed out, insects differ from crustaceans and vertebrates in that genetic factors directly determine sexual differentiation, with hormones playing only a secondary role.

The functioning of hormones in adult insects is by no means confined to reproduction. Two examples of this may be given. *Rhodnius* takes in a large volume

diuretic hormone, which begins within thirty seconds of feeding, is prevented by cutting the ventral nerve cord.

Another example is provided by the regulation of blood-sugar levels in *Periplaneta*. Two hormones are concerned, one more potent than the other, and both released from the corpora cardiaca. Their actions show a remarkable resemblance to the actions of glucagon and adrenaline in vertebrates, for they convert the inactive form of phosphorylase to the active form, the reaction taking place within the fat body. The result is to enhance the breakdown of glycogen, the effect in insects being an increased output of the disaccharide trehalose. Why two hormones are required is not clear, but a curious aspect of this is that they are produced from different sources. In locusts, and presumably also in cockroaches, the more potent of the two hormones comes from the secretory cells of the corpora cardiaca, while the less potent comes from the stored neurosecretion of these organs.

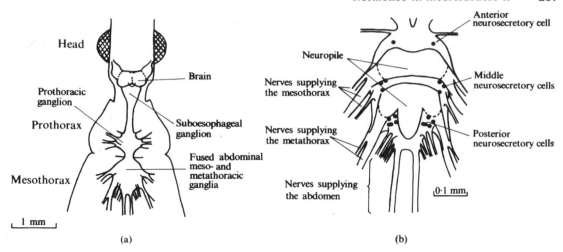

FIG. 14.15. (a) The central nervous system of *Rhodnius*. (b) A diagrammatic representation of the fused ganglionic mass in the mesothorax of *Rhodnius* to show the distribution of the neurosecretory cells. (From Madrell (1963). *J. exp. Biol.* **40**.)

It will be apparent that there are certain basic metabolic activities which are regulated by hormones in crustaceans, insects, and vertebrates, although the details of the mechanisms may differ. Other metabolic actions have also been ascribed to insect hormones, but the evidence is often indirect, and some of the effects demonstrated may well be pharmacological ones. However, it may be expected that with advancing knowledge this evidence will be strengthened, and that we shall find amply illustrated the principle enunciated earlier: that similar needs have called forth the evolution of mechanisms which will be either analogous or homologous, according to the relationship of the groups concerned. Caution is nevertheless needed in developing this concept, for the physiological needs of invertebrates and vertebrates may be very different. For example, it is not obvious that the energy demands of, say, a cockroach are sufficiently like those of a mammal to justify the insect having hormonal regulation of its blood-carbohydrate level. Perhaps hormonal action in this particular instance, however, is associated with some interrelationship of carbohydrate metabolism and other metabolic pathways.

14.7. Colour change in insects

The pigmentation of insects is a familiar enough sight, but colour change, in the sense in which we have considered it in the vertebrates and crustaceans, does not play an important part in their lives, and responses are usually morphological rather than physiological. As with vertebrates, however, hormonal control plays a part in such changes. The larva of *Acrida turrita*, for example, becomes green

in a green and wet meadow, and brown in a dry and yellow one. This is a morphological colour change, which has been shown by implantation experiments to be controlled by the corpora allata. These organs also control the morphological colour change of *Locusta migratoria*; this phenomenon is associated with phase-polymorphism, implantation of corpora allata into brown *gregaria* larvae producing the green colour of the *solitaria* phase. The stick-insect *Carausius* (*Dixippus*) *morosus*, however, is unusual in showing not only a morphological range of colour from green to brown but also physiological changes within this range. These latter changes are not effected by typical chromatophores, as we have already noted, but by the movement of pigment granules within the epidermal cells (Fig. 14.16). The dark condition results from their migration towards the outer surface of the cells, and the light position from their concentration in the deeper regions.

The colour change of this animal is fundamentally an expression of a diurnal rhythm, giving a light colour by day and a dark one by night, but the extent of the reaction depends upon the individual's basic colour. This is determined by the proportions in which the green, orange, and dark brown pigments are present, and the last of these makes the greatest contribution. These colour changes are determined by environmental stimuli through the eyes; if the latter are removed, the responses are lost, and the rhythm does not develop in insects that are kept in the dark from the time of hatching.

In addition to showing this diurnal rhythm, however, the animal, like amphibians, shows a humidity

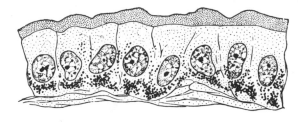

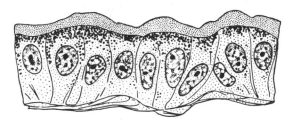

FIG. 14.16. Intracellular migration of pigment in the hypodermal cells of *Carausius morosus*. Light colour during the day (*above*); dark colour during the night (*below*). (From Dupont-Raabe (1957). *Archs Zool., exp. gen.* **94**.)

response, tending to be dark in damp conditions and pale in dry ones. Nervous and endocrine factors co-operate in bringing about this reaction. For example, if the abdomen is placed in a moist chamber, but the head and thorax left outside in a dry environment, darkening will normally begin in the head region and spread over the whole body. This response can be prevented in two ways, either by ligation of the thorax or by section of the central nervous system between the sub-oesophageal and thoracic ganglia. The first of these operations results in the backward spread of darkening being arrested at the ligature, presumably because this is preventing the further diffusion of a hormone. The second operation results in the whole of the anterior region remaining pale, presumably because the normal reaction is mediated by the passage to the brain of nerve impulses arising from receptors in the abdomen. That the capacity for reacting is still present is shown by placing the head end of such an animal into the moist chamber; there is now no barrier to the transmission of nerve impulses from receptors to the brain, and darkening of the head region is immediately initiated.

Ablation and injection experiments show that two hormones may be involved in these changes, one located particularly in the tritocerebral region of the brain, where there is cytological evidence for neurosecretory activity, and the other in the corpora cardiaca. The two supposed hormones are not identical in their effects, and this raises the question of the relationship between the corpora cardiaca and the brain. This we have so far interpreted on the basis of the corpora cardiaca acting as a release centre for neurosecretion produced in the pars intercerebralis of the brain. That a similar possibility exists also in the present case is shown by the presence of a third pair of corpora cardiaca nerves, running from the tritocerebrum. However, if these do, in fact, convey a secretory product to the corpora cardiaca, it must undergo some further processing there to account for the change in its properties. On the other hand, there are secretory cells in the corpora cardiaca, so that the possibility of them producing their own independent secretion is a very real one.

An additional complication in the interpretation is that the corpora cardiaca do not seem to have any function in determining the normal diurnal colour change. Removal of the deuto-tritocerebral region of the brain eliminates this response, the animal then taking on a pale grey colour owing to the inward migration of the brown granules, but removal of the pars intercerebralis, or of this together with the corpora cardiaca, has no effect at all. It may be, then, that a secretion of the corpora cardiaca is concerned with the maintenance of an intermediate coloration, or it may have quite other functions, its influence upon colour being an unimportant by-product of these.

The activity associated with the tritocerebral secretion can be detected in other parts of the central nervous system also, more particularly in the sub-oesophageal ganglion, and it seems possible that this is a result of diffusion or transport of a secretion through the circum-oesophageal connectives. It is not clear whether the secretion is released directly from its point of origin in the brain or from other points elsewhere in the nervous system, but it is clear that there is no specialized release centre comparable with those of the crustaceans. The corpora cardiaca would have been expected to fulfil this function, but in this instance their precise role is difficult to interpret.

Although the colour responses of *Carausius* constitute a behaviour pattern unusual amongst insects, it would be of the greatest interest to determine how far its hormonal basis shares common features with the Crustacea. This problem has been investigated, using the techniques of differential extraction and separation to which we have already referred. The results have shown, amongst other things, that the corpora cardiaca of *Carausius* contain a substance similar to one present in extracts of the sinus gland and postcommissure organs of *Palaemon* (*Leander*), in that it causes contraction of the red pigments of the latter animal. On the other hand, the brain extracts of *Carausius* contain a substance that is not present in *Palaemon*; it has no effect upon the pigment of that animal, but produces darkening in *Carausius* itself, as would be expected, and concentrates the dark pigments of *Crangon*.

It would seem that the pigment effector systems of these animals may eventually prove to have something in common, but it is impossible to judge the physiological significance of either the resemblances or the differences in the absence of precise chemical information. It needs to be remembered that the effector cells themselves are quite different in the two groups, and, having regard to this, and to the early separation of their evolutionary paths which we have commented on earlier, such resemblances as exist between them need cautious evaluation before they can be ascribed to homology.

14.8. Pheromones

Pheromones, which we have defined in connection with mammalian reproduction (p. 133), play a particularly important part in insect life; indeed, it was in this group that they were first intensively studied, and where they gained their name (from the Greek roots *pherein*, to bear, and *hormaein*, to excite); etymologically unattractive, but now in general use. Obviously the investigation of these externally secreted substances constitutes more a field of comparative exocrinology than of comparative endocrinology, but it would be foolish to press the distinction. Hormones and pheromones are better regarded as two regions of a continuous spectrum of chemical communication, often illustrating similar principles.

Progress in this field has depended upon a close correlation of chemical and biological research. The preparation of crude extracts of the animals is one obvious starting point, preferably after the identification of the glands in which the pheromones originate. An alternative method of collection is to 'milk' the animals by passing air over them and condensing its pheromone content. Using *Periplaneta americana* in this way, 12·2 mg of sex attractant has been obtained from many thousands of females over a period of nine months. Separation, characterization, and synthesis of insect pheromones obtained by these procedures, combined with study of their biological properties, has made it possible to show that they constitute an extraordinarily well-developed system of chemical communication, usually functioning by stimulation of antennal receptors. Not the least remarkable feature of the system is the range of information that can be conveyed by one or a very few chemicals, and the very high potencies of the secretions concerned.

Pheromones can function in one or other of two ways. They may produce an immediate and well-defined change in the behaviour of the recipient, presumably by acting upon the nervous system; this is termed a 'releaser' action. Alternatively, pheromones may set up physiological changes, which may influence reproductive maturation, for example, and may then lead to new patterns of behaviour being evoked by later stimuli. This is termed a 'primer' reaction. We have seen an example in the influence of male mice upon the oestrous cycle of the female (p. 134).

Examples of releaser pheromones in insects are provided by sex attractants. These have been specially studied in Lepidoptera, where they are often long-chain unsaturated alcohols or their esters, but their use is widespread in other groups as well, including Orthoptera, Coleoptera, Hymenoptera, and Diptera. The female of the silkworm moth, *Bombyx mori*, secretes an attractant from abdominal glands, extracts of which induce great excitement in males, accompanied by erratic dancing and attempts to copulate with test objects. This substance, an alcohol termed bombykol (Fig. 14.17), was chemically characterized by Butenandt and his colleagues, an achievement which demanded 30 years work, and the extraction of bombykol esters from some 250 000 moths.

The identification of bombykol led to intensive research which has resulted in sex attractants being demonstrated in many other insect species, and notably in Lepidoptera, although their chemical characterization has not always been a straightforward operation. Gyptol (Fig. 14.7), for example, is a compound earlier thought to be a pheromone of the female gypsy moth, *Porthetria dispar*, which is a devastating pest of foliage. The actual sex attractant of this species has proved to be a different compound, but gyptol, and an even more attractive homologue called gyplure, well illustrate the remarkable properties of these substances. Gyptol is so potent that in laboratory conditions it can attract males in amounts of no more than 10^{-12} mg. In the field it is less effective, but even so, males are attracted to traps containing only 10^{-7} mg. Data from other species are no less impressive. For example, a single caged virgin sawfly, *Diprion similis*, has been reported to have lured over 11 000 males in five days. However, pheromones are not an extragavant encouragement to nymphomania; the capacity of the female sawfly to attract males declines rapidly after copulation.

FIG. 14.17. Pheromones, natural and artificial.

$$CH_3 — CH_2 — CH_2 — CH = CH — CH = CH — (CH_2)_8 — CH_2OH$$

Bombykol

$$CH_3 — (CH_2)_5 — \underset{\underset{COOCH_3}{|}}{CH} — CH_2 — CH = CH — (CH_2)_5 — CH_2OH$$

Gyptol

$$CH_3 — (CH_2)_5 — \underset{\underset{COOCH_3}{|}}{CH} — CH_2 — CH = CH — (CH_2)_7 — CH_2OH$$

Gyplure

$$CH_3 — \underset{\underset{O}{||}}{C} — (CH_2)_5 — CH = CH — COOH$$

9-oxodecenoic acid

$$CH_3 — \underset{\underset{OH}{|}}{CH} — (CH_2)_5 — CH = CH — COOH$$

9-hydroxydecenoic acid

This, in fact, is a field in which chemically based studies need cautious biological evaluation, for the maximal attractiveness of females may not be shown by pure compounds. This is well demonstrated by experiments with the sex attractant (propylure) of the pink bollworm moth, *Pectinophora gossypiella*. This substance, an acetate of an unsaturated alcohol, excites males in laboratory cages, but does not attract them to traps in the field, although crude extracts of the females are able to do so. The reason is that the extracts also contain *N,N*-diethyl-*m*-toluamide (known as Deet), which is needed to activate the pheromone. The two substances must be mixed if they are to lure males to field traps. Even so, they are less efficient than the crude extracts; perhaps, then, the latter contain also a second activator. It is of singular interest that Deet had not been reported from a natural source prior to its discovery in *Pectinophora*, although it had been earlier known as an effective repellant of mosquitoes.

Sex pheromones are not confined to females; they are also produced by males, which use them as attractants or aphrodisiacs. Three examples must serve. The male cockroach, *Leucophaea maderae*, secretes a pheromone which causes the female to mount its abdomen and lick its tergum. Male flower-visiting beetles of the family Machilidae saturate their body hairs with a secretion that both attracts the females and excites them. Males of the butterfly genus *Lycorea* use their pheromone in a more positive way. Flying in pursuit of the female, they sweep her antennae with protrusible brushes, called hair pencils. These carry a secretion that induces the female to alight and to acquiesce in copulation.

With insects sensitive to such minute amounts of pheromone (1–200 molecules may be the threshold in some instances), how do they contrive to orientate towards the source? The answer is thought to be that they fly upwind, perhaps from distances of 100 m, until the concentration of material is sufficient to enable them to discriminate and to detect the direction of origin. Whatever the method, however, this is a biological situation lending itself to more than one approach to the control of insect pests. For example, it is possible to disturb orientation by permeating the atmosphere with a synthetic pheromone.

Applied to the control of the cabbage loper moth, *Trichoplusia ni*, 17 mg of synthetic pheromone placed on each of 100 stakes spaced over a plot of 27 m² has proved sufficient to prevent males from homing on the females. It has been calculated, indeed, that less than 0·2 g/acre would be sufficient to control the insect over large areas. Another promising method is to mask the pheromone by distributing other chemicals in the area. Formaldehyde vapour can block the action of attractants on males; Chanel No. 5 has also proved effective, and may commend itself as being more elegant.

The use of pheromones reaches a particularly high level of specialization in the social insects (Isoptera and Hymenoptera), where they play a fundamentally important role in the integration of social organization. These insects possess a variety of glands discharging chemical secretions that carry a diversity of information which is decoded by the particular members of the colony that are the specific targets. Here, as with internally secreted hormones, there is close adaptation between the secretions and their targets. As a result, a very small number of chemical products (sometimes called sociohormones), discharged separately or in combination, is adequate to provide for complex patterns of social interrelationship.

Ants have developed, along many independent lines of evolution, the secretion of pheromones to form odour trails. These secretions, which are highly specific, so that no species disturbs the movements of another, may originate in various ways; in the alimentary tract, for example, or in specialized glands. In the fire ant, *Solenopsis saevissima*, the trail pheromone originates in a specialized gland, Dufour's gland, and is discharged from this through the sting; sometimes a poison gland secretion may be used. The action of these secretions is nicely adjusted to the needs of the colony. For example, the trail secretion of *Atta texane* contains a volatile component which loses its potency after 60 minutes; this is used for the rapid recruitment of other workers. In addition, however, there is a non-volatile component which remains active for many days; this provides for a persistent trail which can be reinforced with additional secretion while it continues in use.

The behaviour of the fire ant, moving up a trail leading to a source of food, illustrates particularly well the efficiency of this means of communication. The pheromone is very volatile, but individuals that obtain food will add more secretion to the trail on their homeward journey. The intensity of the trail is thus an index of the amount of food available, and a high level of secretion increases the number of individuals that react to it. Once the food has been exploited, however, the trail will no longer be reinforced, and so the efforts of the colony will not be wasted.

Odour trails leading to food sources are also laid by many species of stingless bees. Scout bees deposit droplets of a pheromone at regular intervals; these droplets volatilize, providing an aerial trail which recruits other bees and leads them to the food. As with the ants, those bees that return with food add to the trail, and this reinforcement results in rapid recruitment of other individuals. It is said that this mechanism can achieve an efficiency fully comparable with that achieved by the combination of dancing and chemical information provided by the communication system of the honey bee. Moreover, it has the advantage that it can be used to lead stingless bees to flowers in tall trees, whereas the honey bee is restricted by its mode of communication to the exploitation of ground flora. This, of course, is not a disadvantageous limitation. It illustrates how chemical communication can be specialized to provide for non-competitive exploitation of the environment by different species.

Pheromones also serve as alarm substances, (analogous ones are produced by fish), and these, too, are well adjusted to the needs of the colony. The alarm pheromone of the harvesting ant, *Pogonomyrmex badius*, is a short-lived volatile substance which loses its potency within 35 s. At the periphery of its diffusion range its concentration is sufficiently low to attract the workers, while centrally it is high enough to evoke their alarm response. So the arrival of a foreign worker, for example, is rapidly and efficiently dealt with by a small local group of ants, the rest of the colony being left undistracted.

Another illustration is provided by termites, in which trail-laying behaviour may be released by alarm stimuli operating at more than one level. The discovery of breaks in the structure of the nest releases high-level alarm behaviour, accompanied by the laying of a trail which leads other ants to the repair of the break. The discovery of a food source produces low-level alarm behaviour, resulting in the laying of a trail from the food back to the nest.

Honey bees, as is well known, make use of dance patterns to give information regarding food and nest sites, but these are supplemented by pheromones. Workers encountering a new food source release a terpene, geraniol, from their abdominal Nassanoff glands, which they expose while they fan their wings. This provides information additional to that given by the 'waggle dance'. When they sting an intruder, they also release, with the poison, a secretion from adjacent glands. This attracts other workers to the same spot, and greatly increases the force of this defensive mechanism, as is well known to those who have the misfortune to arouse this response.

An especially striking feature of the honey bee, however, is the variety of information and instruction which it draws so economically from a minimal range of secretions. One substance that is of critical importance to these bees has been characterized as *trans*-9-keto-2-decenoic acid (9-oxodecenoic acid) (Fig. 14.17). This pheromone, which is produced in the mandibular glands of the queen, but is not secreted by workers, is remarkably versatile; electrophysiological studies have shown that certain antennal receptors on all three castes are sensitive exclusively to it. It is the sex attractant of the queen honey bee, which attracts the drone during the nuptial flight, and which also functions as an aphrodisiac, stimulating the drone to mount the queen. It also acts within the hive, being one component of queen substance; this is licked from the queen by the workers, who then distribute it throughout the colony by the regurgitation of their food. It inhibits queen rearing by the workers (i.e. the construction of queen cells), and it partially inhibits their ovarian development. It is estimated to be present at $130 \mu g$ per queen throughout life, its concentration falling off towards the end, and thus permitting the rearing of new queens.

9-Oxodecenoic acid, to be fully effective, has to act in conjunction with a second compound, *trans-*

9-hydroxy-2-decenoic acid (9-hydroxydecenoic acid). This substance, formerly called inhibitory scent, is a volatile compound which is also produced in the mandibular glands of the queen. It does not act as a sex attractant, but is essentially a primer, the two pheromones together completely inhibiting ovarian development in the workers, and so completing the arrest of queen rearing. Both substances are also used in swarming, and this well illustrates the interaction of pheromones to bring about adaptive behaviour. The ketoacid activates restless bees, while the hydroxyacid tranquillizes them after they have settled, and thus ensures economy of effort.

Another substance secreted by honey bees, closely related in structure to 9-oxodecenoic acid, is 10-hydroxydecenoic acid. This is present in the royal jelly, which is secreted by the mandibular glands of worker bees, and is an important nutritive factor in determining the production of queens. It would appear, therefore, that this is another example of the evolution of substances with different regulatory properties and modes of action from some common molecular pattern. It will not escape notice, either, that there is here a certain degree of analogy between the fabrication of orally administered contraceptives by man (p. 131) and the mechanism of sexual regulation practised in the beehive.

With pheromones, as with other aspects of chemical communication, there are resemblances between insects and crustaceans. The Pacific crab,

Portunus sanguinolentus, provides an example of a crustacean sex pheromone. Males carry females for up to six days before the female moults, for copulation must occur immediately after the moult, while the new exoskeleton is still soft. The placing of premoult females in a tank results in the males beginning display and search behaviour, and becoming so excited that they pull at any crab with which they come into contact. Tests in which males are placed in water in which females have previously been maintained show that this response is due to a sex attractant which is present in the urine of the premoult female.

Such signals are not confined to reproduction. For example, much chemical communication takes place between lobsters (*Homarus americanus*). Individuals fed to satiation on flounder, so that their feeding responses are negligible, respond by upstream movement to water from tanks containing moulted females, or intermoult or moulted males, but they do not respond to water occupied by intermoult females, or by cast shells. It is thought that these responses, which are presumably mediated by one or more pheromones, are not sexual, but are primarily of social significance. As emphasized earlier, they cannot be sharply distinguished from responses to metabolic or other chemical products in the environment, so that chemical characterization is needed to establish their truly pheromonal status.

15

Some evolutionary implications

15.1. The evolution of hormones

We are now in a position to judge how fruitful the comparative method has been in yielding up the general principles which we hoped might emerge from its application. One set of problems to which we have made repeated reference revolves around the origin and evolutionary history of hormones. In this connection, comparisons are often drawn with vitamins, for the two groups of substances resemble each other in being required only in very minute quantities and in influencing the activities of the body without providing energy for them. The obvious difference between them is that in general the hormones can be synthesized from the raw materials provided in the food, whereas vitamins must be made available from external sources, and from this point of view the latter substances have sometimes been referred to as exogenous hormones. This, however, is a simplification which obscures some important considerations.

If we look at this matter with particular reference to the B vitamins, we find these to be a group of substances which are essential at all levels of plant and animal life. This is because they are obligatory components of fundamental biochemical mechanisms which must be almost, if not quite, as old as life itself, and we are able to define their function with some precision because we are able to analyse those mechanisms. The B vitamins can be synthesized by the autotrophic plants, and it has been plausibly suggested that the inability of animals to do so is a consequence of the loss of synthetic capacity during the course of evolution. The dependence of animals upon their hormones, however, seems to be of a character quite different from this, although the distinction is obscured by the fact that while the green plant as a whole can synthesize its requirements of B vitamins, this capacity is not shared equally by all the parts of it. For example, roots are in general unable to synthesize thiamine, and so we find that this substance has to be formed in the leaves and transported down to the roots, where it then exerts a specific physiological effect upon their growth. Thereby it clearly satisfies our formal definition of a hormone, a point that we return to below.

Hormones, however, differ fundamentally from the B vitamins in that they do not appear to be essential components of biochemical machinery, for life can often proceed in their absence, even if with reduced efficiency. They seem rather to have been evolved *pari passu* with the development of the increasing complexity of animal organization, and probably with a great deal of independent evolution, at least in the major phyla, although we do not yet know enough to feel sure of this. Their function appears to be to serve as the regulators of specialized reactions rather than as primary components of these, and the difficulties that we encounter in trying to define their individual modes of action are surely a consequence of their relatively late introduction into these complex relationships. There seems here to be some resemblance to the fat-soluble vitamins, which are a characteristic requirement of the vertebrates, and the history of which must therefore have differed from that of the B vitamins. Vitamin A, in fact, offers an interesting parallel with the catechol hormones for, like those substances, it is present in certain invertebrates although its physiological significance in them remains obscure. As regards vitamin D_2, it is of particular interest to find that its molecular structure is based upon the steroid nucleus which has been turned to such profitable use by vertebrates in their endocrine systems. In fact, it is difficult to see why they should be able to synthesize a variety of steroid hormones and yet have to rely upon ultra-violet irradiation for the transformation of 7-dehydrocholesterol into calciferol. It is possible that this reflects some biochemical limitation in the higher forms, for the accumulation of the vitamin in certain fish shows no obvious correlation with their diet or with their exposure to sunlight, and there is some slight evidence that complete synthesis may occur in this group.

We may consider animal hormones, then, as products of biological progress, a term which we use in the broad sense of an increasing improvement of adaptation, leading to an increasing mastery of the environments which have been available for exploitation. Hormones are essential, too, for the maintenance of this progress, as is made even more apparent by the existence of comparable systems in plants. Four categories of plant hormones are known: auxins, gibberellins, cytokinins, and inhibitors. They must have evolved independently of animal hormones, and their chemical constitution (Fig. 15.1) shows no close affinity with these, although the

differentiation, and they also retard senescence by preventing the breakdown of protein and the destruction of chlorophyll. Finally, the various growth inhibitors have a variety of actions, including the promotion of leaf-fall and the development of dormancy in buds.

In addition to satisfying what is clearly a fundamental requirement in living organisms for chemical regulation, the mode of operation of plant hormones has some similarity in principle to that of certain animal hormones, in that modification of RNA synthesis and metabolism seems often to be involved. But even more striking resemblances are seen in

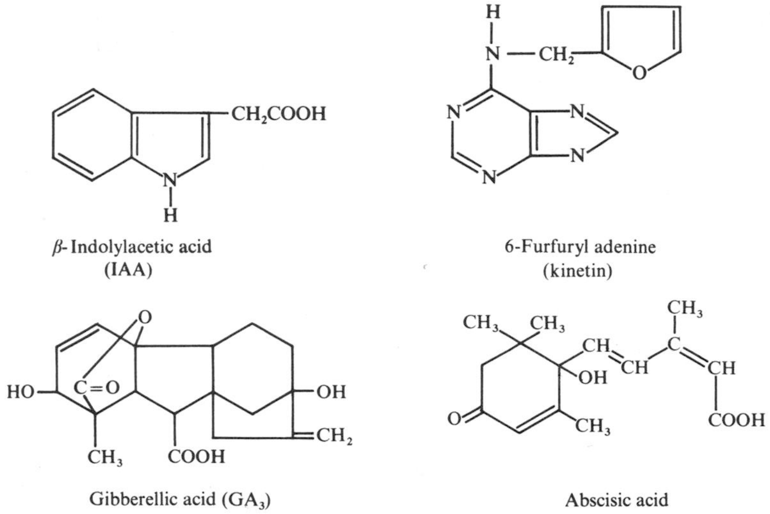

β-Indolylacetic acid
(IAA)

6-Furfuryl adenine
(kinetin)

Gibberellic acid (GA₃)

Abscisic acid

FIG. 15.1. Plant hormones.

synthetic pathways of the gibberellins are associated with those of steroids and terpenoids. Moreover, there is obviously no vascular transmission in the animal sense of that term, but nor is there in *Hydra* and other lower invertebrates. These substances, therefore, like thiamine, satisfy the classical definition of hormones, in that they are produced in one region and pass from it in small amounts to evoke adaptive responses elsewhere.

Auxins (e.g. indolylacetic acid, IAA) are formed at the tip of the coleoptile, and then pass to the growing region, where they promote longitudinal growth by evoking elongation of the coleoptile cells. Gibberellins, which are abundant in seeds, and are also present in young leaves and in roots, promote the growth of main stems after moving up from the roots in the xylem. Cytokinins, which are derivatives of adenine, are synthesized in roots, and move up in the xylem to the leaves and fruit. There, in association with auxins, they promote normal growth and

examples of hormonal interaction, one being illustrated in the germination of cereal seeds. Gibberellin, formed after water inhibition of water, induces breakdown of food reserves, with the release of tryptophan. This moves to the coleoptile tip, where it is metabolized to form indolylacetic acid, which then moves down to the growing zone. Given, then, the profound differences between the organization of plants and animals, their endocrinology shows a considerable degree of unity in their operation of chemical regulation.

Studies of animal endocrinology shed a little light on some of the ways in which hormones might have originated. We have seen that the evolution of endocrine systems may sometimes have depended on animals making use of molecules which happened to be available, either in the external medium or as a result of their own metabolism. The wide distribution of iodine binding, the appearance of which clearly antedated the origin of vertebrates, is one illustration of this possibility, and another suggestive fact is the presence of acetylcholine and adrenaline in *Paramecium*. Even more significant is the wide distribution of the steroid-ring system, which has led to the suggestion that it may perhaps be of abiotic origin. The new techniques mentioned earlier have shown it to be present in blue–green algae, bacteria, fungi, and the higher plants, as well as throughout the animal kingdom. This distribution is accompanied by remarkable uniformity in the associated biosynthetic pathways. Fungi, for example, can metabolize exogenous progesterone to C_{19} steroids, although, unlike higher plants, they have not yet been shown to form pregnenolone by the side-chain cleavage of cholesterol. All of this certainly suggests that the wide-ranging possibilities implicit in steroid synthesis had been well sifted before the vertebrates began to exploit them. Indeed, this would seem to follow from the fact that a greater variety of them is synthesized in the lower forms than in the higher ones.

Such modes of origin, however, can hardly be applicable to all hormones, for the complex protein secretions of the adenohypophysis seem to be largely peculiar to it, and we have found reason to suspect an entirely different course of events here. It is possible to conceive that this particular organ began as an externally secreting gland, concerned, perhaps, in the type of ecological interrelationship which we discussed earlier (p. 1), and that its diverse secretions might have arisen by molecular evolution of protein products that were already complex in character. We have noted, too, that insulin and the other hormones of the gastro-intestinal tract might similarly have evolved out of the secretory activity of a primarily digestive epithelium, while thyroglobulin, essential for the biosynthesis of the thyroid hormones, must surely have evolved out of the secretions of the endostyle.

We can thus see that to ask whether the establishment of endocrine systems has involved the evolution of hormones or merely the evolution of their effects is to raise a question which permits of no simple answer. Hormones are parts of evolving systems and in some instances, as with the thyroid hormones, they seem to have retained a fixed molecular structure while natural selection has modified their relationships with their so-called target organs. In other instances, as with the steroid hormones and hypothalamic polypeptides, there has equally clearly been an evolution of molecular pattern, although here, too, the modification of the effects of the hormones must have been an important element in adaptive evolution. In other instances again, as where we find polypeptide hormones sharing a common sequence of amino acids, we suspect that hormones have evolved by divergence after gene duplication; the equivalent at the molecular level of the principle of adaptive radiation. On this view, the potential variability of the structure of the more complex protein hormones has provided a basis for natural selection to achieve a close adaptive relationship between the secretion and the evolving effectors that it regulates.

15.2. Neurohormones and neuroendocrine integration

If we turn now to consider the principles that underlie the integration of endocrine systems, we cannot fail to be struck by the important part played by neurosecretory cells, and by the dominant position that they occupy in invertebrate endocrine systems. This, as we have already seen, is not surprising. Neurosecretion, which may perhaps have evolved as a development of the secretory capacity of conventional nerve cells, could have provided in early Metazoa, as it does in the lower forms today, a convenient mechanism for transducing evolutionary cues into widely distributed chemical signals. There-

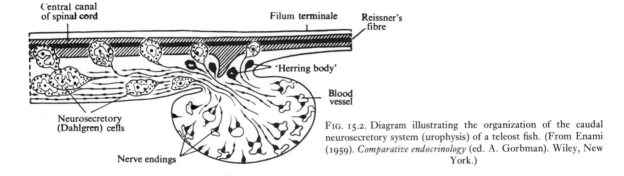

FIG. 15.2. Diagram illustrating the organization of the caudal neurosecretory system (urophysis) of a teleost fish. (From Enami (1959). *Comparative endocrinology* (ed. A. Gorbman). Wiley, New York.)

after, and especially with the evolution of vascular transmission, neurosecretory systems must have evolved independently along many lines in different groups, yet always with the exploitation of the same underlying principles of organization. This is clearly true of the arthropods and vertebrates, and may even be true within the arthropods themselves.

FIG. 15.3. An axon associated with the urophysis of the eel, *Anguilla rostrata*. Neurosecretory materials are present, forming both clusters and granules (arrows). Bouin's fluid, Heidenhain's haematoxylin. (From Holmgren (1959). *Anat. Rec.* 135.)

Indeed, the situation in the central nervous system of fish shows how such a pattern can develop independently in different parts of the same body.

The existence of large neurosecretory cells (Dahlgren cells) in the spinal cord of fish has already been mentioned (p. 57). In elasmobranchs, these cells tend to accumulate at the hind-end, but their axons run to a diffuse vascular bed which forms only an inconspicuous neurohaemal organ. In teleosts the system is more compact, and forms a well-defined lobate structure (Fig. 15.2) which constitutes the urophysis, or urohypophysis (the former name is preferred). The neurosecretion is passed down axons (Fig. 15.3) into a neurohaemal centre which forms a conspicuous ventral swelling of the spinal cord, sometimes projecting to the outside through the protective meninx. The parallelism of organization, both structural and ultrastructural, with that of the neurohypophysial system is thus very striking. Extracts of the urophysis affect a number of structures, including smooth muscle and the cardiovascular system, but its function remains uncertain.

In looking for unity of principle underlying the diversity of the major neurosecretory systems, it is worth noting that they have some association with the body surface and with receptor organs. This is true, for example, of the sensory pore X-organ of crustaceans, which has been thought to represent the transformed receptor cells of a sensory pore or papilla. The same may be true of the secretory cells of the pars intercerebralis of insects, for in the Apterygota these are said to be represented by a group of cells lying dorsal to the brain and separate from it, and corresponding in position with the lateral frontal organs of lower crustaceans. From these cells, which have contents staining with chrome-alum–haematoxylin, axons pass through the brain to enter the corpora cardiaca. We have seen evidence, too, that the pituitary gland may well have evolved out of a sensory pit, which seems to be a fundamental characteristic of the ciliary-feeding hemichordates and protochordates.

It is not yet possible to bring these thoughts into a single pattern, if, indeed, such a pattern exists. We have mentioned the view that neurosecretory cells evolved out of the inherent secretory capacity of the neuron. Another view, however, is that they could have evolved independently from secretory cells in the ependyma, or in the ectoderm, from which the nervous system itself is derived, and from which, perhaps, it inherited its secretory capacity. Perhaps some general principle has determined the development of major endocrine centres around receptor

TABLE 15.1

Examples of different types of interrelationship in endocrine systems (partly after, B. Scharrer (1959). In *Comparative endocrinology* (ed. A. Gorbman). Wiley, New York.

Source	First-order effects on:	Second-order effects on:	Third-order effects on:
X-organ/sinus gland	→Chromatophore activation		
Hypothalamus/ Neurohypophysis	→milk ejection; →antidiuresis		
X-organ/sinus gland	→inhibition of Y-organ	→initiation of moult after removal of inhibition of Y-organ	
Pars intercerebralis/ corpora cardiaca	→activation of prothoracic gland	→initiation of moult	
Hypothalamus/ neurohypophysis	→pars intermedia	→chromatophore activation	
Hypothalamus	→pars distalis	→adrenocortical tissue	→water; salt-electrolytes, etc.
Hypothalamus	→pars distalis	→thyroid gland	→metabolism, etc.
Hypothalamus	→pars distalis	→gonads (endocrine cells)	→sex characters, etc.

organs associated with the brain. Such a receptor organ might have been responsible, perhaps by means of its own secretions, for evoking responses to pheromones or other external stimuli. Thereafter, it might have become sensitive to endogenous stimuli, and so have evolved into an organ that was purely internal and endocrine in its functional relationships.

These comparisons and speculations are difficult to formulate in detail in the imperfect state of our present knowledge; their chief value at this stage lies in the stimulus that they can give to the planning of further investigations. We may conclude, however, by examining briefly the types of functional relationships involved in endocrine integration. Examples of these, some better established than others, are illustrated in Table 15.1, from which it may be seen that they comprise causal chains of varying lengths, corresponding to what have been called systems of the first order, second order, and third order.

First-order systems are those in which the secretory and release components of the neurosecretory complex discharge a hormone that acts directly upon its target tissues. Examples are the chromatophore responses evoked by the X-organ/sinus gland complex, and the milk-ejection response evoked by the hypothalamus/neurohypophysis complex.

Second-order systems are those in which the complex discharges a hormone that acts upon another endocrine gland, which then evokes a response in its target tissue. Examples are the moult-initiation action of the pars intercerebralis/corpora cardiaca complex, mediated through the prothoracic gland, and the chromatophore responses evoked by the pars intermedia. Thus we see that colour change may be regulated in the vertebrates through a second-order system while in the crustaceans it is regulated through a first-order one. We see, too, that the second-order system which controls the initiating of the moult in insects is a stimulating (or positive) one, while in crustaceans the corresponding system, although also a second-order one, exerts an inhibiting (or negative) action. Such comparisons could be extended usefully to all the systems that we have studied, but it will suffice now to note only one further example, that of the pars distalis, the tropic effects of which differ from those that we have so far enumerated in constituting a third-order system.

15.4 Envoi

The significance of all such comparisons is that they present a warning against allowing fascinating similarities of pattern to blind us to differences that may be of the greatest importance in the final analysis of function. In this connection it is particularly instructive to examine another illustration from the molluscs. The maturation of the gonads in *Octopus* is regulated by the optic glands, paired structures lying on the optic stalks on either side of the brain (Fig. 15.4). Prior to sexual maturity, the secretory activity of these glands is inhibited by a controlling system which is neural and not neurosecretory. This is shown by its localized action; if the optic

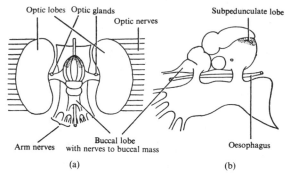

FIG. 15.4. Anatomy of the brain of *Octopus* (a) as it would be seen from above after removal of the cartilage surrounding the central mass and (b) in vertical longitudinal section. The subpedunculate lobe is stippled in both diagrams. (From Wells (1960). *Symp. Zool. Soc. Lond.* **2**.)

nerve is cut on one side there results an enlargement of the gland on that side, while the gland on the other side is unaffected. The eventual onset of sexual maturity, whether this be normal or induced by experimental treatment, is preceded by an enlargement of the optic glands resulting from a release of this inhibition; they then discharge a gonadotropic secretion which influences the gonads after transmission through the blood stream.

Transection experiments in these animals have shown that the inhibitory nerve supply originates in the subpedunculate lobes (Fig. 15.4) situated in the supra-oesophageal region of the brain mass, for a central lesion involving these lobes results in an increase in the secretory activity of the optic glands and a rapid enlargement of the ovary (Fig. 15.5). Here, then, as in the other groups that we have just considered, sexual maturation is under the control of the higher nerve centres, but the interesting difference is that there is no indication that neurosecretory nerves are concerned in *Octopus*. Evidently, therefore, nature does not always work through similar sets of blueprints, and it is prudent not to assume too confidently the existence of a particular type of design until this has actually been proved to exist.

This is not, of course, an argument against the comparative method as such, but merely a warning to show the caution with which it should be used. Indeed, it must be hoped that its value has by now been sufficiently demonstrated to justify us in ending our argument, as we began, with William Harvey, who once remarked that if only anatomists 'had been as conversant with the dissection of the lower animals as they are with that of the human body, many matters that have hitherto kept them in a perplexity of doubt would, in my opinion, have met them freed from every kind of difficulty'. Biologists will not doubt the fundamental truth of this, even when they find difficulties to be more in evidence than the prospect of overcoming them, as may sometimes seem to be true of comparative endocrinology at the present time. Such difficulties are not, however, to be regretted; rather should they be readily accepted as an indication that the subject is growing up, and welcomed as a tribute to the range and penetration

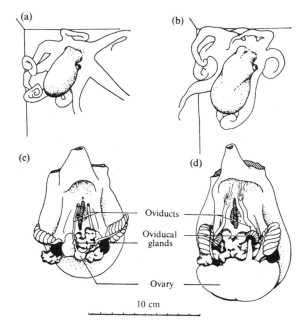

FIG. 15.5. Experimental modifications of the condition of the ovary in *Octopus*. (a) Unoperated female and (c) the same dissected to show the contents of the mantle cavity. (b) Animal in which a central brain lesion including the subpedunculate lobe had been made and (d) the same dissected; note the enlargement of the ovary and oviducts. (From Wells and Wells (1959). *J. exp. Biol.* **36**.)

of the investigations that are contributing to its maturation.

Time alone will reveal what form that maturity will take. We cannot now attempt to judge which of our favourite hypotheses will survive, which will collapse in ruins, and what new ones will emerge. *Darum sahe ich, dass nicht bessers ist, denn das der Mensch frölich in seiner Arbeit; den das ist sein Teil. Denn wer will ihn dahin bringen, dass er sehe, was nach ihm geschehen wird?*

Suggestions for further reading

These suggestions are intended to give some insight into the development of the subject, and to provide paths of entry into the more specialist current literature. They are restricted therefore mainly to books, reviews, and reports of symposia, all of which contain extensive bibliographies. Many of them are relevant to several chapters other than those for which they are cited, but it has usually seemed unnecessary to mention them more than once.

Many references to individual research papers will be found in the legends to text figures. These are often not repeated in the separate reading lists, so that they constitute what is, in effect, an additional bibliography.

GENERAL

BARRINGTON, E. J. W. (1964). *Hormones and evolution.* English Universities Press, London.
—— (1968). *The chemical basis of physiological regulation.* Scott, Foresman and Co., Glenview, Illinois.
—— (ed.) (1975). Trends in comparative endocrinology. *Am. Zool.* **15**, suppl.
—— and JØRGENSEN, C. B. (eds) (1968). *Perspectives in Endocrinology.* Academic Press, New York.
BELL, G. H., DAVIDSON, J. N., and ENSLIE-SMITH, D. (1972) *Textbook of physiology and biochemistry* (8th edn). Churchill Livingstone, Edinburgh and London.
FRIEDEN, E. and LIPNER, H. (1971). *Biochemical endocrinology of the vertebrates.* Prentice–Hall, Englewood Cliffs, New Jersey.
GORBMAN, A. and BERN, H. A. (1962). *A textbook of comparative endocrinology.* Wiley, New York.
HARINGTON, C. R. (1946). The scientific foundations of endocrinology. *J. Endocrin.* **5**, Proc., ii–xi.
HIGHNAM, K. C. and HILL, L. (1969). *The comparative endocrinology of the invertebrates.* Edward Arnold, London.
HOAR, W. S. and BERN, H. A. (eds) (1972). Progress in comparative endocrinology. *Gen. comp. Endocrin.*, suppl. 3.
—— and RANDALL, D. J. (eds) (1969–71). *Fish physiology* (6 volumes). Academic Press, New York.
IDLER, D. R. (ed.) (1972). *Steroids in nonmammalian vertebrates.* Academic Press, New York.
KARLSON, P. (ed.) (1965). *Mechanisms of hormone action.* Academic Press, New York.

PRASAD, M. R. N. (ed.) (1969). Progress in comparative endocrinology. *Gen. comp. Endocrin.*, suppl. 2.
SAWIN, C. T. (1969). *The hormones: endocrine physiology.* Little, Brown, and Company, Boston.
TEPPERMAN, J. (1968). *Metabolic and endocrine physiology: an introductory text* (2nd edn). Year Book Medical Publishers, Inc., Chicago.
TOMBES, A. S. (1970). *Introduction to invertebrate endocrinology.* Academic Press, New York.
TURNER, C. D. and BAGNARA, J. T. (1971). *General endocrinology* (5th edn). University of Chicago Press, Philadelphia.
VARIOUS AUTHORS (1959 *et seq.*). *Handbook of physiology; a critical, comprehensive presentation of physiological knowledge and concepts.* American Physiological Society, Washington, D.C.
YOUNG, F. G. (1970). The evolution of ideas about animal hormones. In *The chemistry of life* (ed. J. Needham). Cambridge University Press.
ZARROW, M. X., YOCHIM, J. M., and McCARTHY, J. L. (1964). *Experimental endocrinology.* Academic Press, New York.

CHAPTER 2

ANDERSSON, S. (1973). Secretion of gastrointestinal hormones. *A. Rev. Physiol.* **35**, 431–52.
BABKIN, B. P. (1950). *Secretory mechanisms of the digestive glands* (2nd edn). Hoeber, New York.
BARRINGTON, E. J. W. (1971). Evolution of hormones. In *Biochemical evolution and the origin of life* (ed. E. Schoffeniels), pp. 174–90. North-Holland, Amsterdam.
BAYLISS, W. M. and STARLING, E. H. (1902). The mechanism of pancreatic secretion. *J. Physiol. Lond.* **28**, 325–53.
DUPRE, J. (1972). Gastro-intestinal hormones. In *Modern trends in endocrinology* (eds. F. T. G. Prunty and H. Gardiner-Hill), Vol. 4, pp. 278–301. Butterworths, London.
GREGORY, R. A. (1966). Memorial Lecture: The isolation and chemistry of gastrin. *Gastroenterology* **51**, 953–9.
—— (1968). Gastrin—the natural history of a hormone. *Harvey Lectures Ser.* **64**, 121–55.
GROSSMAN, M. I. (1950). Gastrointestinal hormones. *Physiol. Rev.* **30**, 33–90.
—— (1967). Neural and hormonal stimulation of gastric

secretion of acid. In *Handbook of physiology* (eds F. Code and W. Heidel), Section 6, Vol. 2, pp. 835–63. American Physiological Society, Washington D.C.

—— (1970). Spectrum of biological actions of gastrointestinal hormones. In *Frontiers in gastrointestinal hormone research*. Nobel Symposium XVI.

JORPES, J. E. (1968). Memorial Lecture: The isolation and chemistry of secretin and cholecystokinin. *Gastroenterology* 55, 157–63.

MUTT, V. (1972). Some recent developments in the field of intestinal hormones. In *Endocrinology 1971* (ed. S. Taylor), pp. 250–6. Heinemann, London.

SMIT, H. (1968). Gastric secretion in the lower vertebrates and birds. In *Handbook of physiology* (eds F. Code and W. Heidel), Alimentary Canal V, Chap. 135, pp. 2791–805. American Physiological Society, Washington D.C.

CHAPTERS 3 and 4

BARRINGTON, E. J. W. (1973). The pancreas and intestine. In *The biology of lampreys* (eds M. W. Hardisty and I. C. Potter), Vol. 2, pp. 135–69. Academic Press, London and New York.

BEST, C. H. (1959). A Canadian trail of medical research. *J. Endocrin.* 19, Proc., i–xvii.

BLUNDELL, T. L., DODSON, G. G., DODSON, E., HODGKIN, D. C., and VIJAYAN, M. (1971). X-ray analysis and the structure of insulin. *Recent Prog. Horm. Res.* 27, 1–40.

BROLIN, S. E., HELLMAN, B., and KNUTSON, H. (eds) (1964). *The structure and metabolism of the pancreatic islets*. Pergamon Press, Oxford.

EPPLE, A. (1969). The endocrine pancreas. In *Fish physiology* (eds W. S. Hoar and D. J. Randall), Vol. 2, pp. 275–319. Academic Press, New York.

FALKMER, S. (1967). Comparative endocrinology of the islet tissue. *Exc. Med. Int. Cong. Ser.* 172, 55–66.

—— and MARQUES, M. (1972). Phylogeny and ontogeny of glucagon production. In *Glucagon* (eds P. J. Lefebvre and R. H. Unger). Pergamon Press, Oxford and New York.

FOA, P. P. (1964). Glucagon. In *The hormones* (eds G. Pincus, K. V. Thimann, and E. E. Astwood), Vol. 4, pp. 531–56. Academic Press, New York.

GREENWOOD, F. C. (1967). Immunological procedures in the assay of protein hormones. In *Modern trends in endocrinology* (ed. H. Gardiner-Hill), Vol. 3, pp. 288–322. Butterworths, London.

LANGERHANS, P. (1869). Beiträge zur mikrosopischen Anatomie der Bauchspeicheldrüse. Reprinted in *Bull. Inst. Med.* 5, 259.

LEFEBVRE, S. E. and UNGER, R. H. (eds) (1972). *Glucagon: molecular physiology, clinical and therapeutic implications*. Pergamon Press, Oxford.

LI. C. H. (1969). Recent studies on the chemistry of human growth hormone. In *La spécificité zoologique des hormones hypophysaires et de leurs activités* (ed. M. Fontaine), pp. 175–9. Centre National de la Recherche Scientifique, Paris.

—— (1972). Aspects of the comparative chemistry of human pituitary growth hormone and chorionic somatomammotropin. In *Growth and growth hormone* (eds A. Pecile and E. E. Müller), pp. 17–24. Excerpta Medica, Amsterdam.

MAIN, I. H. M. (1972). Prostaglandins: are they circulatory or local hormones. In *Modern trends in endocrinology* (eds F. T. G. Prunty and H. Gardiner-Hill), Vol. 4, pp. 302–26. Butterworths, London.

MURPHY, B. E. P. (1969). Protein binding and the assay of nonantigenic hormones. *Recent Prog. Horm. Res.* 25, 563–610.

PECILE, A. and MÜLLER, E. E. (eds) (1972). *Growth and growth hormone. Proceedings of the Second International Symposium on growth hormone*. Excerpta Medica, Amsterdam.

RHOTEN, W. B. (1971). Light and electron microscopic studies on pancreatic islets of the lizard, *Lygosoma laterale*. I. *Gen. comp. Endocrin.* 17, 203–19.

ROBISON, G. A. (1972). Cyclic AMP. In *Modern trends in physiology* (ed. C. B. B. Downman), Vol. 1, pp. 143–61. Butterworths, London.

SMITH, L. F. (1966). Species variation in the amino acid sequence of insulin. *Am. J. Med.* 40, 662–6.

YOUNG, F. G. (ed.) (1960). Insulin. *Br. med. Bull.* 16, 175–259.

WILHELMI, A. E. and MILLS, J. B. (1961). The chemistry of the growth hormone of several species. In *La spécificité zoologique des hormones hypophysaires et de leurs activités* (ed. M. Fontaine), pp. 165–73. Centre National de la Recherche Scientifique, Paris.

CHAPTER 5

BALL, J. N., OLIVEREAU, M., SLICHER, A. M., and KALLMAN, K. D. (1965). Functional capacity of ectopic pituitary transplants in the teleost *Poecilia formosa*, with a comparative discussion of the transplanted pituitary. *Phil. Trans. R. Soc. Lond.* B 249, 69–99.

BARGMANN, W. and SCHARRER, B. (eds) (1970). *Aspects of neuroendocrinology*. Springer-Verlag, New York.

BENOIT, J. and DALAGE, C. (eds) (1963). *Cytologie de l'adénohypophyse*. Centre National de la Recherche Scientifique, Paris, No. 128.

DODD, J. M., FOLLETT, B. K., and SHARP, B. J. (1971). Hypothalamic control of pituitary function in submammalian vertebrates. *Adv. comp. Physiol. Biochem.* 4, 114–223.

DONOVAN, B. T. (1970). *Mammalian neuroendocrinology*. McGraw-Hill, London.

EVERETT, J. W. (1964). Central neural control of reproductive functions of the adenohypophysis. *Physiol. Rev.* 44, 373–431.

FONTAINE, M. (ed.) (1969). *La spécificité zoologique des hormones hypophysaires et de leurs activités*. Centre National de la Recherche Scientifique, Paris.

GABE, M. (1966). *Neurosecretion*. Pergamon Press, Oxford.

KOBAYASHI, H. and MATSUI, T. (1961). Fine structure of

the median eminence and its functional significance. In *Frontiers in neuroendocrinology* (eds W. F. Ganong and L. Martini) Vol. 3. Oxford University Press, New York.

MEITES, J. (ed.) (1969). *Hypophysiotropic hormones of the hypothalamus: assay and chemistry.* Williams and Wilkins, Baltimore.

OLIVEREAU, M. and BALL, J. N. (1964). Contributions a l'histophysiologie de l'hypophyse des téléostéens, en particulier de celle de *Poecilia* species. *Gen. comp. Endocrin.* 4, 523–32

PICKFORD, G. E. and ATZ, J. W. (1957). *The physiology of the pituitary gland of fishes.* New York Zoological Society, New York.

SAGE, M. and BERN, H. A. (1971). Cytophysiology of the teleost pituitary. *Int. Rev. Cytol.* 31, 339–76.

SCHARRER, B. (1969). Neurohumours and neurohormones: definitions and terminology. *J. Neuro-Visc. Rel.*, Suppl. 9, 1–20.

SCHARRER, E. and SCHARRER, B. (1963). *Neuroendocrinology.* Columbia University Press, New York.

VAN OORDT, P. G. W. (1968). The analysis and identification of the hormone-producing cells of the adenohypophysis. In *Perspectives in endocrinology* (eds E. J. W. Barrington and C. B. Jørgensen), pp. 405–67. Academic Press, London and New York.

WINGSTRAND, K. G. (1951). *The structure and development of the avian pituitary.* C. W. K. Gleerup, Lund.

CHAPTER 6

ACHER, R. (1971). The neurohypophysial hormones: an example of molecular evolution. In *Biochemical evolution and the origin of life* (ed. E. Schoffeniels), pp. 43–51. North-Holland, Amsterdam.

BARGMANN, W. (1960). The neurosecretory system of the diencephalon. *Endeavour* 19, 125–33.

GESCHWIND, I. I. (1969). The main lines of evolution of the pituitary hormones. In *La spécificité zoologique des hormones hypophysaires et de leurs activités* (ed. M. Fontaine), pp. 385–406. Centre National de la Recherche Scientifique, Paris.

HELLER, H. (1963). Neurohypophysial hormones. In *Comparative endocrinology* (eds U. S. von Euler and H. Heller), Vol. 1, pp. 25–80. Academic Press, New York.

—— (1974). Molecular aspects in comparative endocrinology. *Gen. comp. Endocrin.* 22, 315–32.

—— and PICKERING, B. T. (eds) (1970). Pharmacology of the endocrine system and related drugs: the neurohypophysis. In *International encyclopaedia of pharmacology and therapeutics*, § 41, Vol. 1. Pergamon Press, Oxford.

—— and SPICKETT, S. G. (1967). The polymorphism of the neurohypophysial hormones. *Mem. Soc. Endocrin.* 15, 89–106.

OHNO, S. (1970). *Evolution by gene duplication.* Allen and Unwin, London.

SAWYER, W. H. (1961). Neurohypophysial hormones. *Pharmacol. Rev.* 13, 225–77.

—— (1965). Evolution of neurohypophysial principles. *Archs. Anat. microsp. Morph. exp.* 54, 295–312.

VLIEGENTHART, J. F. G. and VERSTEEG, D. H. G. (1967). The evolution of the vertebrate neurohypophysial hormones in relation to the genetic code. *J. Endocrin.* 38, 3–12.

CHAPTERS 7 and 8

AMOROSO, E. C. (1955). Endocrinology of pregnancy. *Br. med. Bull.* 11, 117–25.

ASDELL, S. A. (1964). *Patterns of mammalian reproduction* (2nd edn). Comstock, New York.

AUSTIN, D. R. and SHORT, R. V. (eds). *Reproduction in mammals*, Book 4. *Reproductive patterns.* Cambridge University Press.

BERN, H. A. and NICOLL, C. S. (1968). The comparative endocrinology of prolactin. *Recent Prog. Horm. Res.* 24, 681–720.

—— and —— (1969). The taxonomic specificity of prolactins. In *La spécificité zoologique des hormones hypophysaires et de leurs activités* (ed. M. Fontaine), p. 193, Centre National de la Recherche Scientifique, Paris.

BRUCE, H. M. (1970). Pheromones. *Br. med. Bull.* 26, 10–13.

HALL, K. (1960). Relaxin: a review. *J. Reprod. Fertil.* 1, 368–84.

HISAW, F. L. (1959). Endocrine adaptations of the mammalian oestrous cycle and gestation. In *Comparative endocrinology* (ed. A. Gorbman), pp. 533–52. Wiley, New York.

LACY, D. (1967). The seminiferous tubule in mammals. *Endeavour* 26, 101–8.

NALBANDOV, A. V. (1964). *Reproductive physiology* (2nd edn). W. H. Freeman and Company, San Francisco.

NICOLL, C. S. and BERN, H. A. (1971). On the actions of prolactin among the vertebrates: is there a common denominator? In *Ciba Foundation Symposium on lactogenic hormones* (eds G. E. W. Wolstenholme and J. Knight), pp. 299–324. Churchill–Livingstone, London.

PARKES, A. S. (ed.) (1952–66). *Marshall's physiology of reproduction*, Vols 1–3. Longmans, London.

REITER, R. J. (ed.) (1970). Symposium on comparative endocrinology of the pineal. *Am. Zool.* 10, 187–267.

SCHALLY, A. V., ARIMURA, A., and KASTIN, A. J. (1973). Hypothalamic regulatory hormones. *Science* 179, 341–50.

TYNDALE-BISCOE, H. (1973). *Life of marsupials.* Edward Arnold, London.

WURTMAN, R. J., AXELROD, J. and KELLY, D. E. (1968). *The pineal.* Academic Press, New York.

YOUNG, J. Z. (1973). The pineal gland. *Philosophy* 48, 70–4.

CHAPTER 9

AURBACH, G. D., KEUTMANN, H. T., NIALL, H. D., IREGEAR, G. W., O'RIORDAN, J. L. H., MARCUS, R., MARX, S. J., and POTTS, J. T., Jr. (1972). Structure, synthesis and mechanism of action of parathyroid hormone. *Recent Prog. Horm. Res.* **28**, 353–98.

BARRINGTON, E. J. W. (1964). Hormones and evolution. *Experientia* **18**, 201–10.

ETKIN, W. and GILBERT, L. I. (1968). *Metamorphosis; a problem in developmental biology.* Appleton–Century–Crofts, New York.

GAILLARD, P. J., TALMAGE, R. V., and BUDY, A. M. (eds) (1965). *The parathyroid glands.* University of Chicago Press, Chicago.

HOAR, W. S. (1953). Control and timing of fish migration. *Biol. Rev.* **28**, 437–52.

MacINTYRE, I. (1968). Calcitonin: a review of its discovery and an account of purification and action. *Proc. R. Soc. Lond.* B **170**, 49–60.

MILLER, J. F. A. P. (1964). The thymus and the development of immunological responsiveness. *Science* **144**, 1544–51.

PEARSE, A. G. E. (1969). The cytochemistry and ultrastructure of polypeptide hormone-producing cells of the APUD series and the embryologic, physiologic and pathologic implications of the concept. *J. Histochem. Cytochem.* **17**, 303–13.

PITT-RIVERS, R. and TATA, J. R. (1959). *The thyroid hormones.* Pergamon Press, London.

POTTS, J. T., JR., KEUTMANN, H. T., NIALL, H. D., TREGEAR, G. W., HABENER, J. F., O'RIORDAN, J. L. H., MURRAY, T. M., POWELL, D., and AURBACH, G. C. (1972). Comparative biochemistry of parathyroid hormone and calcitonin. *Gen. comp. Endocrin.*, Suppl. 3, 405.

RASMUSSEN, H. (1961). The parathyroid hormone. *Scient. Am.* **204**, 56–63.

—— SZE, Y.-L., and YOUNG, R. (1964). Further studies on the isolation and characterization of parathyroid polypeptides. *J. Biol. Chem.* **239**, 2852—7.

TATA, J. R. (1969). The action of thyroid hormones. *Gen. comp. Endocrin.*, Suppl. 2, 385–97.

CHAPTERS 10 and 11

BUTLER, D. G. (1973). *Structure and function of the adrenal gland of fishes. Am. Zool.* **13**, 839–79.

CHESTER JONES, I. (1957). *The adrenal cortex.* Cambridge University Press, London.

CHRISTIAN, J. J. and DAVIS, D. E. (1964). Endocrines, behaviour, and population. *Science* **146**, 1550–8.

COPE, Z. (1964). Jane Austen's last illness. *Br. med. J.* 18 July, 182.

COUPLAND, R. (1965). *The natural history of the chromaffin cell.* Longmans, London.

—— (1972). The chromaffin system. In *Handbook of experimental pharmacology* (eds H. Blaschko and E. Muscholl), New Series, Vol. 33, pp. 16–45. Springer-Verlag, Berlin, Heidelberg, and New York.

FALCK, B., HILLARP, N.-Å., THIEME, G., and TORP, A. (1962). Fluorescence of catecholamines and related compounds condensed with formaldehyde. *J. Histochem. Cytochem.* **10**, 348–54.

LI, C. H. (1962). Synthesis and biological properties of ACTH peptides. *Recent Prog. Horm. Res.* **18**, 1–40.

—— (1963). The ACTH molecule. *Scient. Am.* **209**, 46–53.

PEART, W. S. (1965). The renin-angiotensin system. *Pharmacol. Rev.* **17**, 143–82.

SANDOR, T. (1969). A comparative survey of steroids and steroidogenic pathways throughout the vertebrates. *Gen. comp. Endocrin.*, Suppl. 2, 285–98.

SCHMIDT-NIELSON, K. (1960). The salt-secreting gland of marine birds. *Circulation* **21** (Part 2), 955–67.

SELYE, H. (1957). *The stress of life.* Longmans, London.

—— (1959). Perspectives in stress research. *Perspect. Biol. Med.* **2**, 403.

VON EULER, U. S. (1963). Comparative chromaffin cell hormones. In *Comparative endocrinology* (ed. U. S. von Euler), Vol. 1, pp. 258–90. Academic Press, New York.

CHAPTER 12

BAGNARA, J. T. (1966). Cytology and cytophysiology of non-melanophore pigment cells. *Int. Rev. Cytol.* **20**, 173–205.

—— TAYLOR, J. D., and HADLEY, M. E. (1968). The dermal chromatophore unit. *J. Cell Biol.* **38**, 67–79.

BRADSHAW, S. D. and WARING, H. (1961). Comparative studies on the biological activity of melanin-dispersing hormone (MDH). In *La spécificité zoologique des hormones hypophysaires et de leurs activités*, pp. 135–59. Centre National de la Recherche Scientifique, Paris.

FINGERMAN, M. (1963). *The control of chromatophores.* Pergamon, Oxford.

GESCHWIND, I. I. (1959). Species variation in protein and polypeptide hormones. In *Comparative endocrinology* (ed. A. Gorbman), pp. 421–43. Wiley, New York.

GORDON, M. (ed.) (1959). *Pigment cell biology.* Academic Press, New York.

HOGBEN, L. (1942). Chromatic behaviour. *Proc. R. Soc. Lond.* B **131**, 111–36.

HÖRSTADIUS, S. (1950). *The neural crest.* Oxford University Press, London.

LI, C. H. (1969). β-lipotropin, a new pituitary hormone. In *La spécificité zoologique des hormones hypophysaires et de leurs activités* (ed. M. Fontaine), pp. 93–101. Centre National de la Recherche Scientifique, Paris.

LOWRY, P. J. and CHADWICK, A. (1970). Interrelationships of some pituitary hormones. *Nature, Lond.* **226**, 219–22.

PARKER, G. H. (1948). *Animal colour changes and their neurohumours.* Cambridge University Press, London.

VARIOUS AUTHORS. (1969). Cellular aspects of the control of colour changes. *Am. Zool.* **9**, 427–540.

WARING, H. (1963). *Color change mechanisms of cold-blooded vertebrates.* Academic Press, New York.

CHAPTER 13

BERN, H. A. and KNOWLES, F. G. W. (1966). Neurosecretion. In *Neuroendocrinology* (eds L. Martini and

W. F. Ganong), Vol. 1, p. 139. Academic Press, New York.

CHARNIAUX-COTTON, H. (1965). Contrôle endocrinien de la différenciation sexuelle chez les crustacés supérieurs. *Archs. Anat. microsp. Morph. exp.* **54**, 405–15.

CLARK, R. B. (1969). Endocrine influences in annelids. *Gen. comp. Endocrin.*, Suppl. 2, 572–81.

DURCHON, M. and SCHALLER, F. (1964). Recherches endocrinologiques en culture organotypique chez les annélides polychètes. *Gen. comp. Endocrin.* **4**, 427–32.

FINGERMAN, M. (1966). Neurosecretory control of pigmentary effectors in crustaceans. *Am. Zool.* **6**, 169–79.

HAGADORN, I. R. (1966). Neurosecretion in the Hirudinea and its possible role in reproduction. *Am. Zool.* **6**, 251–61.

KANATANI, H. (1972). Adenine derivatives and oocyte maturation in starfishes. In *Oogenesis* (ed. J. D. Biggers and A. W. Schuetz). University Park Press, Baltimore, Maryland.

KLEINHOLZ, L. H. (1961). Pigmentary effectors. In *The physiology of crustacea* (ed. T. H. Waterman), Vol. 2, pp. 133–69. Academic Press, New York.

—— (1970). A progress report on the separation and purification of crustacean neurosecretory pigmentary-effector hormones. *Gen. com. Endocrin.* **14**, 578–88.

PASSANO, L. M. (1961). Molting and its control. In *The physiology of crustacea* (ed. T. H. Waterman), Vol. 2, pp. 473–536. Academic Press, New York.

RALPH, C. L. (1967). Recent developments in invertebrate endocrinology. *Am. Zool.* **7**, 145–60.

SCHARRER, B. and WEITZMAN, M. (1970). Current problems in invertebrate neurosecretion: Neurosecretion in invertebrates. In *Aspects of Neuroendocrinology* (eds W. Bargmann and B. Scharrer). Springer-Verlag, New York.

TIEGS, O. W. and MANTON, S. M. (1958). The evolution of the Arthropoda. *Biol. Rev.* **33**, 255–337.

CHAPTER 14

BEROZA, M. (1970). *Chemicals controlling insect behaviour.* Academic Press, New York.

DAHM, K. H., TROST, B. M., and RÖLLER, H. (1967). Synthesis of the racemic juvenile hormone. *J. Am. chem. Soc.* **89**, 5292–4.

FRAENKEL, G. and HSIAO, C. (1965). Bursicon, a hormone which mediates tanning of the cuticle in the adult fly and other insects. *J. Insect Physiol.* **11**, 513–56.

GERSCH, M. (1961). Neurosecretory phenomena in invertebrates. *Gen. comp. Endocrin.*, Suppl. 2, 553–64.

GILBERT, L. I. (1964). Hormones regulating insect growth. In *The hormones* (eds G. Pincus, K. V. Thimann, and E. B. Astwood), Vol. 4, pp. 67–134. Academic Press, New York.

GOLDSWORTHY, G. J. and MORDUE, W. (1974). Neurosecretory hormones in insects. *J. Endocrin.* **60**, 529–58.

SCHARRER, B. (1965). Recent progress in the study of neuroendocrine mechanisms in insects. *Archs. Anat. microsp. Morph. exp.* **54**, 331–42.

THOMAS, P. J. and BHATNAGER-THOMAS, P. L. (1968). Use of juvenile hormone analogue as insecticide for pests of stored grain. *Nature, Lond.* **219**, 949.

WIGGLESWORTH, SIR V. B. (1970). *Insect hormones.* Oliver and Boyd, Edinburgh.

WILLIAMS, C. M. (1968). Ecdysone and ecdysone-analogues: their assay and action on diapausing pupae of the cynthia silkworm. *Biol. Bull.* **134**, 344–55.

—— and LAW, J. H. (1965). The juvenile hormone: its extraction, assay and purification. *J. Insect Physiol.* **11**, 569–80.

WILSON, E. O. (1963). Pheromones. *Scient. Am.* **208** (5) 100–14.

CHAPTER 15

BLACK, M. and EDELMAN, J. (1970). *Plant growth.* Heinemann, London.

FRIDBERG, G. and BERN, H. A. (1968). The urophysis and the caudal neurosecretory system of fishes. *Biol. Rev.* **43**, 175–99.

LEDERIS, K. (1970). Trout urophysis: Biological characterization of the bladder-contracting activity. *Gen. comp. Endocrin.* **14**, 427–39.

WELLS, M. J. (1960). Optic glands and the ovary of *Octopus. Symp. Zool. Soc. Lond.* **2**, 87–107.

Index